AN ATLAS OF ULTRASOUND COLOR FLOW IMAGING

AN ATLAS OF ULTRASOUND COLOR FLOW IMAGING

Edited by

Barry B Goldberg MD

Professor of Radiology
and Director, Jefferson Ultrasound Research and Education Institute
and Division of Ultrasound, Department of Radiology
Thomas Jefferson University Medical College and Hospital
Philadelphia, PA, USA

Daniel A Merton BS RDMS

Technical Coordinator of Research
Jefferson Ultrasound Research and Education Institute
and Division of Diagnostic Ultrasound, Department of Radiology
Thomas Jefferson University Medical College and Hospital
Philadelphia, PA, USA

Colin R Deane PhD

Principal Clinical Scientist
Department of Medical Engineering and Physics
King's College Hospital
London, UK

MARTIN DUNITZ

First published in the United Kingdom in 1997 by

Martin Dunitz Ltd
The Livery House
7–9 Pratt Street
London NW1 0AE

A CIP catalogue record for this book is available from the British Library.

ISBN 1-85317-063-1

Composition by Scribe Design, Gillingham, Kent
Printed in Singapore

This book is dedicated first to my wife, Phyllis, whose advice and editorial assistance has been invaluable. In addition, I dedicate this book to the numerous students from around the world who have provided me with the stimulus to produce it.

BBG

I dedicate this book to my wonderful wife Ruth and sons Daniel ('DJ') and Henry, and to the memory of Susan.

DAM

To my wife Anne.

CRD

Contents

Contributors

Colin R Deane PhD
Principal Clinical Scientist, Department of Medical Engineering and Physics, King's College Hospital, London SE5 9RS, UK.

Flemming Forsberg PhD
Head of Research, Jefferson Ultrasound Research and Education Institute, and Assistant Professor of Radiology, Division of Diagnostic Ultrasound, Department of Radiology, Thomas Jefferson University Medical College and Hospital, Philadelphia PA 19107, USA.

Barry B Goldberg MD
Professor of Radiology and Director, Jefferson Ultrasound Research and Education Institute, and Division of Ultrasound, Department of Radiology, Thomas Jefferson University Medical College and Hospital, Philadelphia PA 19107, USA.

Beth R Gross MD
Assistant Professor of Radiology, Department of Radiology, North Shore University Hospital, New York University School of Medicine, Manhasset NY 11030, USA.

Ji-Bin Liu MD
Research Assistant Professor of Radiology, Division of Diagnostic Ultrasound, Department of Radiology, Thomas Jefferson University Medical College and Hospital, Philadelphia PA 19107, USA.

Daniel A Merton BS RDMS
Technical Coordinator of Research, Jefferson Ultrasound Research and Education Institute, and Division of Diagnostic Ultrasound, Department of Radiology, Thomas Jefferson University Medical College and Hospital, Philadelphia PA 19107, USA.

William D Middleton MD
Associate Professor of Radiology and Chief, Diagnostic Ultrasound, Mallinckrodt Institute of Radiology, Washington University School of Medicine, St Louis MO 63110, USA.

Tina L Nack MPE RVT RDMS
Clinical Coordinator of Vascular Ultrasound, Division of Diagnostic Ultrasound, Department of Radiology, Thomas Jefferson University Medical College and Hospital, Philadelphia PA 19107, USA.

John S Pellerito MD
Chief, Division of US/CT and MRI, Department of Radiology, North Shore
University Hospital, Cornell University Medical College, Manhasset NY
11030, USA.

Philip W Ralls MD
Professor of Radiology and Chief, Body Imaging and Interventional
Radiology, Department of Radiology, University of Southern California
School of Medicine, Los Angeles, CA 90033, USA.

Preface

The growth of ultrasound from its beginnings in the late 1940s has been almost exponential. Ultrasound has gone from simple A-mode through M-mode, B-scan (both bi-stable and gray-scale), real-time imaging and Doppler (both pulsed and color), and has become established throughout the world. In fact, it has been estimated that one out of every three imaging studies now performed worldwide is an ultrasound examination.

While the predominant uses of ultrasound involve gray-scale real-time imaging, the ability of color Doppler imaging to detect and display blood flow in two dimensions has led to a significant increase in its usefulness in a wide variety of areas, including the heart and blood vessels. More recently, other forms of display using formats that lead to increased sensitivity, known as amplitude, power or energy Doppler, have shown the potential for increasing the utilization and importance of Doppler in a wide variety of scanning procedures. In the near future, the use of ultrasound contrast agents will further increase the importance of this mode of display.

While gray-scale ultrasound imaging is understood by many and is appropriately used globally, it is more difficult, in general, to obtain adequate color Doppler images. In addition, the importance of this modality in a wide variety of diagnostic procedures is only now being established; of course, its usefulness with ultrasound contrast agents is still investigational. This Atlas is designed to provide a full understanding of the established and potential uses of color flow imaging throughout the body. No attempt has been made to make this an all inclusive text but, instead, the more important uses of this form of display are emphasized. In addition, there are chapters that are devoted to an understanding of the physics of ultrasound and instrumentation, as well as to the understanding of artifacts which can make interpretation difficult. This book should prove of interest not only to those physicians and sonographers currently using color flow imaging, but also to students, including residents, fellows and technologists, who want to learn more about this rapidly developing area of ultrasound imaging.

BBG
DAM
Philadelphia, 1997

CRD
London, 1997

Acknowledgments

We acknowledge the help of all the sonographers and sonologists who have contributed images used throughout this Atlas. Their contributions have resulted in a thorough compilation of clinical cases and normal examples. We also thank Alan Burgess and Ian Mellor of Martin Dunitz Ltd for their continual support and patience, and commitment to the final product. Daniel Merton wishes to express his gratitude to Dr Barry Goldberg for his advice as friend and mentor throughout his career. Colin Deane thanks Dr David Goss of King's College Hospital, London, for help and advice.

Chapter 1 Physical principles of Doppler ultrasound and color flow imaging

Flemming Forsberg

INTRODUCTION

For over 30 years, ultrasound scanners have exploited the Doppler effect to detect echoes scattered by moving blood. The clinical uses of bloodflow imaging systems have expanded immensely since the first measurement of flow in the heart was performed by Satomura in 1956. Currently available techniques include continuous wave Doppler, pulsed wave Doppler, color flow imaging, color velocity imaging and, as the newest, color amplitude imaging.

Many texts are available detailing the principles and signal processing of color flow imaging. However, recent developments in signal processing and displays have produced new imaging parameters, many of which are used in the clinical chapters of this book. The aim of this chapter is to summarize the principles that contribute to the images. For a more thorough analysis of the subject, texts are recommended at the end of the chapter.

THE DOPPLER EFFECT IN MEDICAL ULTRASOUND

The Doppler principle was first formulated in 1842 by the Austrian physicist Johann Christian Doppler (1805–1853). This phenomenon affects all types of waves when the source and the receiver are moving relative to each other, even though Doppler in his original paper specifically studied the changing color of the light from a double star.

Assuming the speed of the source to be much lower than the speed of sound, one proceeds as follows. If a sound source is moving towards a stationary listener, the listener hears a higher number of sound waves per unit time and, consequently, a higher frequency than the frequency (f_s) emitted by the source. Thus, the perceived wave has undergone a shift in frequency, which will be proportional to the velocity of the source. This frequency shift (f_D) is known as the Doppler shift frequency. This will be positive when the distance between the source and the listener diminishes, as in this case. Conversely, for an increasing distance a negative Doppler shift is produced, since fewer waves per time unit are received; see Fig. 1.1.

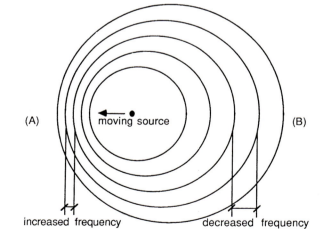

Figure 1.1 *The Doppler principle. A source of sound moves from right to left. A listener at A hears a higher frequency, while a listener at B hears a lower one.*

The general Doppler equation for sound waves is:

$$f_D = \frac{v_l + v_s}{c} f_s, \quad v_s \ll c \qquad (1.1)$$

where the velocity of the listener and the source, respectively, are denoted v_l and v_s. Here a velocity which has a direction bringing source and listener closer together is considered positive. The velocity of sound is designated c. The Doppler principle has been put to practical use in many fields, e.g. radar, underwater sonar and medical ultrasound.

In the field of real-time transcutaneous bloodflow velocity measurements, Doppler ultrasound is the dominant method of choice. Here the reflected ultrasound wave undergoes a Doppler shift in frequency due to the movement of the blood. Blood consists of several components, but it is the red blood cells that act as scatterers, since the other solids (i.e. white blood cells and platelets) are either present in insignificant numbers or are far too small to add to the scattered ultrasound echo.

After insonation of a blood vessel, the Doppler shift frequency f_D will be proportional to the velocity of the erythrocytes v given by:

$$f_D = \frac{2v \cos \theta}{c_t} f_c \qquad (1.2)$$

where f_c is the frequency of the emitted ultrasound wave and c_t is the mean velocity of sound in tissue (approximately 1540 m/s). Since only the movement directly towards or away from the transducer contributes to the Doppler shift, equation 1.2 has been scaled with $\cos \theta$ where θ designates the angle of incidence between the blood velocity vector and the ultrasound beam. The effect of varying the different parameters is given in Table 1.1.

The reason for the discrepancy between the general Doppler equation for sound waves and equation 1.2 is that the erythrocytes act both as transmitters and receivers (i.e. source and listener) of the ultrasound wave. First, the erythrocytes form a receiver in motion and the ultrasound wave from the transducer will be perceived as Doppler shifted. Second, when the ultrasound wave is reflected, the erythrocytes will act as a transmitter in motion relative to the stationary receiving transducer, hence, the factor 2 (for two Doppler shifts) and only one velocity which appear above.

MEASUREMENT TECHNIQUES

The first Doppler blood velocity measurements were performed using a continuous wave (CW) system. Such a system requires a separate transmitter and receiver. For example, one can use two piezoelectric transducers mounted in the same enclosure, as depicted in Fig. 1.2, which shows a simplified block diagram of a CW Doppler system.

The direction of flow is determined via quadrature demodulation. In simple terms the received signal is compared to the transmitted pulse, which allows forward and reverse flow to be separated. This

Table 1.1 Changing parameters in the Doppler equation—the effect on the Doppler shift (f_D).

Parameter	Change	Effect on f_D
Speed of sound	Increase	Decrease
	Decrease	Increase
Transducer frequency	Increase	Increase
	Decrease	Decrease
Angle of incidence	Increase	Decrease
	Decrease	Increase

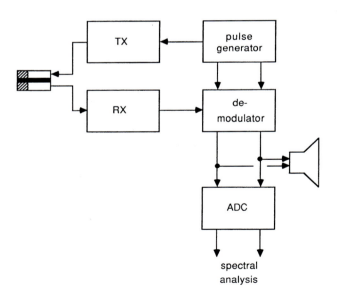

Figure 1.2 Block diagram of a CW Doppler system. Separate transducers and circuitry for transmission (TX) and reception (RX) are used.

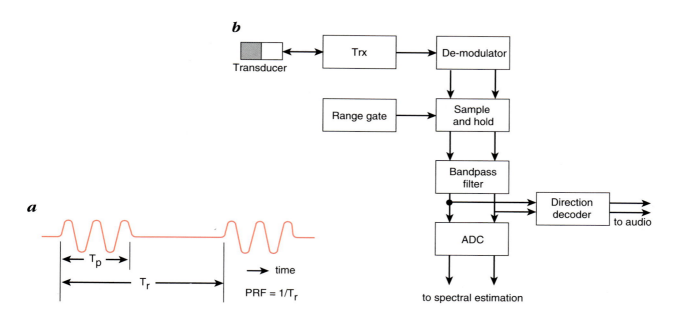

Figure 1.3 *(a) Burst sequence for PW Doppler. A pulse of duration T_P is transmitted at intervals of time T_R. The frequency of pulse transmission, the pulse repetition frequency, is $1/T_R$. (b) Block diagram of PW Doppler system. The single transducer element is used for both transmitting and receiving (Trx).*

process (as well as some filtering) transforms the received data from a high-frequency signal (2–10 MHz) to a Doppler signal (typically 150–20 000 Hz) containing only echoes backscattered from blood.

Since the frequencies used in medical ultrasound and the velocities encountered in the human body combine to produce Doppler frequency shifts in the audible range, it is customary to send the Doppler signal directly to loudspeakers. An experienced sonographer can gain significant diagnostic information from the audio output. Another way of processing the Doppler signal is to digitize it in an analog-to-digital converter (ADC), and then use, for example, a fast Fourier transform (FFT) to extract the spectral information.

A CW system has no limit on the maximum velocity measurable and can, in theory, measure any velocity correctly. However, the technique suffers from one major constraint. Since information is received from the entire ultrasound beam, it is impossible to determine the position of a specific blood vessel. Hence, an erroneous velocity measurement may result if several blood vessels are insonated simultaneously.

The limitation in range resolution of a CW Doppler system can be overcome by emitting short tone bursts with a certain pulse repetition frequency (PRF) as shown in Fig. 1.3a. This is the principle behind pulsed wave (PW) Doppler systems. Here the transducer acts as receiver, when not transmitting, and only one transducer is therefore needed, as depicted in the block diagram of Fig. 1.3b.

In PW mode range discrimination is obtained, since the time of flight of a received echo can be converted into a specific depth (sample volume location). This assumes the propagation velocity of

Table 1.2 CW versus PW Doppler ultrasound measurements.

CW	PW
+ sensitive	+ range resolution
+ inexpensive	+ variable sample volume size
+ high signal/noise ratio	+ stepping stone to more advanced modalities
+ low acoustic output power	- lower signal/noise ratio
- no range resolution	- higher output power
	- range–velocity ambiguity

ultrasound in tissue to be known, and the received signal sampled accordingly (i.e. after a specific delay). One sample per period is acquired until enough data for an accurate estimation of the Doppler shift have been collected (typically 64–128 samples). The technique is known as range gating. A comparison of the CW and PW methods is given in Table 1.2.

LIMITATIONS OF DOPPLER SYSTEMS

The use of CW and PW Doppler ultrasound systems raises a number of problems and ambiguities, all of which influence the performance of color flow imaging (CFI) systems as well. Even when only one vessel is studied and only one frequency is emitted, a range of Doppler frequencies will be received. This phenomenon is known as spectral broadening. It is due either to flow profile variations within the vessel (i.e. many different velocities are detected) or to transit time effects. The latter is a fundamental uncertainty inherent in Doppler measurements. It is due to the finite period of time that each erythrocyte contributes to the backscattered signal, when it passes through the beam. Thus, even a single scatterer moving at a constant velocity will give rise to a spread of frequencies.

An echo must have returned to the receiver before the next burst is transmitted, if the depth of origin is

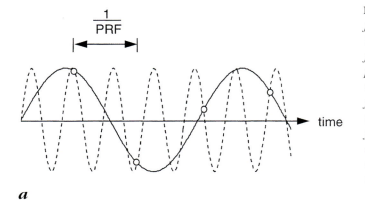

a

Figure 1.4 (a) Aliasing arises because a cyclic function is measured by sampling at intervals of time. The diagram shows what can occur if a high-frequency (dotted line) is sampled at an insufficient pulse repetition frequency (PRF). The sample points are represented by open circles. The reconstructed frequency (solid line) is lower than the true frequency. (b,c) Aliasing in pulsed Doppler. The Doppler frequency at peak systolic velocity is misinterpreted as a low frequency (b). By increasing the PRF, the velocities throughout the waveform are shown unambiguously (c).

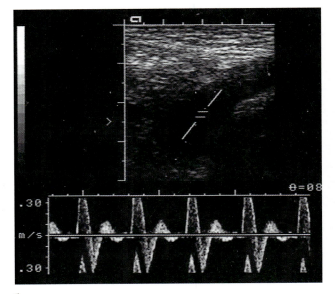

b

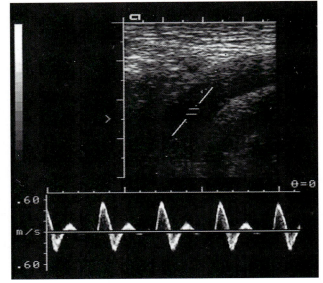

c

Table 1.3 Techniques for avoiding aliasing.

Increase the PRF
Increase the beam/vessel angle
Reduce the depth
Reduce the transducer frequency
Change the baseline
Use CW instead

where f_s is the system's sampling frequency (equal to the PRF). Note that while the maximum velocity measurable, v_{max}, increases with increasing PRF, the maximum depth measurable, d_{max}, decreases. In practice, aliasing can be avoided or at least limited by changing a number of parameters; see Table 1.3 and Fig. 1.4b,c.

The ambiguities in maximum depth and velocity measurable are often combined into one expression (the range–velocity ambiguity):

$$d_{max}v_{max} = \frac{c^2}{8f_c} \tag{1.4}$$

If the flow to be studied is known to be unidirectional, the relationship is altered to $c^2/4f_c$. The maximum depth and velocity are inversely related, and this equation is, therefore, independent of PRF. The trade-off between depth and velocity measurements constitutes an important compromise inherent in PW Doppler systems. The limitations this imposes are demonstrated in Fig. 1.5. The use of higher transducer frequencies is seen to limit the measurable velocity significantly for a given depth. Finally, it should be mentioned that the range–velocity ambiguity is a consequence of the measurement procedure and not a physical limitation. In theory it should be possible to devise processing schemes bypassing this limitation.

to be unambiguously determined. The maximum depth accessible is therefore limited by the propagation velocity and the interpulse duration of the systems (i.e. 1/PRF). Furthermore, there is a limit to the maximum velocity measurable. This is due to the digitizing applied. If the Doppler signal changes too rapidly between samples, it is impossible to reconstruct the correct Doppler shift frequency. This phenomenon is known as (frequency) aliasing, and an example is given in Fig. 1.4a. To avoid aliasing, the Nyquist sampling theorem must be fulfilled. This requires that:

$$f_D \leq \frac{f_s}{2} = \frac{PRF}{2} \tag{1.3}$$

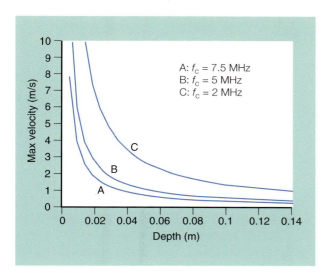

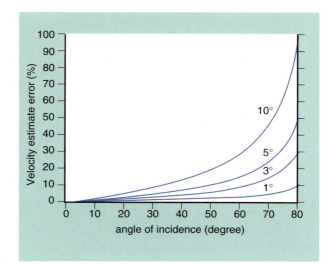

Figure 1.5 *The range–velocity ambiguity limits for ultrasound frequencies of 2, 5 and 7.5 MHz.*

Figure 1.6 *Velocity estimate errors. The x-axis shows the beam/vessel angle. The different lines show the errors due to 1, 3, 5 and 10°.*

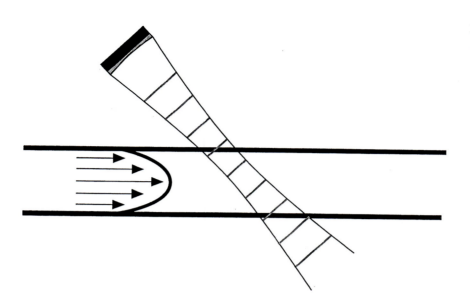

Figure 1.7 *Velocity profile measurement using a multigated (MG) Doppler system.*

An additional problem affecting all Doppler scanners is the angular dependence when converting the Doppler shift from a frequency (in Hz) to a velocity (in m/s). The correct angle of incidence (i.e. θ in equation 1.2) may not be known. Suppose, as an example, that the true angle is 50° but it is estimated to be 45°. The error in the velocity is 10%. At 70° the same uncertainty results in a 25% error, while at angles less than 20% these errors are insignificant, as demonstrated in Fig. 1.6.

MULTIGATED PW DOPPLER SYSTEMS

A PW Doppler system only provides information from one particular location. In order to obtain data from several depths simultaneously, a so-called multigated (MG) PW Doppler system must be employed.

Basically, after demodulation the received signal is directed to a number of parallel processing chains. Each has a slightly different range gate setting. This allows a number of adjacent sample volumes to be positioned across a vessel (Fig. 1.7). The problem of locating a vessel is greatly reduced.

Since the assessment of the bloodflow velocity is performed simultaneously in each sample volume, the velocity distribution along the vessel cross-section can be determined as a function of time. The veloc-

ity profile will be influenced by the presence of, for example, plaques or stenoses and can be, therefore, a useful diagnostic tool.

DUPLEX DOPPLER SYSTEMS

In spite of the advantages afforded by MG Doppler systems, orientation (in general) and locating the desired vessel (in particular) remain a problem. One way to overcome this is to combine two-dimensional B-scans with flow information. The first such combined systems were referred to as duplex Doppler scanners.

In duplex systems a PW Doppler beam is visualized across the B-mode image with the sample volume position indicated by a cursor (i.e. a range gate). This permits vessels to be easily selected for further evaluation. One example is shown in Fig. 1.8, with the duplex image at the top and spectral Doppler data, in the form of a sonogram, at the bottom. Notice how the location of the sample volume alters the measured spectra (low velocity at the vessel walls and higher flow in the center).

An advantage of a duplex system is that the angle of incidence can be estimated from the B-scan. Thus, Doppler frequency shifts can be transformed to flow velocity estimates. The assessment of the angle of

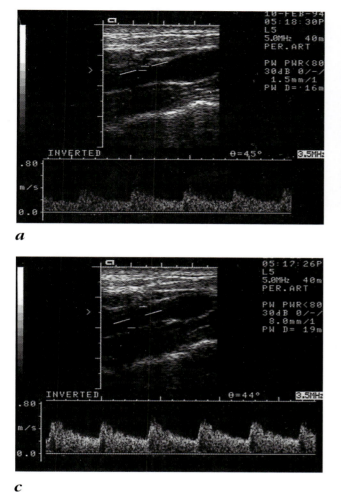

a

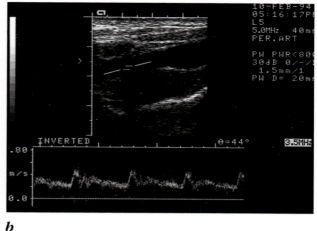
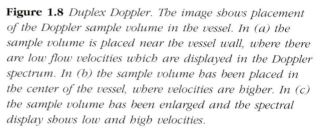

b

c

Figure 1.8 *Duplex Doppler. The image shows placement of the Doppler sample volume in the vessel. In (a) the sample volume is placed near the vessel wall, where there are low flow velocities which are displayed in the Doppler spectrum. In (b) the sample volume has been placed in the center of the vessel, where velocities are higher. In (c) the sample volume has been enlarged and the spectral display shows low and high velocities.*

incidence rests on a number of assumptions, such as flow parallel to the vessel walls and no curvature of the vessel in the scan plane. These assumptions are rarely fulfilled. However, the errors introduced are small, and velocity estimates facilitate comparisons between measurements since one more variable has been excluded. Due to the angular error, mentioned previously, one should always have a beam/flow angle of less than 60°.

Other errors include vessels being off-axis or curving compared to the scan plane (within the sample volume). This problem also occurs in CFI systems. The vessels are being projected onto a plane (Fig. 1.9). The error in velocity measurements due to z-plane misalignment has been found to be less than 5% at optimal settings, but up to 20% error has been measured in non-optimal circumstances.

The significance of the slice thickness or z-plane misalignment problem can be reduced in two ways, either using an annular array, which can be focused both in the z-plane and the lateral plane simultaneously, or by employing recently developed two-dimensional electronic arrays, which allow the slice thickness to be adjusted.

In spite of the name 'duplex', the B-mode and the Doppler scanning do not occur simultaneously. It takes significantly longer to acquire Doppler data than B-mode data, and early duplex scanners (using mechanical transducers) often froze the B-scan completely when obtaining flow information. The loss of real-time imaging was a major drawback. More recent duplex systems employing mechanical transducers might lower the frame rate, but will not freeze the image. It is, however, relatively straight-

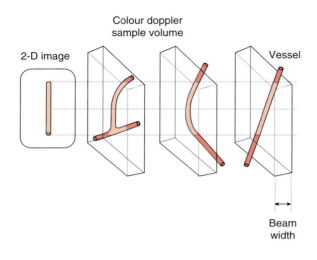

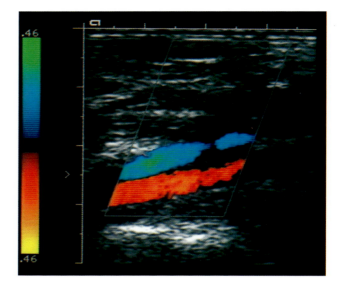

Figure 1.9 *Two-dimensional Doppler image representing different three-dimensional vessel anatomy. (Redrawn from Deane CR, Forsberg F, Thomas N and Roberts VC, J Biomed Eng 1991 volume 13, page 249, Figure 1, with permission from Butterworth-Heinemann, Oxford, England.)*

Figure 1.10 *Color flow image using blue for frequency shifts towards the beam and red away from it. The color represents velocity vectors in the direction of the beam. They are limited to a one-dimensional interpretation of flow. There has been no attempt to correct for the beam/flow angle.*

forward to employ different frequencies for imaging and Doppler (e.g. swapping one crystal out of three in a rotating transducer setup).

Currently, real-time duplex imaging is achieved with an electronically controlled transducer (phased or linear array), which can switch between imaging and Doppler fast enough to maintain an acceptable frame rate. Even though it is more complicated to obtain different transmit frequencies for Doppler and B-mode (it requires employing very broad-band transducers), such systems have many practical advantages when compared to their mechanical counterparts.

COLOR FLOW IMAGING

After devising MG Doppler systems that acquire flow data along an entire scan line, and Doppler systems which overlap a Doppler beam on a B-mode image, the next step seems logical: overlay a B-scan with flow information from all depths, i.e. along the entire A-line, and expand the number of A-lines to cover a region of interest. This is the principle of all CFI systems.

Instead of the Doppler shifts being displayed as a separate entity, the information can be superimposed on the B-scan. The estimated velocity of each sample volume is mapped to a color representing the direction of flow as well as its magnitude (via the color hue). Typically, shades of red and blue are used for flow towards and away from, respectively, the transducer (Fig. 1.10). There are, however, numerous other color maps available from different manufacturers. The variance of the velocity estimate, i.e. the spectral broadening of the Doppler signal, can be included as a third color (often green; Fig. 1.11).

Even though CFI systems may appear to constitute a 'logical' extension of PW Doppler and duplex Doppler, they do in fact represent a fundamentally different hardware structure. The reason for this is time! In a PW system 64–128 samples are acquired per Doppler waveform over approximately 10 ms. Even if each A-line was processed in enough paral-

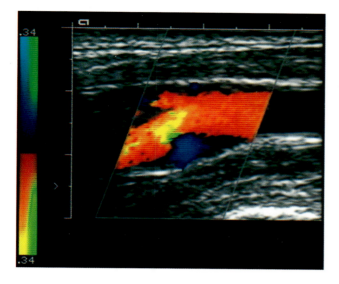

Figure 1.11 *Color flow showing green-labeled variance. There is a small region showing high variance where there is most flow fluctuation between sampling pulses.*

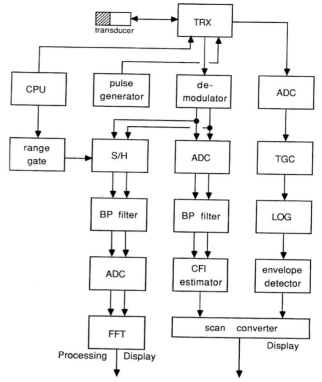

Figure 1.12 *Block diagram of integrated CFI scanner. The second column from the left represents the PW Doppler system, the third the color flow system, and the right-hand column the B-mode system. Abbreviations are explained in the text.*

lel channels to cover all depths along the scan line, there would not be sufficient time to record 128 Doppler A-lines and a B-mode image in real time. Consequently, CFI systems are limited to typically 6–32 samples per range gate, i.e. 6–32 bursts transmitted in each direction. This time limit puts severe constraints on all filters and estimators involved in the processing scheme. Hence, digital filters and early digitizing are essential in CFI systems to get sufficiently fast and short responses.

In Fig. 1.12 a block diagram of a basic CFI system is presented. The leftmost column represents a PW Doppler system (cf. Fig. 1.3), while the middle column is the color Doppler processor. Notice how the digitization (i.e. the ADC) takes place as early as possible. Since the strong stationary and quasistationary echoes are not filtered out before digitization, a very powerful ADC is required. The rightmost column depicts the B-mode circuitry. The time-gain compensation (TGC) is an attempt to compensate for the effect of attenuation, before the signal is logarithmically compressed for envelope detection and display.

Another consequence of the limited processing time available in CFI systems is that the Doppler signal itself is not estimated. Instead, just one parameter, such as the mean Doppler shift, is extracted and shown. Thus, a method for estimating the chosen parameter quickly along the entire A-line, without resorting to parallel processing, must be devised. This is the task of the CFI estimator of Fig. 1.12.

FREQUENCY ESTIMATORS FOR CFI SCANNERS

The estimation technique used in most CFI systems is known as the autocorrelation method. Here the phase of the autocorrelation function is calculated as a function of the interpulse duration time (i.e. 1/PRF).

This is equivalent to comparing echo segments from consecutive A-lines to one another, and allows the phase change caused by the Doppler shift of the erythrocytes to be estimated. The mean Doppler shift and thus the velocity can be calculated from this phase shift.

The autocorrelator can estimate the Doppler shift along an A-line with as few as 3–4 samples. This requires all stationary echoes, which are much stronger than the bloodflow signals, to be removed efficiently. The calculations are performed in approximately 1 ms at a PRF of 4 kHz (compared to the 10 ms of an ordinary PW Doppler system).

An alternative estimator based on time domain correlation has been developed. In this method the velocity estimate is based on maximizing the cross-correlation between small segments of two consecutive A-lines. The delay corresponding to maximum correlation, τ, is related to the axial velocity via:

$$\tau = \frac{2v}{c} T_R \qquad (1.5)$$

where T_R is equal to 1/PRF.

One major advantage of the time domain correlation approach is that it is much less susceptible to aliasing. Remember that it measures time delays and not phase changes. The simple relationship of equation 1.5 provides an indication of the distance a group of scatterers have moved between two consecutive excitation pulses. If their speed is sufficiently high, the group of reflectors being tracked may totally leave the sample volume before the next burst arrives. This renders the velocity estimate meaningless. Hence, aliasing in a time domain system is determined by the PRF and the beam width employed. This constitutes a much more flexible limit on velocity detection than the rigid Nyquist sampling theorem of PW-based systems.

Moreover, recent investigations indicate that the cross-correlation technique as well as the so-called wide-band maximum likelihood estimator (WMLE) are significantly more precise in the presence of intervening tissue (compared to the traditional autocorrelator). While a commercial scanner using time domain correlation is available (under the name color velocity imaging or CVI), no system employing the even more promising WMLE method has yet been launched.

PULSE-ECHO/DOPPLER INTERACTION

To get a real-time B-mode image as well as to visualize rapid flow changes, it is necessary to switch rapidly between imaging and Doppler acquisition. Linear or phased array transducers with their electronic switching and beam-steering capabilities are, therefore, the most common choice for CFI systems. Mechanical transducers have been employed in the past, but these are becoming increasingly rare on today's scanners.

Another problem is how to combine the pulse-echo and Doppler data acquisition. In synchronous systems the received signal is split into two separate processing schemes, one for imaging and one for Doppler. Unfortunately, the requirements for optimal Doppler and optimal pulse-echo imaging are not identical. Therefore, even though very high frame rates are feasible, this is achieved at the expense of resolution and general image quality.

Alternatively, pulse-echo and Doppler data can be acquired independently (an asynchronous system). This scheme allows the B-mode imaging and the Doppler pulses to be optimized separately. However, other compromises are required.

If every other pulse is used for imaging, and alternatively Doppler, the available PRF is halved. This means a reduction in the maximum velocity measurable. On the other hand, if many Doppler bursts are employed interrupted by a single imaging pulse, the possible B-scan frame rate is reduced. Instead, a complete timesharing scheme is used. A whole image scan is performed and Doppler information is then collected over a time period which retains a reasonable frame rate (e.g. 15 frames/s).

Asynchronous data acquisition will mean missing the Doppler signal in periods during which the B-mode image is being formed. Hence, it is necessary to generate a substitute signal. This is done by either repeating the last bit of Doppler data acquired or by synthesizing a Doppler fill-in signal. In CFI systems the period of flow data acquisition can be minimized by reducing the overall number of Doppler scan lines, the axial resolution and the region of interest.

PROBLEMS IN CFI

As described, CFI systems are based on the principles of PW Doppler scanners. Hence, aliasing is a recurring problem. However, aliasing is a bigger problem in CFI systems, since typically a much lower PRF is used. Another problem arises because one simple 'characteristic' Doppler frequency representing the blood velocities in the sample volume over a 1-ms period is displayed, separated by long 'dead times'. A frame rate of 10 is not uncommon in CFI scanners, which means a rate of 10 interrogations and displays per sample volume per second. This should be compared to the approximately 100 spectra per second calculated in a PW Doppler sample volume.

Solid tissue motion is another CFI artifact. This so-called flash artifact is usually of very short duration, which makes it easy to recognize, although the artifact may obscure low flows, particularly in the abdomen.

Since all color coding is performed relative to the transducer, multiple flow/beam angles may constitute a problem. Very tortuous vessels will be color coded in a wide range of hues, often with flow both towards and away from the transducer. This phenomenon is less noticeable in linear arrays, where the angle of incidence (the beam/vessel angle) is constant. In transducers with a sector-shaped field of view (i.e. phased array, annular array, curvilinear array and mechanical transducers) even a straight vessel perpendicular to the transducer surface will be coded in a multitude of hues.

Due to the very limited number of samples available for the CFI estimators, these are inherently more qualitative than their spectral counterparts (FFT-based processors as in CW, PW and MG Doppler systems). Consider a PW Doppler system. The sonogram provides a display of all Doppler frequencies detected in the sample volume in each 10-ms period at a rate of 100 displays per second. Conversely, in a CFI system one Doppler shift is found for each 100 ms. More quantitative blood velocity information is thus obtainable from a PW Doppler system.

COLOR AMPLITUDE IMAGING

Color flow maps based on amplitude information have been available for many years. Much of the early work demonstrated little difference between

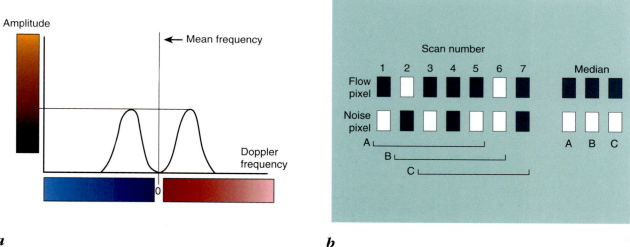

a   *b*

Figure 1.13 *Color amplitude imaging. (a) The output from the color Doppler processor shows the movement signal in terms of a velocity–frequency (blue–red scale) based on the velocity component of the scatterers and an amplitude (yellow scale) based on the received power from the amplitude. The diagram shows two signals, one in the blue range of frequencies and one in the red. Both have the same amplitude. If these two signals resulted from successive pulse pairs, the mean frequency/velocity of the two pulse pairs would be zero and any signal based on the mean would show no color. The mean amplitude would be the amplitude of the individual signals, and there would be color shown on the amplitude scale. (b) Frame averaging to reduce signal noise. The diagram shows the color output from two sample volumes displayed as pixels, one arising from a flow source and one from noise. In successive real-time scans, both signals show intermittent color. By taking the median over five successive scans, the noise signal is removed and flow is shown within the flow sample volume. The median is updated with every successive scan.*

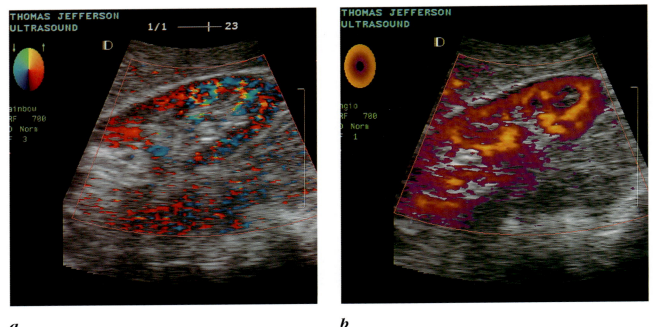

a   *b*

Figure 1.14 *Color amplitude image of a kidney. (a) Conventional color flow image shows the presence of a range of frequency shifts in the cortical region of the kidney and noise in the surrounding tissue. (b) Color amplitude image of the same kidney. The color hue is more uniform and gain has been increased to enhance the flow signal. Frame averaging reduces noise in the tissue.*

this mode and conventional mean frequency-based CFI. Recently, however, color amplitude imaging (CAI) has received much attention due to the reported increase in 'flow sensitivity', which is in fact a result of the increase in display dynamic range achievable by this technique.

In CAI the density of the red blood cells is depicted as opposed to their velocity (Fig. 1.13). The amplitude and, thus, the intensity and power of the backscattered signal depends on the number of red blood cells present within the sample volume, the size of the vessel and the attenuation of the intervening tissue. Since the Doppler frequency shift information is not utilized, amplitude imaging is non-directional, and does not suffer from aliasing. Furthermore, CAI is significantly less angle dependent, which effectively eliminates the multiple-angle artifact often encountered in traditional CFI.

Another advantage of amplitude displays is the improvement in functional lumen definition. The difference between Doppler frequency shifts from a sample volume close to the vessel wall and from one partially overlapping the wall will be very small. However, the number of red blood cells insonated within the two sample volumes will be quite different and, therefore, so will the amplitude of the backscattered signals.

CAI is often referred to as being 'more sensitive' than conventional CFI; 10–15 dB of improvement have been reported. This, however, is a misconception caused by inappropriate terminology. Since both amplitude and frequency shift maps are derived from the same information (the same RF A-lines), one cannot, by definition, be more sensitive than the other. The reason why smaller vessels are visualized in CAI is that the display dynamic range has been increased by sacrificing part of the available information (i.e. velocity and directivity) and by increasing the persistence of the displayed flow signals. This allows the 'color priority' to be increased, thus producing the apparent increase in sensitivity.

CAI differentiates between regions of flow and regions of no flow (Fig. 1.14), but cannot assess effects such as pulsatility and flow reversal.

Table 1.4 Characteristics of color amplitude displays.

Advantages	Disadvantages
Increases display dynamic range ('increased sensitivity')	Susceptible to motion artifacts
No multiple-angle artifact	No direction information
No aliasing	No velocity information
Limited angle dependence	More affected by attenuation
Better vessel wall definition	Limited temporal information

Furthermore, amplitude displays are more susceptible to attenuation effects, i.e. loss of signal strength with increasing depth. However, the most noticeable disadvantage of CAI is the susceptibility to motion artifacts. Amplitude displays can be overwhelmed by the flash artifact, which severely limits their applicability in areas with significant motion (e.g. the heart).

To compensate for the motion-induced artifacts, CAI employs significant weighted temporal averaging (i.e. high frame-to-frame averaging) (Fig. 1.13b). This technique reduces the flash artifact, but also increases the display response time (i.e. the color map seems to lag behind the gray scale image). A summary of the characteristics of amplitude displays is given in Table 1.4.

CONCLUSION

CFI systems are frequently used in conjunction with PW Doppler systems. The color map is used to guide for sample volume placement (i.e. the site for spectral analysis) and for giving an instant overview of the flow conditions in a region of interest. This latter ability is what makes the CFI system such an important (albeit qualitative) diagnostic tool. CAI depicts the density of red blood cells in a vessel and should be used as an adjunct to conventional mean frequency-based Doppler displays.

FURTHER READING

Doppler JC, Uber das farbige licht der Doppelsterne und einiger anderer Gestirne des Himmels, *Abb K Bohm Ges Wissenach (Prague)* (1843) 465–82.

Hein IA, O'Brien Jr WD, Current time-domain methods for assessing tissue motion by analysis from reflected ultrasound echoes—a review, *IEEE Trans Ultrason Ferroelec Freq Contrl* (1993) **40**:84–102.

Kremkau FW, Doppler color imaging. Principles and instrumentation, *Clin Diagn Ultrasound* (1992) **27**:7–60.

Kristoffersen K, Angelsen BAJ, A time-shared ultrasound Doppler measurement and 2D imaging system, *IEEE Trans Biomed Eng* (1988) **35**:285–95.

Leeman S, Roberts VC, Willson K, Quantitative Doppler with ultrasound pulses, *Phys Med Biol* (1986) 134–40.

Magnin PA, Doppler effect: history and theory, *Hewlett-Packard J* (1986) **37**:26–31.

Mitchell DG, Color Doppler imaging: principles, limitations, and artifacts, *Radiology* (1990) **177**:1–10.

Rubin JM, Bude RO, Carson PL et al, Power Doppler US: a potentially useful alternative to mean frequency-based color Doppler US, *Radiology* (1994) **190**: 853–6.

Satomura S, A study on examining the heart with ultrasonics, *Jpn Circul J* (1956) **20**:227.

Shung KK, Siegelman RA, Reid JM, Scattering of ultrasound by blood, *IEEE Trans Biomed Eng* (1976) **23**:460–7.

Chapter 2 Basic principles of and practical hints for color flow imaging

Philip W Ralls and Daniel A Merton

INTRODUCTION

Some terminology commonly used to describe the sonographic detection of blood flow is inaccurate, misused or confusing. For example, both color Doppler and spectral Doppler are pulsed and duplex. The term 'duplex Doppler' describes a combined display of anatomic and flow information, a feature of both color flow imaging (CFI) and pulsed (single sample volume) spectral Doppler images. Additionally, not all CFI is performed using Doppler techniques. The American Institute of Ultrasound in Medicine recommends the term 'pulsed Doppler' be reserved for single sample volume Doppler interrogation *without* a corresponding B-mode image, and 'duplex Doppler' to describe single sample volume Doppler *with* a corresponding B-mode image. In order to avoid confusion and maintain consistency, the term 'duplex Doppler' (DD) will be used in this chapter to indicate single sample volume pulsed Doppler with a corresponding two-dimensional image (with or without a spectral display), and CFI will be used to represent all ultrasonic CFI modes. Specific types of CFI will be indicated when necessary.

All ultrasound flow detection techniques use the pulse-echo principle (distance from the transducer determined by time of flight) to localize flow information. CFI displays bloodflow information superimposed over all or part of the gray scale image (Fig. 2.1). This is distinct from conventional DD, which requires the operator to manually position a relatively small sample volume, or range gate, over a selected portion of the gray scale image in an attempt to obtain flow signals. If an area is not

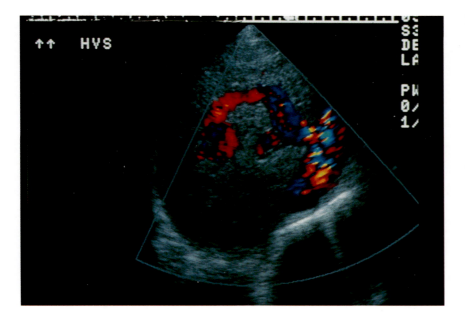

Figure 2.1 *CFI can demonstrate bloodflow superimposed over large anatomic regions. Transverse CFI of the right lobe of the liver demonstrating dilated hepatic veins in a patient with heart failure and tricuspid regurgitation. Notice how the enlarged hepatic veins are shown throughout the visualized portion of the liver.*

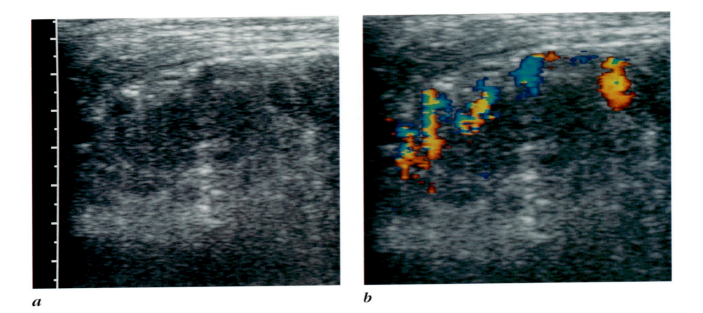

a *b*

Figure 2.2 *Transverse images of the right upper abdomen without (a), and with (b) CFI. Omental varices resulting from portal hypertension are seen only with CFI. CFI enhances the information content of sonographic images by displaying flow that is otherwise not visualized. This is an example of pathology not appreciated by gray scale imaging alone.*

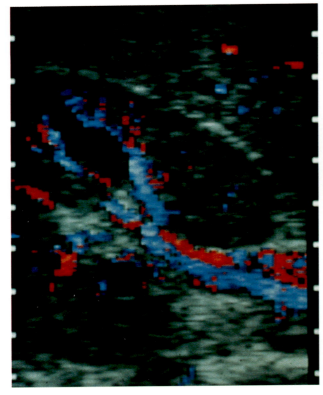

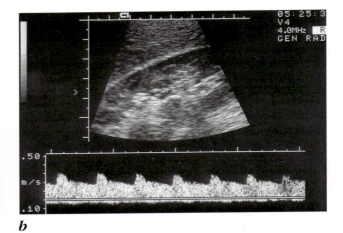

b

Figure 2.3 *When detailed spectral Doppler information is required, CFI can be used to localize the sample volume more quickly and with greater precision than is usually possible without its use. Here a transverse CFI of the right kidney (a) identifies the location of the main renal artery and vein as well as small intrarenal vessels. Intrarenal bloodflow can be obtained using conventional DD with spectral analysis (b), but the information is only obtained by manually positioning the sample volume within the kidney—a process that may be time-consuming, more operator dependent, and tedious.*

a

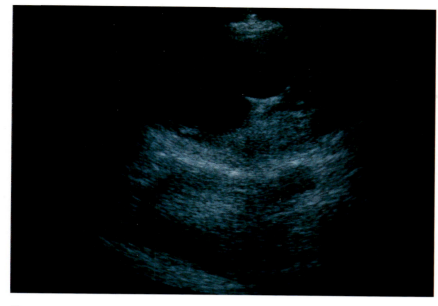

a

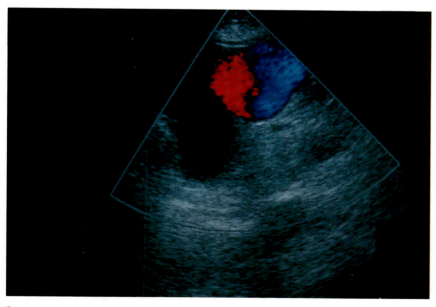

b

Figure 2.4 *In this oblique image of the gallbladder region using gray scale only (a), a fluid collection adjacent to the gallbladder was suspected, and needle aspiration considered. CFI (b) immediately revealed the vascular nature of the structure and a potentially hazardous aspiration was prevented. This was determined to represent a varix of a recannalized paraumbilical vein adjacent to the gallbladder. While this could have been determined using gray scale and/or spectral Doppler, CFI made the diagnosis more quickly and with less operator dependence.*

interrogated, flow in unexpected areas will be missed (Fig. 2.2). Thus, CFI generally provides flow information from a larger portion of the image more quickly, and with less operator dependence than does DD. When detailed quantitative flow information is important, or to better demonstrate temporal changes in bloodflow dynamics, a spectral Doppler display is required. In this case CFI can facilitate quick and accurate sample volume placement by providing a 'road map' of areas with flow, which the operator can use as a guide to position the sample volume and obtain a spectral Doppler display (Fig. 2.3). CFI is invaluable when flow detection or global anatomic information on bloodflow is needed to assist in deriving a diagnosis. CFI's ability to provide a global view of flow in real

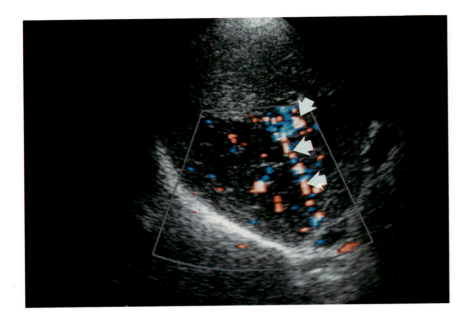

Figure 2.5 *Using CFI of the liver, increased flow at the periphery of a hepatocellular carcinoma (arrows) can be compared to the normal adjacent parenchyma. CFI facilitates comparison of flow between adjacent or even non-adjacent regions.*

time minimizes the chance of missing flow in an unexpected area (Figs 2.2 and 2.4) and facilitates comparison of flow in different anatomic locations (Fig. 2.5). In addition, CFI allows more rapid acquisition of both anatomic and flow information than is usually possible with conventional DD, and the combination of bloodflow information in color with anatomy in gray scale is generally easier to comprehend than a DD display.

BASIC PRINCIPLES

With most conventional CFI systems both flow direction and mean Doppler frequency shifts are color coded. Typically, the colors red and blue represent flow directed toward or away from the transducer respectively (Fig. 2.6). Mean Doppler frequency shifts are often depicted as differences in color saturation,

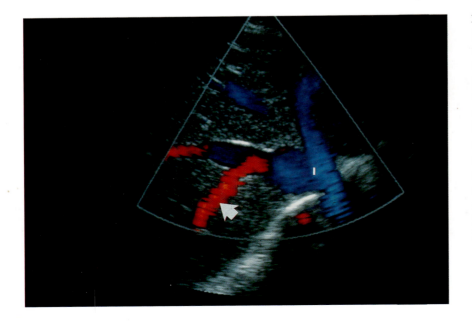

Figure 2.6 *Transverse CFI of the liver at the level of the hepatic vein confluence demonstrates bloodflow directed into the inferior vena cava (I). Typically, flow towards the transducer is coded red (arrow) and flow directed away from the transducer is coded blue. While this display feature can be inverted, using a standard flow direction display allows the operator to become more accustomed to interpreting the flow information, which may allow more rapid determination of flow direction.*

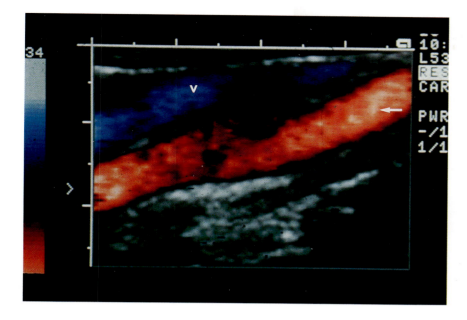

Figure 2.7 *CFI saturation map of the common carotid artery and jugular vein (V). With this color flow map, the more saturated, deeper colors represent lower Doppler frequency shifts (velocities) occurring along the vessel walls, and lighter colors represent the greater Doppler frequency shifts encountered in center stream (arrow).*

with lighter colors representing higher-frequency shifts, and deeper reds and blues corresponding to lower-frequency shifts (Fig. 2.7). An alternative flow display is the color hue map in which different colors (e.g. red to orange, and blue to green) are used to color code different Doppler frequency shifts (Fig. 2.8). Most manufacturers allow the operator to select from a variety of color maps, the choice of which is a matter of operator preference. Consistently utilizing a single color map for a given application may allow users to become more accustomed to interpreting the CFI information.

There are significant differences in the way flow signals are obtained between CFI and DD. With DD the sample volume location is insonated many times, resulting in a comprehensive display of the entire range of Doppler frequency shifts. Since CFI must display, in real time, both flow and gray scale infor-

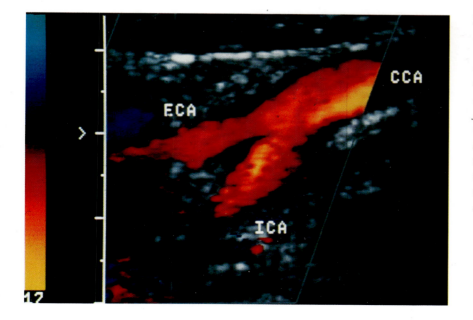

Figure 2.8 *CFI hue map image of the common carotid artery (CCA) bifurcation. With this flow map, different Doppler frequency shifts are displayed as different colors. Note that the lower Doppler frequency shifts along the vessel walls are deep red, and the higher Doppler frequency shifts in midstream progress from orange ultimately to yellow. ECA, external carotid artery; ICA, internal carotid artery.*

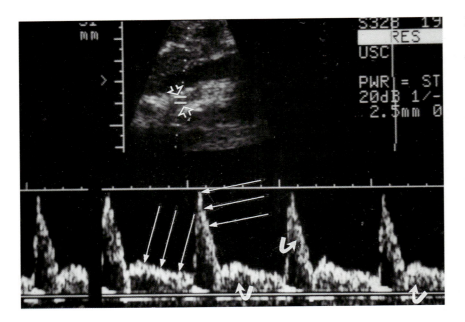

Figure 2.9 *Pulsed Doppler spectral analysis displays not only peak frequency shifts (long thin arrows) but also the lower-frequency shifts (curved arrows) occurring simultaneously. Doppler spectral analysis provides more detailed flow information than CFI, albeit over a much smaller area—in this case a 2.5 mm sample volume (open arrows).*

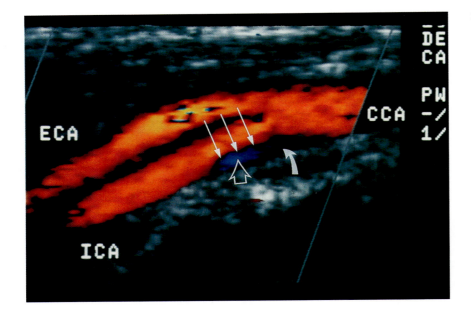

Figure 2.10 *Longitudinal CFI of the common carotid artery (CCA) bifurcation. This color hue map shows mean Doppler frequency shifts throughout the entire color box (indicated by the parallel gray lines). The global display of bloodflow using CFI provides flow information in real time that is usually easier to comprehend than conventional spectral Doppler displays. Antegrade flow is present in the internal (ICA) and external (ECA) carotid arteries. A normal region of flow reversal (open arrow) in the carotid bulb is displayed as blue. Note the black line (thin arrows) separating the adjacent regions of flow in opposite directions. A small area of no flow (curved arrow) is a result of an anechoic vessel wall defect causing narrowing of the functional lumen.*

mation over a relatively large area, flow information derived from each scan line is necessarily more limited; each scan line is insonated only a few times per frame, much fewer than with DD. Thus, as a practical matter, CFI typically can only display mean Doppler frequency shifts and variance (roughly corresponding to spectral broadening), whereas DD displays the peak, as well as all other detectable Doppler shifts (Fig. 2.9). One exception to this is color amplitude imaging (CAI) where the amplitude (also known as 'power', 'energy', or 'intensity') of the color Doppler signal is displayed as opposed to the Doppler frequency shifts. Another exception is a non-Doppler flow detection modality termed Color

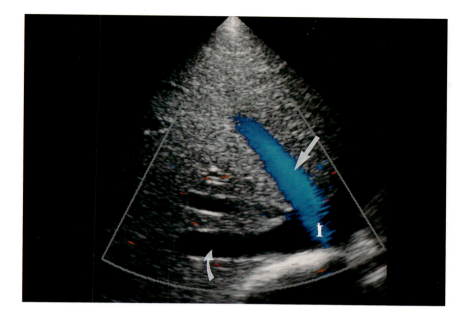

Figure 2.11 *Transverse CFI of the hepatic vein confluence with the IVC (I). Bloodflow in the middle hepatic vein (arrow) is well seen because the low scan angle (near zero degrees) results in an adequate Doppler shift. The right hepatic vein (curved arrow) is being imaged at a nearly perpendicular angle and no flow information is displayed. Using a low angle of insonation is critical to optimize flow detection.*

Velocity Imaging™ (Philips Medical Systems, Santa Ana, Ca) which displays peak flow velocities in color. In essence, regardless of which color modality is used, CFI provides less complete bloodflow information, but with the added benefit of providing a more global and readily obtained depiction of bloodflow in real time (Fig. 2.10).

Color flow images which are not angle corrected by the operator display *mean Doppler frequency shifts*, not *flow velocities*. For this reason, CFI is primarily used for a qualitative assessment of bloodflow and quantification of flow via velocity estimates, or a variety of pulsatility ratios is performed using DD with spectral waveform analysis.

It is important to remember that there is a fundamental technical difference between CFI and conventional gray scale ultrasound. Because Doppler ultrasound typically has a lower signal-to-noise ratio than gray scale imaging, signal attenuation is more of an obstacle. Therefore, the CFI transmit frequency is typically lower than the transmit frequency used to acquire gray scale data. For example, a 3.5 MHz (gray scale) probe will usually use a transmit frequency of 2.0 MHz to obtain CFI data. As with gray scale imaging, CFI transducer frequencies used for superficial (i.e. small parts, and peripheral vascular) applications are higher (4–6 MHz) than those frequencies used for CFI when deeper structures need to be

assessed. For abdominal CFI applications, CFI frequencies typically range from 2 MHz to 4 MHz. Some manufacturers provide, within a single probe, several CFI output frequencies, thereby allowing the operator to select the CFI frequency best suited for a given scanning situation without having to change probes.

A basic principle of all Doppler scanning techniques is that lower scan angles produce greater Doppler shifts. The maximum Doppler shift occurs when blood is flowing directly towards or away from the transducer. Thus, the optimal scan angle is zero degrees (Fig. 2.11). As the scan angle approaches 90°, the Doppler frequency shift decreases. At 90°, cosine τ equals zero. Hence, blood flowing perpendicular to the scan line will often not be detected, since no Doppler shift is generated (Figs 2.11 and 2.12). Attempting to keep the angle of incidence near zero degrees will improve CFI sensitivity and reduce flow direction ambiguities.

With CFI, blood flowing at a uniform velocity in a vessel will be displayed as different colors if imaged at different angles. Thus, bloodflow in a tortuous vessel will be represented by several different colors (Fig. 2.13). Similarly, blood flowing in a vessel parallel to the transducer face of a sector or curved linear array transducer may be displayed as red on one side of the image and blue on the other (Fig. 2.14). This

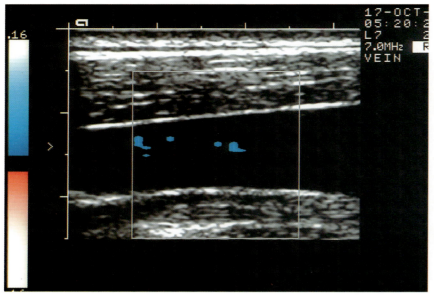

a

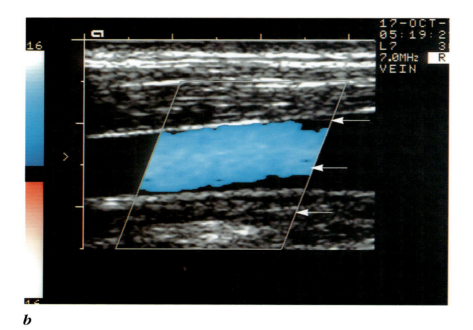

b

Figure 2.12 *Using a flat linear array transducer to image the jugular vein with the CFI beam directed straight down (a), and electronically steered (b) at an angle as indicated by the slant of the color box (arrows). Due to a poor Doppler angle, the flow information obtained in (a) is insufficient and the flow direction ambiguous. In (b) the improved Doppler angle provides an unambiguous display of bloodflow location and direction. When imaging vessels that course parallel to the face of a flat linear array transducer, steering the Doppler beam provides better Doppler angles and will result in the acquisition of improved CFI information.*

results from the divergent scan lines produced by these transducers, and the flow direction relative to the transducer.

When the bloodflow velocity is relatively high and a low pulse repetition frequency (PRF) is used (as, for example, in situations where optimal sensitivity is important), aliasing may result. Aliasing causes ambiguous or confusing color and spectral Doppler displays. Aliasing on spectral Doppler causes a 'wrap-around' display with part of the waveform (usually the peaks of arterial signals) displayed on the wrong side of the baseline (Fig. 2.15). Aliasing on CFI results in a color display in which the color signals will extend from the maximum frequency shift in one

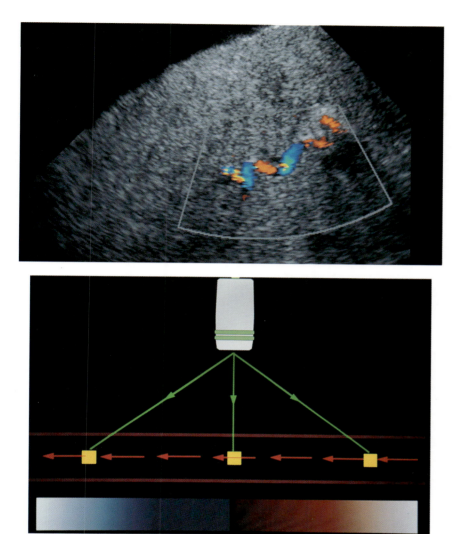

a

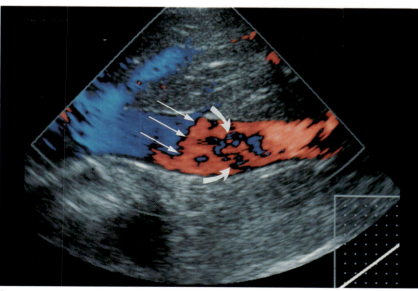

b

Figure 2.13 *Transverse CFI of a hepatic artery branch within a cirrhotic liver. Red and blue indicate flow towards and away from the transducer respectively. In this tortuous 'corkscrew' artery associated with cirrhosis, bloodflow is represented by different colors within the same vessel due to the changes in flow direction relative to the transducer.*

Figure 2.14 *Sketch, sector transducer (a). Longitudinal CFI (b) of the inferior vena cava. (a) demonstrates the phenomenon that is seen when a curved linear or sector transducer is employed for CFI. When a vessel courses parallel to the transducer face, the changing scan angles cause bloodflow to be displayed in varying colors within the same vessel. In (b) blood flows towards the transducer on the right side of image (color coded red) and away from the transducer on the left side (color coded blue). Between these two areas is a transition zone where there is no flow detected, representing a 90° Doppler angle (thin arrows). Near 90°, different colors will be displayed (curved arrows) when bloodflow is not uniform, as is the case in many vessels, especially veins.*

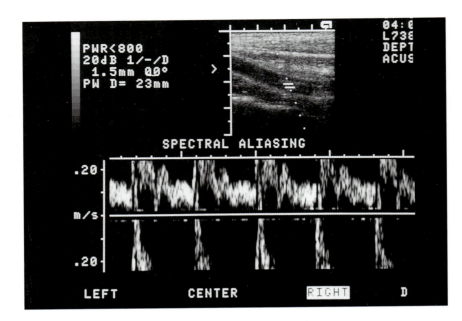

Figure 2.15 *Spectral Doppler aliasing. An inadequate (i.e. too low) pulse repetition frequency (PRF) results in aliasing, with the highest-frequency shifts 'wrapped around' and displayed below the baseline.*

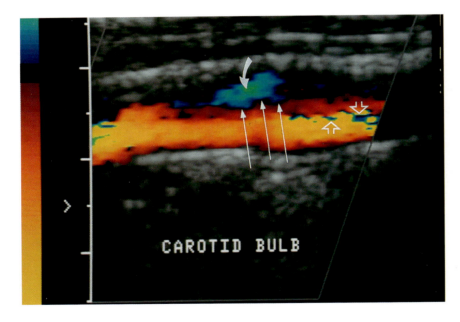

Figure 2.16 *Longitudinal CFI of the carotid bulb demonstrating CFI velocity resolution and color aliasing. Velocity resolution is demonstrated as the ability to visualize focal variations of flow velocities which are occurring across the vessel lumen. The slower flow velocities occurring along the vessel walls are coded deep red, while the higher velocities near center stream are coded orange and yellow. CFI aliasing (open arrows) is identified by the color transition from the highest value in one direction (in this case yellow) adjacent to the highest value in the opposite direction (green), while true flow reversal occurring in the bulb (curved arrow) is identified by flow coded blue separated from flow coded red by a black line (thin arrows).*

direction into the maximum frequency shift in the opposite direction ('wrap-around') and, if the aliasing is severe, progressively further into the color shades related to lower-frequency shifts in the opposite direction of the flow (Figs 2.16 and 2.17). This can potentially result in a confusing CFI representation of flow in a vessel. To avoid aliasing, a CFI system must sample at a rate at least two times higher than the mean Doppler frequency shift. Increasing the PRF or changing the baseline position eliminates aliasing by displaying the flow in a single color. Less severe color aliasing may simulate flow reversal, potentially causing a diagnostic error (Fig. 2.18). However, a true change in flow direction is displayed as a color

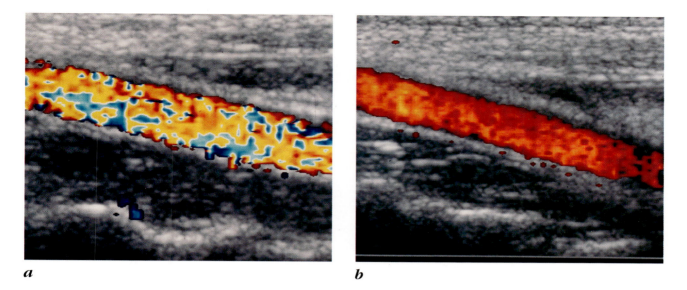

a *b*

Figure 2.17 *Severe CFI aliasing. When a low PRF is utilized (a) CFI displays a mixture of colors within the vessel. Increasing the PRF (b) eliminates aliasing and provides an image with unambiguous flow direction.*

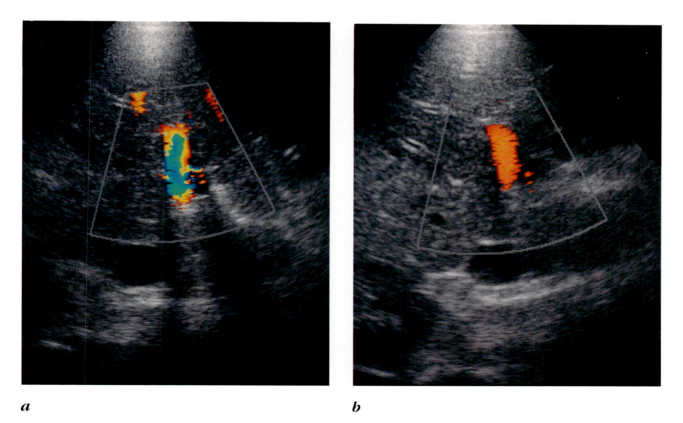

a *b*

Figure 2.18 *Transverse CFI of the left portal vein. Color aliasing (a) initially led to an erroneous diagnosis of flow reversal within the left portal vein. Increasing the PRF (b) eliminated the aliasing and demonstrated flow in a normal direction.*

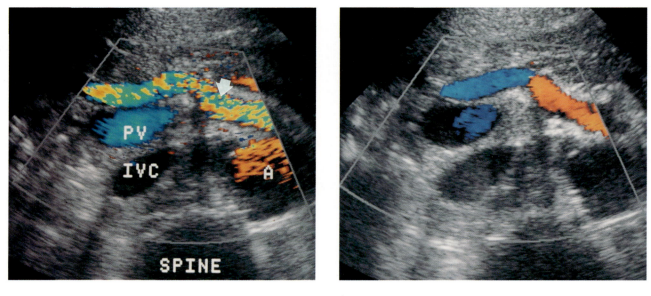

a   *b*

Figure 2.19 *Transverse CFI of the common hepatic artery with a low PRF (a) and higher PRF (b). Aliasing can be a useful artifact in abdominal scanning. At settings frequently used for abdominal scanning, flow within arteries is aliased (arrow), while flow within veins is not. This may allow the examiner to distinguish arteries from veins, often obviating the need to perform spectral Doppler to make this determination. When flow direction must be determined, the PRF can be increased (b) to eliminate the aliasing. While this will accurately display flow direction in the artery, a higher PRF will also reduce the CFI sensitivity to slower flow found in the inferior vena cava (IVC), portal vein (PV) and aorta (A). Note the change in color within the common hepatic artery, caused by the changing angle of flow in relation to the ultrasound beam (see Fig. 2.14).*

transition between the colors representing the lowest-frequency shifts in opposite directions, separated by a black line (Figs 2.10 and 2.16). The black line, not present in color transitions related to aliasing, is the region where no flow is displayed; the Doppler frequency shift is low and thus filtered out by the wall filter. In abdominal CFI aliasing can, at times, actually be a helpful artifact. At PRF settings often used, flow within arteries is aliased, while flow within veins is not. This may allow the examiner to more easily distinguish arteries from veins, without having to perform spectral Doppler analysis (Fig. 2.19). Of course, aliasing can be avoided, and flow direction better determined, by increasing the sampling rate (i.e. the PRF) or shifting the color baseline position. When evaluating flow in relatively large vessels such as the common carotid artery or abdominal aorta, a properly adjusted PRF and baseline position will provide good velocity resolution (the ability to demonstrate local variations of flow velocities occur-

ring across the vessel lumen) as well as a sufficient level of flow sensitivity to detect the slower velocities occurring along the vessel walls, and in diastole when looking at arterial bloodflow. When evaluating flow in smaller vessels, such as those within the renal cortex or small tumor vessels, using a low PRF will increase flow sensitivity and facilitate detection of flow (Fig. 2.20). As a reminder, while reducing the PRF will increase the sensitivity to low flow velocities, it will also reduce the frame rate and, therefore, temporal resolution.

Other significant factors influencing CFI sensitivity include: (1) the trade-off between tissue penetration and echo intensity; and (2) the impact of beam characteristics on Doppler information. When superficial organs or vessels are scanned, penetration is not a problem. It is better to use high-frequency CFI transducers for these applications, as higher echo intensity and superior resolution are obtained (Fig. 2.21). In abdominal and other deep Doppler

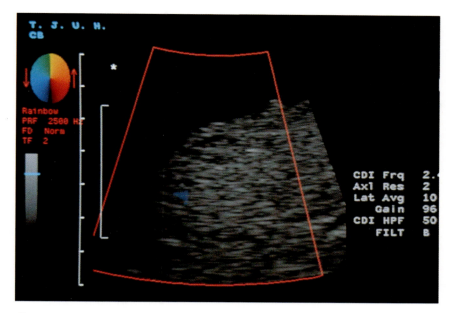

a

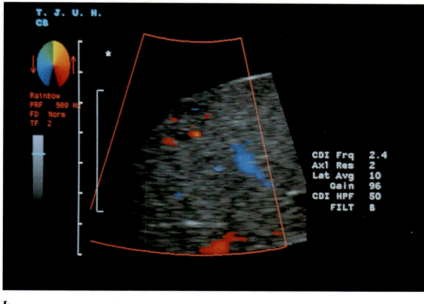

b

Figure 2.20 *Magnified transverse CFIs of a liver lesion (a) with a PRF of 2500, and (b) with a PRF of 900. (All other color parameters remain the same.) Note the increased sensitivity obtained with the lower PRF which enables detection of slow flow within vessels at the tumor periphery.*

applications, however, the need for adequate tissue penetration dominates (Fig. 2.22). Obviously, if adequate tissue penetration does not occur, no information will be provided. Thus, in many applications, penetration/attenuation effects dominate, and lower CFI frequencies should be used even at the cost of lower echo intensity and spatial resolution.

PRACTICAL CFI SCANNING TECHNIQUES

The acquisition of Doppler information and gray scale information requires significantly different technical approaches. Gray scale imaging is best

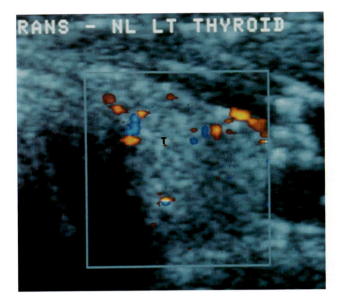

a

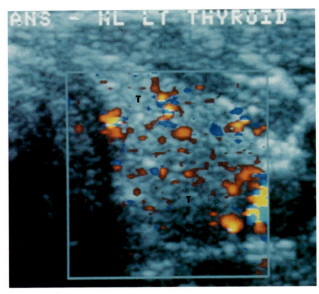

b

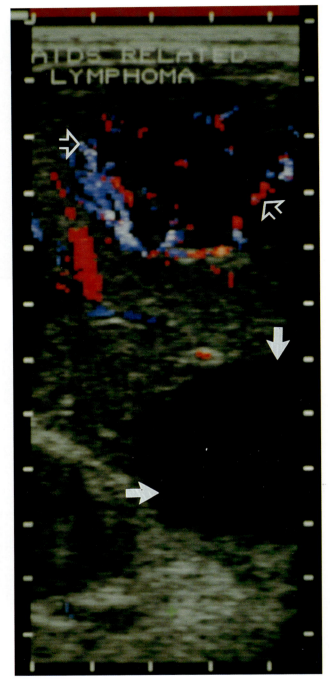

Figure 2.21 *Transverse CFI of the thyroid gland (T) obtained using a 5 MHz Doppler output frequency (a) reveals flow primarily located at the surface of the gland. Using a 7.5 MHz Doppler frequency (b), reveals more internal thyroid flow, a result of the greater Doppler frequency shifts provided by the higher Doppler output frequency. Use of a higher Doppler frequency is the dominant factor which provides higher sensitivity to flow in superficial structures. In deeper structures tissue penetration becomes more important and lower Doppler frequencies will usually provide better flow information.*

Figure 2.22 *AIDS-related lymphoma with focal liver masses. Flow is detected in the superficial hepatic lesion (open arrows), but tissue penetration is insufficient to detect flow in a deeper lesion (arrows), even though both are identical histologically. If a high-frequency transducer does not provide the necessary flow information, a lower-frequency CFI probe will often provide the tissue penetration needed.*

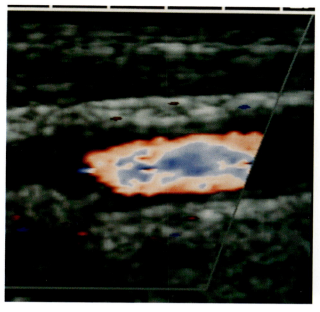

a

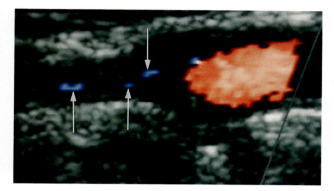

b

Figure 2.23 *Longitudinal CFI of a high-grade stenosis of the internal carotid artery. When scanning superficial structures, a higher CFI frequency is advantageous. An image obtained at 5 MHz for CFI (a) suggests complete obstruction of the internal carotid artery. However, using 7 MHz CFI (b), flow is detected through a high-grade carotid stenosis (arrows).*

performed using a 90° angle of insonation (perpendicular to structures), a narrowly focused beam, and short ultrasound pulses to optimize spatial resolution. In contrast, the Doppler frequency shift is maximum at zero degrees (parallel to the vessel axis) and the frequency response is most uniform when a relatively unfocused beam and a long pulse length are used. Frequency requirements also differ. A higher frequency is generally better for gray scale, where resolution needs dominate, whereas with CFI penetration is often the primary requirement and use of a lower frequency results in improved flow detection. These conflicting requirements make it easy to appreciate the engineering challenges involved in producing a state-of-the-art real-time CFI system. Several different approaches to this problem have been used in today's commercially available instruments. In many cases, performing all or most gray scale imaging prior to attempting to acquire Doppler information will allow the operator to concentrate on obtaining optimal resolution in gray scale, while concentrating on flow angles during the Doppler evaluation. In practice, obtain the two types of information (i.e. gray scale and Doppler) separately, but combine the results to form a diagnosis.

COMMON TECHNICAL CFI PROBLEMS AND THEIR SOLUTIONS

PROBLEM 1: LACK OF FLOW IN A VESSEL, OR POOR VESSEL FILL-IN: 'WHAT DO I DO WHEN I DON'T SEE FLOW?'

Many factors are important when CFI sensitivity is a problem. Good acoustic access is a prerequisite. To ensure this, the examiner must often try various patient positions, acoustic windows, and different transducer configurations. When scanning intercostally, a phased sector or curved linear array transducer with a small radius of curvature will usually afford better access than does a flat linear array probe. Scan angles close to zero degrees will also maximize sensitivity to flow by maximizing the Doppler frequency shifts. There is a trade-off between higher resolution provided by high frequencies, and penetration provided by lower frequencies. In superficial applications, a higher frequency is generally best (Fig. 2.23). In most other situations, penetration is usually the dominant requirement, and a lower frequency improves flow detection (Fig. 2.24). Once good acoustic access at a low scan angle

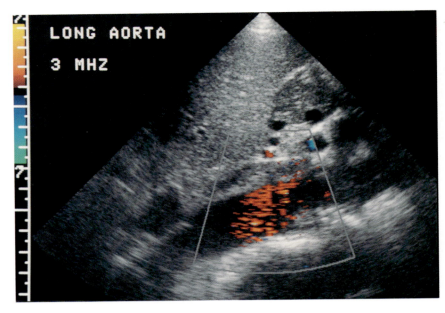

a

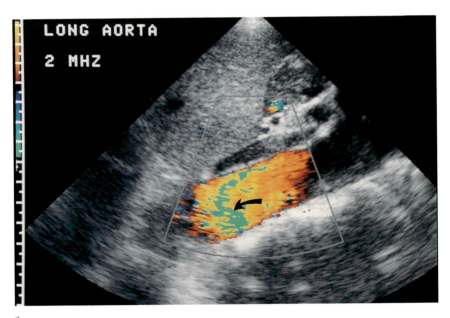

b

Figure 2.24 *Longitudinal CFI of the abdominal aorta. When scanning deeper structures, tissue penetration requirements dominate over the higher-frequency shifts provided by higher-frequency CFI transducers. While the image obtained at 3 MHz (a) demonstrates some flow within the aorta, an image obtained at 2 MHz (b) demonstrates flow much better. Some aliasing is present (curved arrow). The lack of flow information in the higher-frequency image is due to suboptimal penetration.*

and the correct frequency transducer have been obtained, the CFI system parameters must be optimized. The lowest PRF that provides flow information without aliasing will increase CFI sensitivity, as well as reduce acoustic power exposure (Fig. 2.25). As mentioned, shifting the CFI baseline to avoid aliasing instead of increasing the PRF will maintain a higher degree of CFI sensitivity. When evaluating slow bloodflow, a low wall filter (also known as a 'high-pass filter') will improve sensitivity (Fig. 2.26); however, color flash artifacts may be encountered if too low a wall filter and/or PRF are used (Figs 2.25 and 2.27). Additionally, measures that increase the signal-to-noise ratio should be used. A

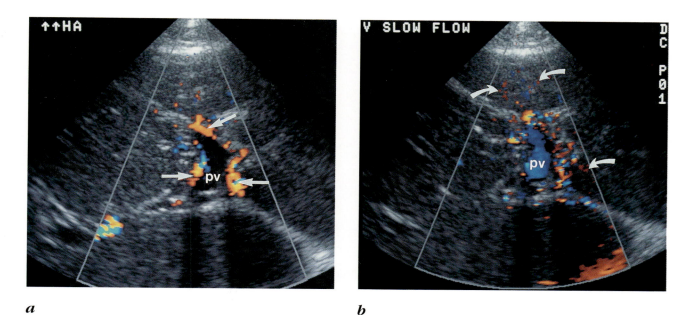

Figure 2.25 *Transverse CFI of the left portal vein (pv) in a patient with hepatic cirrhosis. Initially no flow is demonstrated within the left portal vein (a) when a moderate PRF is employed. Note the prominent hepatic artery branches (straight arrows). A lower PRF increases CFI sensitivity to slow flow (b) and allows detection of abnormal (hepatofugal) flow in this vessel. The higher level of sensitivity achieved by utilizing a lower PRF also may increase the likelihood of introducing color artifacts associated with tissue motion (curved arrows).*

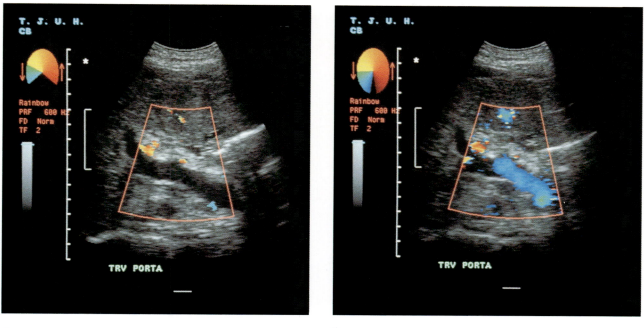

Figure 2.26 *Transverse CFI of the portal vein with the color wall filter set at (a) 100 Hz and (b) 25 Hz in a patient with portal hypertension. In cases of very slow bloodflow, lowering the wall filter will provide increased CFI sensitivity, which in this case enabled the system to display the hepatofugal flow present in this vessel.*

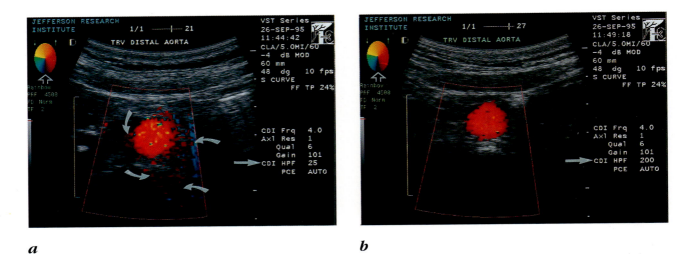

a   *b*

Figure 2.27 *Transverse CFIs of the distal aorta during cardiac systole using low (a) and high (b) wall filter (high-pass filter, HPF) levels (straight arrows). The other color flow parameter values remain the same in these two images. Note the color artifacts (curved arrows) in (a) due to vessel wall motion. These low-frequency Doppler shifts (indicated by a color assignment of deep shades of red and blue) are eliminated by applying a higher level of wall filtering (25 Hz versus 200 Hz). The relative level of wall filtering is also indicated as a black area on the color dynamic range wheel (open arrows).*

larger effective sample volume can do this. Features that increase dwell time (more samples per display line), such as using a higher ensemble length (also known as 'color quality', 'color sensitivity', and 'packet size'), will adversely affect frame rate but will increase color flow sensitivity (Fig. 2.28). A narrower color box will often increase line density and may also prove useful in improving flow sensitivity and spatial resolution.

The receiver color gain should be optimized by increasing the gain level until color artifacts are created over stationary tissues, and then slowly reduced until they no longer interfere with image interpretation. If too high a color gain is used, color 'noise' will appear. Often this noise will first be displayed within anechoic areas (Fig. 2.29), due to the system attempting to write color flow data where it does not detect gray scale information. If questions arise regarding the validity of flow information in these cases, a pulsed Doppler sample volume should be positioned within the region of concern to acquire a spectral Doppler waveform. If no flow is detected

by an optimized DD spectral trace, the color information is probably artifactual.

Most but not all color flow ultrasound systems can be adjusted to preferentially display color or gray scale data. Common nomenclature used for this parameter include 'priority', and 'color versus two-dimensional echo priority'. This is a *CFI-exclusive parameter* that even individuals with extensive DD experience may overlook. This control will 'prioritize' the display of either CFI or gray scale data based on the information desired. A high color priority will increase the likelihood of displaying flow information, whereas a low color priority will reduce the display of flow and prioritize the display of gray scale data. A high color priority is beneficial any time a vessel lumen is either too small to be resolved on gray scale or artifactually filled with gray scale echoes. Therefore, this parameter is important to optimize CFI sensitivity for small-parts applications such as thyroid and testicular examinations, where the vessels within these tissues are too small to be seen on gray scale (Fig. 2.30), or in deep abdominal

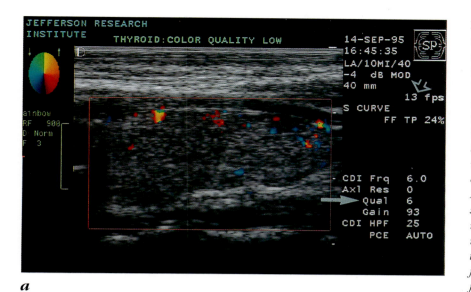

a

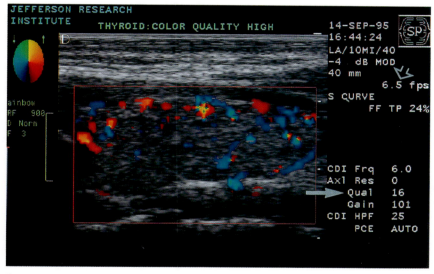

b

Figure 2.28 *Longitudinal CFIs of a normal thyroid gland with the ensemble length ('color quality') (arrows) adjusted (a) low and (b) high. Note the dramatic improvement in color flow information obtained in (b). The increase in sensitivity results from the higher signal-to-noise ratio which then allows use of a higher color gain (93 versus 101). However, the improved flow sensitivity comes at a cost of frame rate (open arrows), and spatial resolution. This is one example of the trade-offs which exist between flow sensitivity, resolution, and frame rate optimization.*

applications when artifacts introduce gray scale echoes within a vessel lumen (Fig. 2.31).

Finally, and only as a last resort after maximizing the parameters already discussed, the acoustic power output level can be increased to improve CFI sensitivity. Although energy deposition with CFI is much less than with single sample volume Doppler, prudent use of acoustic power output is always advised, especially in ophthalmologic, obstetric and pediatric applications. Table 2.1 summarizes common system parameter adjustments and scanning techniques which will optimize CFI sensitivity.

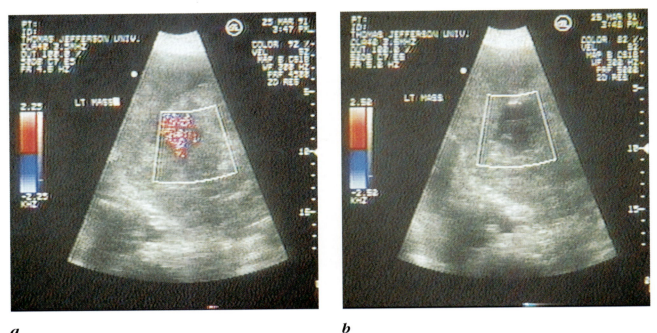

a   *b*

Figure 2.29 *In this transverse view of an abdominal mass (a) the color gain was erroneously adjusted too high, which created artifactual color data in a hypoechoic region of the tumor. When the color gain is correctly adjusted (b), no flow is displayed in this location. An optimized pulsed Doppler spectral waveform (not shown) revealed no flow in this area, which was later determined to represent a region of central tumor necrosis. Typically, more sensitive, pulsed Doppler spectral analysis should be utilized to confirm or rule out the presence of flow in cases of ambiguous color flow data.*

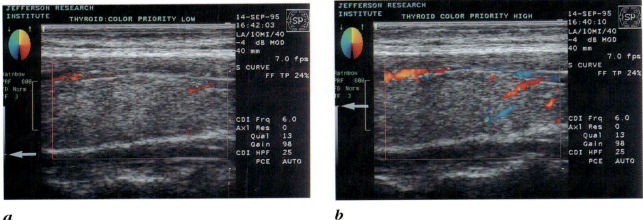

a   *b*

Figure 2.30 *Color priority changes in small-vessel applications. Longitudinal CFIs of a normal thyroid gland with the color priority (arrows) adjusted (a) low and (b) high and all other color parameters unchanged. Note the improved flow information obtained with a high color priority which enables the system to write color data where flow is detected. For small-parts applications such as thyroid, breast and testicular CFI (when the vessels are beyond the resolution of the gray scale image), a high priority will improve CFI displays.*

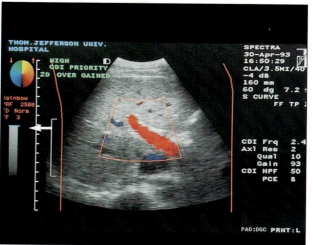

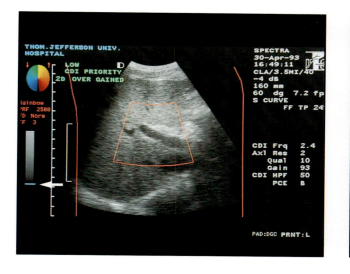

a

b

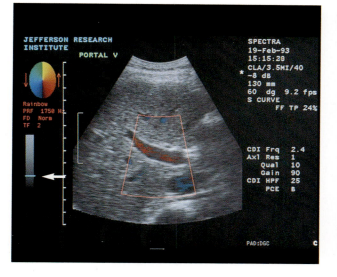

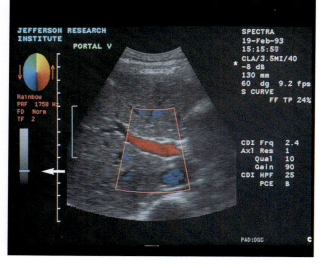

c

d

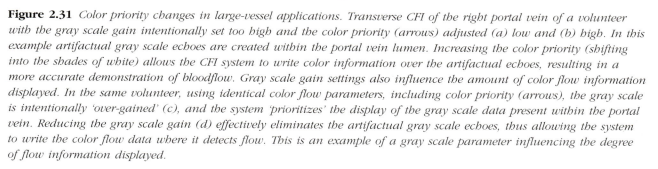

Figure 2.31 *Color priority changes in large-vessel applications. Transverse CFI of the right portal vein of a volunteer with the gray scale gain intentionally set too high and the color priority (arrows) adjusted (a) low and (b) high. In this example artifactual gray scale echoes are created within the portal vein lumen. Increasing the color priority (shifting into the shades of white) allows the CFI system to write color information over the artifactual echoes, resulting in a more accurate demonstration of bloodflow. Gray scale gain settings also influence the amount of color flow information displayed. In the same volunteer, using identical color flow parameters, including color priority (arrows), the gray scale is intentionally 'over-gained' (c), and the system 'prioritizes' the display of the gray scale data present within the portal vein. Reducing the gray scale gain (d) effectively eliminates the artifactual gray scale echoes, thus allowing the system to write the color flow data where it detects flow. This is an example of a gray scale parameter influencing the degree of flow information displayed.*

PROBLEM 2: SLOW CFI FRAME RATES: OPTIMIZING FRAME RATES WITHOUT SIGNIFICANTLY IMPAIRING FLOW SENSITIVITY

A high frame rate is necessary to obtain sufficient temporal resolution to demonstrate physiologic events in real-time. An insufficient CFI frame rate results in the display of bloodflow that is visually disturbing to the operator and can give misleading or inaccurate flow information. CFI of arterial flow with low frame rates will display only a portion of the cardiac cycle, with entire portions being missed, resulting in a portion of the cycle on one frame and an out-of-sequence portion of the cycle on the next frame.

To maintain high frame rates and obtain good temporal resolution in a CFI mode will inevitably result in some reduction in the amount and/or the sensitivity of flow information obtained. Two parameters that significantly influence frame rates in CFI modes are the size of the color box (also known as 'color window' and 'region of interest') in the lateral dimensions, and the overall image field of view (FOV). Therefore, using as small a lateral size of the color box and as short a FOV as will adequately

Table 2.1 System parameter adjustments and scanning techniques that optimize CFI sensitivity.

Optimize angle of incidence
Decrease pulse repetition frequency
Position focus to area of interest
Increase color gain
Increase color priority
Decrease wall filter
Increase ensemble length
Increase output power

display the area of interest will have a beneficial effect on frame rate. Other CFI parameters which affect the frame rate are PRF and ensemble length. Increasing the PRF will result in an increase in frame rate but a reduction in CFI sensitivity. Reducing the ensemble length (the number of bursts used to produce one line of color information) will increase the frame rate, also at the cost of some loss of CFI sensitivity. One can appreciate, therefore, that performing CFI is a continuous process of balancing

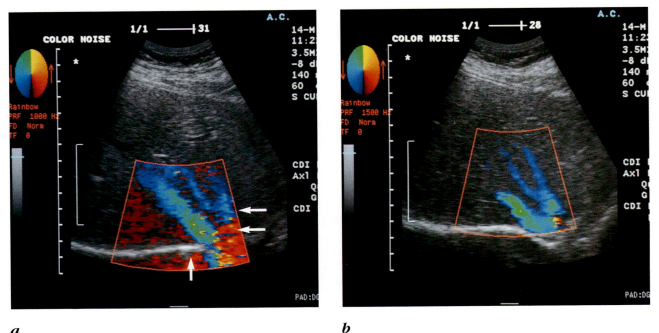

a

b

Figure 2.32 *Color artifacts. Transverse CFI of the hepatic vein confluence and IVC (a) before and (b) after CFI parameter optimization. In this case adjusting the color gain and color box size and position, and increasing the PRF, helped to reduce the color artifacts (arrows) associated with cardiac motion.*

Table 2.2 CFI system parameter adjustments to optimize frame rates.

Parameter	Adjustment
Pulse repetition frequency	Increased
Ensemble length	Decreased
Color box size	Decreased (in lateral dimensions)
Line density	Decreased
Field of view	Decreased
Color persistence*	Decreased

*Decreased color persistence does not actually increase frame rate, but will give what is *perceived* to be a higher frame rate.

between optimal sensitivity to bloodflow and adequate temporal resolution for a real-time image presentation. Because it is difficult to demonstrate in a still image the dynamic nature of frame rate effects, operators should investigate how the parameters mentioned here increase or decrease frame rates and affect flow sensitivity on their own systems, to become accustomed with the trade-offs which exist. Most manufacturers provide a numerical value of the frame rate on their graphics display. The frame rate may be displayed in Hertz (Hz) or frames per second (FPS). Table 2.2 summarizes parameter changes that can help to optimize CFI frame rates.

PROBLEM 3: ARTIFACTS ASSOCIATED WITH COLOR INFORMATION DISPLAYED WHERE THERE IS NO BLOODFLOW— 'COLOR NOISE' OR 'CLUTTER'

When a color flow image becomes degraded by artifactual information in the form of color in areas without flow ('color noise'), the amount of useful information and ease of image interpretation may be compromised. This type of artifact may be caused by tissue motion, inadequate parameter adjustments, or physiologic events · such as bowel peristalsis or cardiac motion. The techniques used to overcome these problems are as varied as the causes, and each scanning situation will have its own set of potential solutions. If, for example, peristalsing bowel causes interference, changing the patient's position to have the bowel move away from the area of interest may

result in adequate CFI visualization of bloodflow. Simple patient instructions, such as asking the patient to hold his or her breath, can reduce tissue motion artifacts associated with respiration. Changing the position and/or the size of the color box to avoid the cause of the artifact (such as the beating heart) can also improve the CFI display. When scanning highly pulsatile structures such as the heart or abdominal aorta, increasing the CFI wall filter can reduce CFI motion artifacts associated with these structures (Fig. 2.32). Other CFI parameter changes that may help reduce these color artifacts include decreasing the color gain and increasing the PRF, both of which will also reduce CFI sensitivity. Usually a compromise must be made in the selection of CFI parameter settings by choosing those that will adequately reduce color artifacts, while providing a satisfactory level of flow sensitivity.

DESIRABLE QUALITIES FOR CFI INSTRUMENTS

Most manufacturers of CFI systems provide pre-assigned parameter packages ('Examination Type', 'Icon', 'Application', 'Setup') to get the operator 'in the ball park' for specific applications. We will refer to them here as 'presets'. While most experienced sonographers are proficient at optimizing a gray scale image, CFI may pose a new challenge for those with limited experience and present difficulties in obtaining diagnostically acceptable CFI examinations. In these cases selecting the proper preset will undoubtedly allow the examination to be performed in a more expedient and thorough fashion.

Selecting the proper manufacturer's preset will:

1 Reduce the operator dependence of performing a technically adequate study.
2 Speed the examination process by reducing the amount of parameter adjustments necessary to optimize the color flow data.
3 Optimize parameters that the operator may overlook or does not have access to.
4 Adjust the acoustic output power to the FDA recommended levels.
5 Select the relevant calculation and annotation packages, further reducing examination time.

For these reasons it is strongly suggested that the user develop a habit of routinely selecting the proper

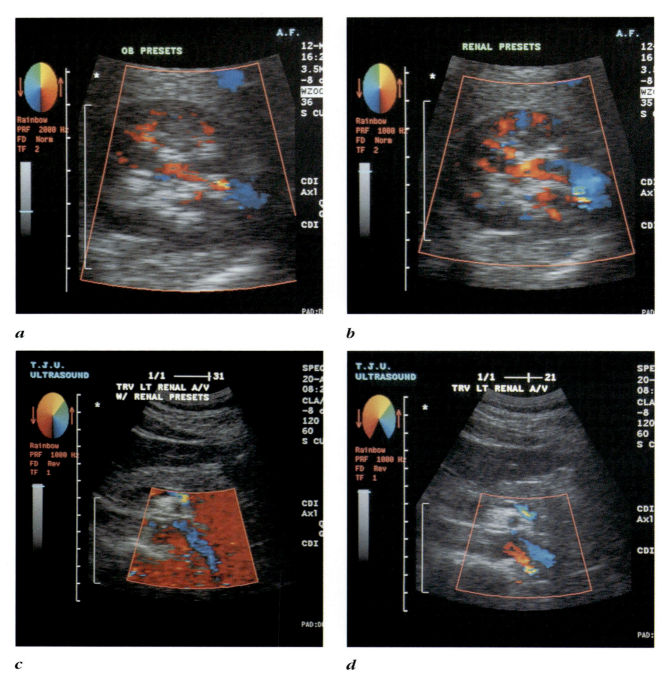

Figure 2.33 *Manufacturer's preset selection. Magnified transverse CFIs of the right kidney using the (a) 'obstetric' and (b) 'renal' presets. Note the improvement in flow information obtained by using the correct (renal) preset for this application. Transverse CFI of the aorta and left renal artery origin using (c) the renal preset parameters, and (d) after CFI parameter optimization. The combination of a low wall filter and high color gain used in the renal preset package is necessary to optimize for flow in vessels within the kidney as originally designed, but these parameter settings are not appropriate for evaluation of the higher flow states encountered at the renal artery origins. Knowledge of the specific applications for which the preset was designed can help the operator to determine which preset to select for a given application.*

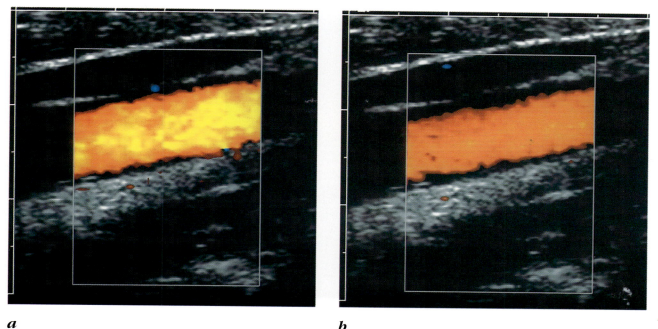

a *b*

Figure 2.34 *Longitudinal CFI of the common carotid artery demonstrating velocity resolution. Note the change in color display between (a) systole and (b) diastole. The higher-frequency shifts occurring in systole (color coded yellow) indicate a higher systolic velocity, while the deep shade of red in diastole indicates a lower velocity. These images also illustrate the ability of CFI to provide an indication of flow pulsatility. The continuous forward flow in diastole indicates that this vessel is subject to low peripheral resistance. Spectral Doppler analysis is required for a more precise measurement of pulsatility.*

preset prior to beginning each examination. In order to use the presets to their maximal benefit, however, the operator must know what the preset package was designed to do. If, for example, a preset for 'renal imaging' was designed to display color flow information from within the renal parenchyma, choosing this preset to evaluate the aorta and renal artery origins will result in inadequate CFI settings and a poor display of flow within these vessels (Fig. 2.33). Although in recent years manufacturers have made significant progress in determining what parameter settings work best for their systems, optimal CFI sensitivity usually requires some alteration from the presets to accommodate the specific demands of each scanning situation.

Certain CFI system features are needed to perform good CFI. The most valuable clinical use of CFI is to enhance the overall diagnostic power of modern ultrasound imaging by adding flow information to the real-time gray scale image. This 'survey' CFI mode is most important for general scanning. In survey CFI mode, one scans a large area relatively quickly to detect areas of unsuspected flow or to quickly differentiate vascular from non-vascular structures. A system needs excellent CFI sensitivity, a near real-time frame rate and good motion discrimination to perform effective survey CFI. Color flow sensitivity is important if unsuspected flow is to be reliably detected. Near real-time frame rates are useful to survey large areas expeditiously, and to obtain adequate temporal resolution to observe pulsatility and flow patterns within vessels (i.e. to differentiate among arteries and veins). Aliasing, which can make it impossible to immediately determine flow direction, is tolerated for this type of CFI scanning. Good motion discrimination, which allows differentiation of bloodflow from moving soft tissue, is important to avoid CFI artifacts that might obscure flow information.

Once unsuspected or abnormal bloodflow has been detected, it can be analyzed more closely by

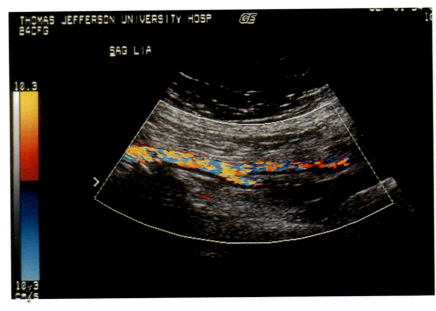

a

Figure 2.35 *Longitudinal color flow images of the left iliac artery (LIA) obtained in conventional (mean Doppler frequency shift) color (a) and color amplitude (b) modes. Due to the low PRF necessary to detect flow in the conventional color mode, significant color aliasing is present. Due to the non-directional nature of the color amplitude mode, aliasing is not present. Also note on the CAI image the improved detection of flow in the internal iliac artery (arrow), which is not seen on the conventional color image.*

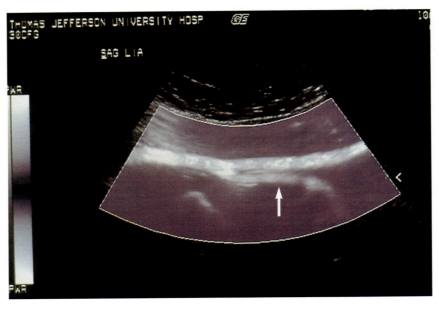

b

using 'quality' CFI. In this CFI scanning mode, sensitivity and motion discrimination are again important. Color aliasing is avoided by using a sufficiently high PRF or proper baseline position. Velocity and spatial resolution are other key features. Spatial resolution is the accuracy with which a system displays the location of flow on the image. As stated earlier, velocity resolution is the ability to depict small local variations in flow (Figs 2.7, 2.8 and 2.34). A properly adjusted PRF is achieved by using the lowest PRF that does not produce aliasing. A PRF adjusted too high will result in poor velocity resolution and under-utilization of the CFI dynamic range. Quality CFI is used initially in most vascular applications, since the

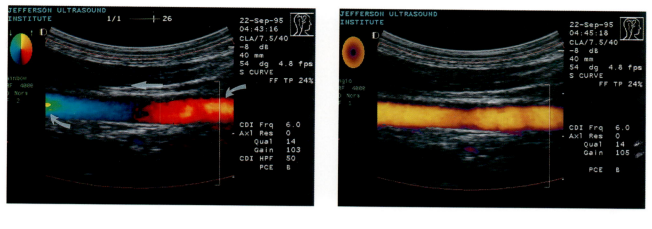

a *b*

Figure 2.36 *The image of the common carotid artery obtained with conventional CFI (a) contains the 'multiple-angle artifact' but demonstrates flow directivity (straight arrow). The more acute Doppler angle at the edges of the image (curved arrows) results in higher Doppler shifts (displayed as shades of yellow on the red side of the color scale, and aliasing on the blue side of the scale) in these locations. The lack of flow in the center of the image is due to the perpendicular angle to flow in this location. In the image acquired using CAI (b), flow is displayed more uniformly with no multiple-angle artifacts and an improved display of flow from the center of the image due to the reduced angle dependence of this flow modality. However, no flow-directional information is provided with CAI.*

location of the vessel to be evaluated is already known, and the area to be examined is relatively limited. Therefore, for these applications frame rates are often not an issue. Finally, as stated earlier, one of the most useful applications of CFI is to localize bloodflow for sample volume placement, when the detailed quantitative information provided by spectral Doppler is required.

COLOR AMPLITUDE IMAGING

A relatively new CFI mode displays the Doppler signal amplitude (also known as 'power', or 'energy') in color as opposed to the mean Doppler frequency shift displayed by conventional CFI. Because implementation primarily requires software revisions it has been widely incorporated into many currently available color-flow-capable systems. Although each manufacturer has adopted its own nomenclature for this type of CFI, we have generically termed this mode color amplitude imaging (CAI). By sacrificing

the display of directional information, extending the dynamic range, and using higher levels of temporal processing, CAI typically has a higher signal-to-noise ratio and appears to have some benefits over conventional CFI. Also, because the color signals of CAI are dependent on the signal amplitude as opposed to the mean Doppler frequency shift, CAI does not alias (Fig. 2.35), and is not affected by multiple-angle artifacts as bloodflow changes direction in relation to the insonating beam (Fig. 2.36). However, primarily due to the high levels of temporal averaging and persistence, CAI has some significant limitations. These include an inability to function in a survey type of CFI scanning mode (which requires relatively high frame rates), in situations where there is considerable tissue motion, such as in echocardiography, and when directional flow information is necessary, such as in the evaluation of portal vein hemodynamics and many peripheral vascular applications. The advantages of CAI lie in its ability to demonstrate flow in very small vessels, flow at a suboptimal Doppler angles, vessel continuity, and very slow bloodflow (Fig. 2.37). Some early reports have indicated that this

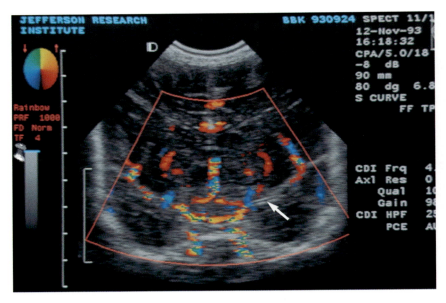

a

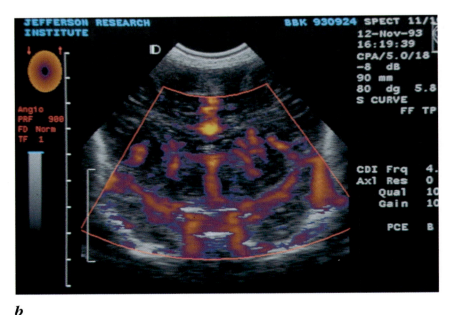

b

Figure 2.37 *Coronal conventional color (a) and color amplitude (b) images of a newborn's brain. In (a) the lack of flow information in the middle cerebral artery (arrow) is due to the poor Doppler angle to flow in this location; however, due to the perpendicular angle of insonation the vessel is visualized with gray scale as two parallel lines. Due to the reduced angle dependence of CAI, flow is detected in this portion of the vessel. Other notable attributes present on the color amplitude image are: the lack of aliasing artifacts, allowing use of a lower PRF (1000 Hz versus 900 Hz); improved signal-to-noise ratio, allowing use of a higher color gain (98 versus 107), which demonstrates flow in more vessels; and overall better vessel continuity due to the combination of all of these factors.*

color flow mode also may prove useful in demonstrating regional differences in bloodflow within organs and tumors. Preliminary results indicate that in many applications the information obtained with CAI is complementary to that of conventional CFI (see Table 1.4). Specific clinical and research applications of CAI are discussed elsewhere in this book.

COLOR AMPLITUDE IMAGING SCANNING TECHNIQUES

Simply changing from conventional CFI to CAI without changing any color flow parameters usually will not optimize flow sensitivity using this new color modality. Although many of the basic principles are

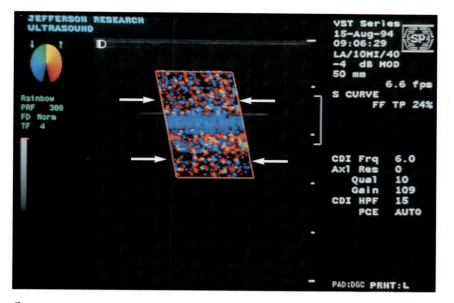

a

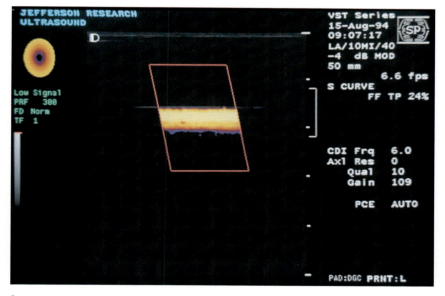

b

Figure 2.38 *Conventional color (a) and color amplitude (b) images of a flow phantom using identical color parameter levels. In (a) color artifacts are present in regions without flow (arrows). Due to the improved signal-to-noise ratio of CAI, there are no color artifacts, and there is an improvement in functional lumen definition.*

the same, because the two flow imaging modes differ significantly in the way the flow data is acquired the operator must optimize each color mode independently. As in conventional CFI mode, selection of the proper manufacturer's preset will often allow more time-efficient and thorough CAI evaluations while at the same time reducing operator dependence.

In general, when scanning with CAI it is beneficial to use lower PRFs, a higher color gain, and a slower scanning technique than used for conventional CFI. The use of a lower PRF is suggested because, due to the non-directionality of the flow information, there are no aliasing artifacts with CAI. A slower scanning technique is recommended due

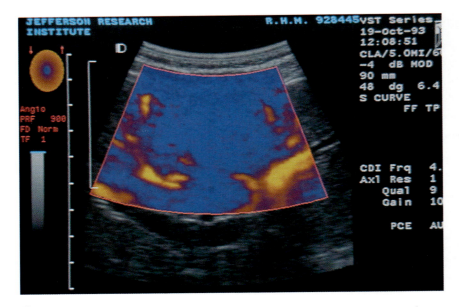

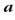

a

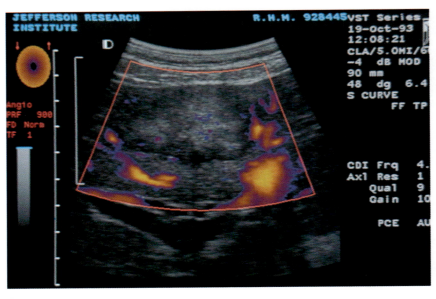

b

Figure 2.39 *Color amplitude images of a hypovascular liver lesion with the blue background (i.e. 'noise level') (a) on and (b) off. The blue background obscures visualization of the mass and the anatomic location of the flow signals which are present. Removing the blue background (which on this system is a post-processing feature) provides information on these anatomic relationships and facilitates image interpretation.*

to the use of lower PRFs which usually will reduce frame rates, and the high levels of temporal processing utilized by most manufacturers of units with CAI capability. Limiting the size of the color box (especially in the lateral dimensions) to include only the region of interest will optimize frame rates. A higher color gain can be used in CAI because there is a higher signal-to-noise ratio in CAI than in CFI (Fig. 2.38).

Two other helpful scanning strategies that facilitate technically adequate, and more easily interpreted, CAI evaluations involve the procurement and display of flow data. Regarding the display features, many manufacturers provide a means of removing the blue (or other color) background when in CAI mode. This can be especially helpful on single, as opposed to dual, monitor systems by allowing visualization of the anatomic landmarks, which may otherwise be obscured by the background noise level (Fig. 2.39). Secondly, when using CAI it is essential to have good patient cooperation. Motion that results from patient movement or breathing will seriously degrade a CAI image with color artifacts. Due to the high levels of color persistence and frame averaging often employed with CAI, motion artifacts are significantly more degrading to image quality and interpretation, because they remain on the system monitor for a longer period of time. Many of these artifacts can be reduced or eliminated by having good patient cooperation, or employing some of the other techniques discussed previously in the section on reducing color artifacts.

Finally, as a reminder, many of the CFI parameters discussed in this chapter are either not relevant in CAI mode, or not typically available to the operator. These include controls such as the baseline shift, color wall filter, directional invert control, and others depending on the specific system used. The current forms of CAI have significant limitations on their applicability in many parts of the body (e.g. the heart), and scanning situations (e.g. uncooperative pediatric patients). However, similar to the way that technological improvements have contributed to expanding the role of conventional CFI, further improvements in CAI can be expected to reduce many of the current limitations that exist today.

GLOSSARY OF COLOR FLOW IMAGING PARAMETERS

Baseline shift This control determines how the range of color flow frequency shifts (as determined by the PRF) are displayed. Shifting the baseline (displaying more frequency shifts in one direction than the other) does not affect the PRF level. At times color aliasing can be avoided by shifting the baseline up or down accordingly, thereby providing a higher degree of flow sensitivity than would be provided by using a higher color PRF to avoid aliasing artifacts.

Beam steering Only available on flat linear array transducers. Allows the operator to direct (steer) the color flow beams at a preset angle (usually fixed at ± 20–30°) which is different from the angle used to acquire gray scale information. Beam steering allows the acquisition of color flow information from vessels which are parallel to the skin surface.

Color box (*color window, color field, region of interest*) The portion of the gray scale image in which color flow information is displayed.
> **Position** Operator adjusted by a trackball or similar control to position color box over a desired area. Color box depth will influence the maximum usable color PRF.
> **Size** Can be adjusted laterally and axially. Large color box sizes (especially in the lateral dimension) result in slower frame rates and suboptimal temporal resolution.

Color gain The color gain control amplifies the strength of the received color flow signal. This control should be adjusted so that color flow information is displayed from moving blood and does not overwrite gray scale information of stationary tissues. If the color gain is too high, artifactual color information often will first appear in anechoic spaces.

Color maps The selection of a color map is usually determined by operator preference. 'Rainbow'-type maps (e.g. blue to green and red to orange) may allow color aliasing to be more readily apparent than does a red–blue map. Variance maps display the degree of deviation from the mean Doppler frequency shift and are primarily used in echocardiographic applications.

Ensemble length (*color sensitivity, packet size, color quality*) Determines how many pulses are transmitted in each scan line of color flow information. High ensemble lengths improve the color signal-to-noise ratio, which allows higher color gain settings and provides better flow sensitivity but reduces frame rates. Low ensemble lengths result in a lower signal-to-noise ratio, but provide better temporal resolution of flow.

Line density This term refers to the lateral spacing of scan lines (A-lines) being transmitted to acquire color flow information. A higher (or tighter) line density will improve spatial resolution but reduce image frame rate, whereas a lower line density will increase the frame rate, but will necessitate a higher degree of interpolation of flow information (i.e. bigger pixels), thereby reducing spatial resolution. Often manufacturers will sacrifice line density when large color boxes are used in order to maintain adequately high temporal resolution (frame rate).

Persistence *(smoothing, temporal filtering)* Determines how long a period of time the color flow information remains on the monitor before new information is displayed. Some systems update color flow information only when a new signal has a greater frequency shift than the one currently displayed. High color persistence can provide better (aesthetically pleasing) vessel fill-in but also results in what is *perceived* to be a slower frame rate. Low persistence typically provides better temporal resolution of flow dynamics.

Power output *(acoustic output)* Refers to the amount of acoustic power transmitted from the transducer into body tissues. Increased power output results in greater flow sensitivity. Caution should be exercised when adjusting power output, especially when performing ophthalmologic, obstetric or pediatric examinations. The acoustic output power should be increased only as a last resort to obtain adequate image quality.

Priority *(two-dimensional echo versus color write priority)* This control is not available on all color flow systems. The priority level is usually indicated on the image gray scale dynamic range bar. The priority control allows the operator to 'prioritize' the display of either gray scale or color flow data. In scanning situations where the vessel lumen is either not seen (beyond the resolution of the two-dimensional image, i.e. thyroid or testicular scans) or has artifactually created low-level gray scale echoes (i.e. abdominal imaging), the color priority should be set high (i.e. into the shades of white) to allow color flow information to be superimposed (given priority) over the gray scale information. Color priority is exclusively a color flow parameter which has no equivalent duplex Doppler counterpart.

Pulse repetition frequency (PRF) *(scale, velocity scale)* Usually adjusted by the velocity or frequency 'SCALE' control. The PRF level determines how often (frequently) a new color flow pulse is transmitted. Higher PRFs allow a greater range of color Doppler shifts to be displayed without aliasing. Lower PRFs provide greater sensitivity to slow bloodflow but may reduce frame rates. A properly adjusted PRF will provide good velocity resolution without color aliasing. Remember that conventional CFI displays only **mean** Doppler frequency shift information in color within a given pixel of the image.

Wall filter *(threshold, high-pass filter)* The wall filter determines the minimum level (mean frequency shift) for color flow information to be displayed by eliminating lower-frequency shifts. The wall filter extends from the baseline to a selected frequency level in both directions, and is often displayed as a black portion on the color dynamic range scale bar equivalent to the selected wall filter level. For venous imaging, the wall filter should be set at a low level to provide greater sensitivity to slow blood flow. High wall filter levels may help to reduce artifacts related to vessel wall motion ('wall thumps'), which are typically low-frequency and high-amplitude signals.

FURTHER READING

Burns PN, The physical principles of Doppler and spectral analysis, *J Clin Ultrasound* (1987) **15**:567–90.

Hendrick WR, Hykes DL, Starchman DE, *Ultrasound Physics and Instrumentation*, 3rd edn (Mosby: St Louis, MO, 1995).

Kremkau FW, *Diagnostic Ultrasound: Principles and Instruments*, 4th edn (WB Saunders Company: Philadelphia, 1993).

Merritt CRB, Doppler color flow imaging, *J Clin Ultrasound* (1987) **15**:591–7.

Merritt CRB (ed), *Doppler Color Imaging*, Clinics in Diagnostic Ultrasound **27** (Churchill Livingstone: New York, 1992).

Mitchell DG, Color Doppler imaging: principles, limitations, and artifacts, *Radiology* (1990) **177**:1–10.

Nelson TR, Pretorius DH, The Doppler signal: where does it come from and what does it mean? *AJR* (1988) **151**:439–47.

Powis RL, Powis WJ, *A Thinker's Guide to Ultrasonic Imaging* (Urban & Schwarzenberg: Baltimore, Munich, 1984).

Wolf KJ, Fobbe F (eds) *Color Duplex Sonography: Principals and Clinical Applications* (Thieme Medical Publishers: New York, 1994).

Chapter 3   Doppler ultrasound – measurement of bloodflow

Colin R Deane

INTRODUCTION

In order to understand and use Doppler ultrasound images, the radiologist, sonographer or technician should be aware of the way in which bloodflow phenomena contribute to the images. Doppler ultrasound essentially provides a measurement of bloodflow velocity which, depending on the mode used and the setup of ultrasound parameters, may be presented in one of several ways. The aim of this chapter is to describe how Doppler ultrasound images and measurement of velocity may be used to quantify physiologic changes in bloodflow and to assist in the interpretation of images in the clinical chapters of the book.

DOPPLER ULTRASOUND MEASUREMENT OF VELOCITY

Current color flow ultrasound techniques, including color Doppler and velocity imaging, utilize one-dimensional imaging of flow velocity. As described in

previous chapters, the measured phase or time shift is derived from the **velocity component** in the direction of the ultrasound beam. The relationship of the beam to the direction of bloodflow is sometimes estimated, e.g. to obtain angle-corrected velocities in the plane of the image. It should always be remembered, however, that blood flows in three dimensions within vessels, and that the accuracy of the angle correction is a limiting factor in calculations of absolute bloodflow velocity.

Even if quantitative measurements of bloodflow velocities are not being attempted, the three-dimensional nature of flow can give rise to images which are, at first, not readily interpreted. Velocity vectors may give rise to strong color flow signals when images are obtained in one plane but weak or absent signals if viewed in another. The way in which velocity vectors interact with the Doppler beam to provide flow images is illustrated in Figs 3.1 to 3.3.

In addition to the errors in Doppler beam/bloodflow angle, errors in velocity estimation can arise due to inherent physical and instrumentation errors, as described in previous chapters. Practitioners of Doppler ultrasound should be aware of possible errors when conducting examinations both in order to minimize them and to establish error ranges for specific measurements.

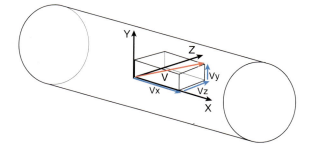

Figure 3.1 *Bloodflow velocity in a vessel. The red arrow represents a bloodflow vector. The blue arrows represent the velocity components of that vector in three orthogonal axes, in the axial direction X and in transverse directions Y and Z. These velocity components contribute to the color flow image, depending on the scan plane and beam steering used.*

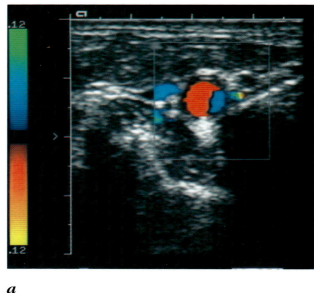

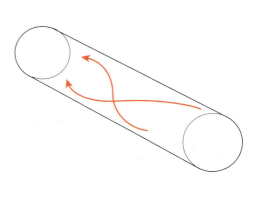

a   *b*

Figure 3.2 *(a) Transverse image of a distal common carotid artery. (The transducer is almost perpendicular to the artery.) The vessel contains velocity components both towards and away from the transducer. Flow is predominantly axial along the common carotid artery. The changing colors reflect the presence of secondary flows (non-axial flows) in the artery. (b) Illustration of secondary flow in an artery. The velocities are predominantly along the vessel but the spiraling nature produces non-axial flow components.*

ULTRASOUND FLOW-MEASURING MODES—FLOW INFORMATION

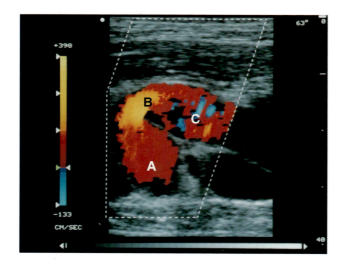

Figure 3.3 *Multidirectional flow within an image. Flow in a hemodialysis fistula. The flow direction is from left to right. At A the vessel comes into the plane of the scan and there is possibly a large flow component orthogonal to the scan plane. Flow velocities are aligned to the ultrasound beam at B. At C, the velocity vectors are almost at right angles to the beam as demonstrated by poor color filling.*

The presentation of flow information by color or spectral display requires different approaches to signal acquisition and processing. Color flow imaging is typically used to investigate flow in a large area within the image but information and temporal resolution are limited (the frame rate may range from 4 frames/s in abdominal applications to 24 frames/s in peripheral vascular examinations). In some systems, it is possible to make an angle correction in order for colors to represent velocities. It is common, however, for an area of flow investigation to contain flow vectors of several directions, in which case angle correction may be misleading.

Spectral Doppler, usually obtained by pulsed wave Doppler in color Doppler scanners, provides detailed flow information within a small sample volume at a high temporal resolution (typically 50–100 Hz). Because the region of interest is small, velocity vectors are more likely to be uniform and beam/flow angle corrections can often be estimated reliably. The sonogram display provides a measure of the time-

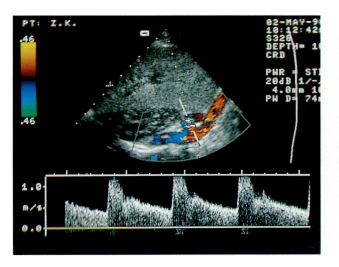

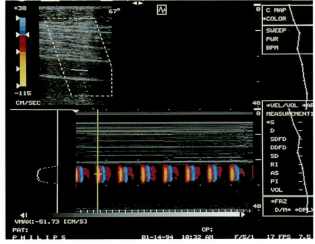

Figure 3.4 *Color flow imaging used in conjunction with spectral Doppler. The color image shows the course of an external iliac artery and renal transplant artery anastomosis. The image allows accurate positioning and angle correction of the pulsed Doppler cursor to obtain the velocity waveform from the renal artery.*

Figure 3.5 *Color velocity imaging combined with an M-mode display gives a time-varying color representation along the line shown in the two-dimensional image. The temporal resolution of the color image is approximately 50 Hz.*

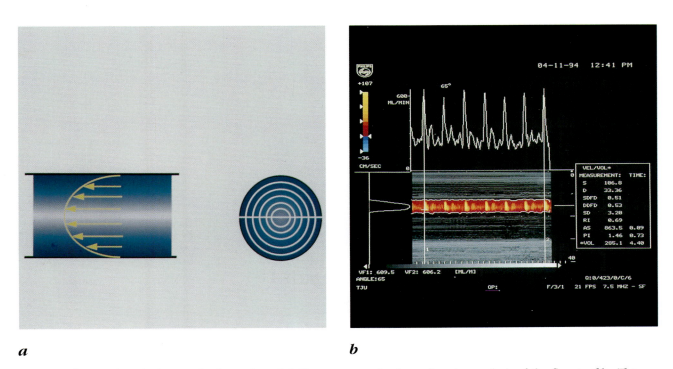

a *b*

Figure 3.6 *M-mode calculation of volume flow. (a) Measurement of volume flow by analysis of the flow profile. The assumption is made that measured velocities within a vessel are representative of a semi-annulus of identical velocity. The velocities are integrated, with appropriate weighting for each semi-annulus. (b) The flow is calculated at 20 ms intervals. The process allows calculation of both velocity and instantaneous effective arterial diameter.*

Table 3.1 Summary of characteristics of ultrasound flow imaging modes.

	Color flow/ velocity imaging	PW spectral Doppler	Color M-mode	Color amplitude imaging
Region of interest	Large	Small	A-line	Large
Spatial resolution	Fair	Poor	Fair	Fair
Temporal resolution	Fair/poor	Good	Good	Very poor
Sensitivity	Fair	Good	Fair	Good
Flow information	Fair	Detailed	Detailed	Poor

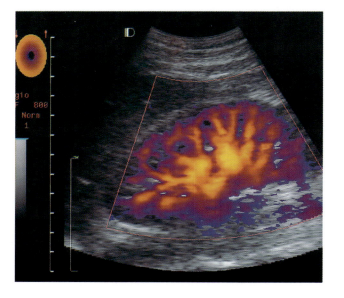

Figure 3.7 *Amplitude color flow. The image is averaged over several frames. This allows for higher receiver gain and thus better sensitivity to low velocities. Color assignment is based on the amplitude of the Doppler signal within sample volumes.*

varying nature of flow and, to a more limited degree, of the range of velocities within the sample volume. The different data provided by the two methods are complementary and in clinical scanning the modes are used as such (Fig. 3.4).

Other techniques available include the use of color-coded M-mode to give high temporal resolution of velocity components along one A-line of the image

(Fig. 3.5). The resulting time-changing flow profile can be integrated to provide an estimate of volume flow (Fig. 3.6). Another method, color amplitude imaging, displays the amplitude of the processed Doppler signal (rather than the frequency shift) as the color scale. Because amplitude varies little during the cardiac cycle, the technique can use high gain and frame averaging within the color image to give greater sensitivity to blood motion at the expense of a dynamic image and directionality (Fig. 3.7). The characteristics of each technique are summarized in Table 3.1.

Bloodflow in arteries and veins is complex and a thorough analysis is beyond the scope of this chapter. Despite its complexity, and despite the limitations of Doppler ultrasound in describing bloodflow information, Doppler techniques have proved to be reliable indicators of a wide range of bloodflow changes, from flow through stenoses to changes in peripheral resistance. These changes to bloodflow are described here in terms of their Doppler characteristics. For those who wish to study bloodflow theory in more detail, further reading is suggested at the end of the chapter.

FLOW WAVEFORMS AND FLOW PROFILES

FLOW WAVEFORMS

The action of the heart produces pulsatile flow in arteries. The resulting time-changing flow can be investigated in terms of the resulting arterial velocities by Doppler techniques. The shape of the flow waveform in an artery is dependent on the pulsatile

Table 3.2 Some common flow waveform descriptive indices.

Index	Definition	Index derived from Fig. 3.10
Resistive index (RI)	$\dfrac{Peak\ systolic\ velocity - minimum\ diastolic\ velocity}{Peak\ systolic\ velocity}$	$\dfrac{S-D}{S}$
Pulsatility index (PI)	$\dfrac{Peak\ systolic\ velocity - minimum\ diastolic\ velocity}{Time\text{-}averaged\ maximum\ velocity}$	$\dfrac{S-D}{M}$
S/D ratio	$\dfrac{Peak\ systolic\ velocity}{End\text{-}systolic\ velocity}$	$\dfrac{S}{D}$

pressure wave at the site of measurement acting on the vascular impedance. Thus, the flow waveform can be altered by upstream, local and distal factors. Highly pulsatile flow is evident in color flow by rapid changes of color hue throughout the cardiac cycle; low-pulsatility flow exhibits little or no change (Fig. 3.8). In spectral Doppler, changes in flow waveform shape are readily appreciated in the spectral display, which typically shows the velocity component within the sample volume over several cardiac cycles (Fig. 3.9).

The shape of the spectral display flow waveform can be characterized by one of several indices, of which the most common are pulsatility index, resistive index and S/D ratio, defined in Table 3.2 (Fig. 3.10). These are all based on the outline shape of the waveform, the maximum frequency envelope, and are, at best, crude measures of flow waveform shape. They do serve to put numerical values on the flow waveform in order to categorize gross changes in flow. They have the advantage that they are non-dimensional, and so are not affected by errors in measuring absolute velocities. Other descriptive measurements of the flow waveform shape include the acceleration of the systolic upstroke, and noting of a feature, e.g. a postsystolic 'notch' in the waveform.

Arteries leading to specific vascular beds have characteristic flow waveform shapes which can be altered as a result of normal physiologic change (Fig. 3.11). Changes can also occur because of anomalous changes to the proximal or distal vasculature. An increase in distal resistance generally leads to an increase in flow waveform pulsatility, with decreased, or even reversed, flow in late systole/early diastole.

(As an approximate guide, very low distal resistance leads to a flow waveform similar in shape to the pressure waveform P; very high distal pressure results in a flow waveform corresponding in shape to the pressure differential dP/dt.) A raised proximal resistance, e.g. due to a stenosis, results in a dampening of the flow waveform, with low pulsatility caused by the diminished pressure pulse through the stenosis and distal vasodilation. The wide range of flow waveforms which can occur in an organ are illustrated by the variation which can occur in renal transplants due to change in downstream resistance (vascular rejection, thrombosis, the presence of arteriovenous fistulas) and upstream resistance (renal artery stenosis) (Fig. 3.12).

FLOW PROFILES

Flow velocity varies across a vessel. Because of viscous friction, flow is slowest close to the vessel wall and is usually fastest in the center of the vessel (Fig. 3.13). This may be seen in the color image of flow as different hues across the vessel image (Fig. 3.14). If the vessel is large enough, the size and placement of the pulsed wave spectral Doppler sample volume may influence the appearance of the spectrum, depending on the range of velocities insonated (Fig. 3.15).

The flow profile and flow waveform are closely interrelated. Low-pulsatility waveforms (e.g. renal, internal carotid and umbilical arteries) leading to low-resistance vascular beds have low acceleration and produce flow profiles that can approximate to parabolic in section. Highly pulsatile waveforms (e.g.

_____ ʃʃʃ ____ _____ ____ ʃʃʃ pulsatile flow pattern is seen as a cyclic red–blue–red pulse on M-mode. Calculated flow volume is approximately 90 ml/min. (d) Color velocity M-mode following vigorous exercise. Volume flow has increased to over 1500 ml/min, and there is high forward flow throughout the cardiac cycle.

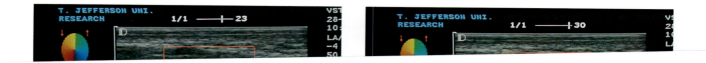

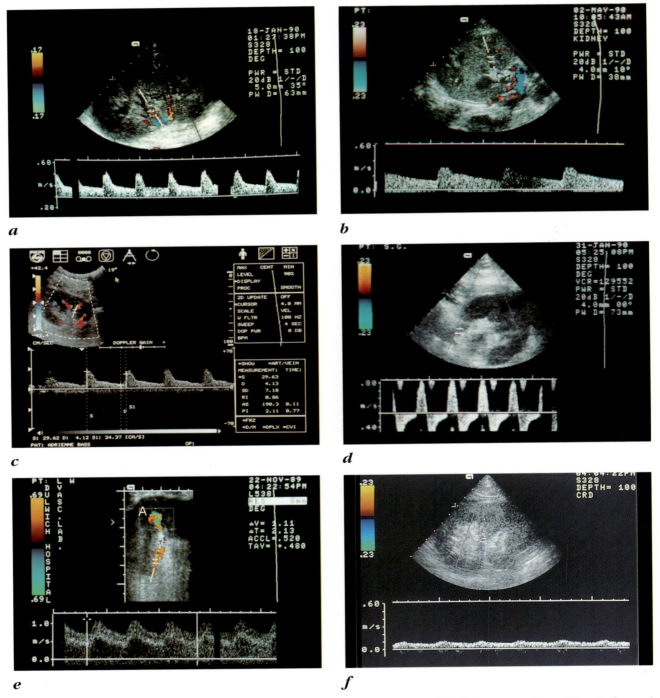

Figure 3.12 *Flow waveforms in renal transplants. (a,b) Flow waveforms in healthy kidney transplants. There is forward flow throughout the cardiac cycle. The appearances of the two waveforms are slightly different because of normal physiologic variation. For example, the heart rate in (b) is slower than that in (a). (c) Vascular rejection. There is diminished diastolic flow due to increased distal resistance. (d) Renal vein thrombosis. There is no net flow. Blood is pumped into the arteries during systole. As arterial pressure falls, blood is ejected back out of the kidney. The renal vascular bed acts as a compliant 'dead end'. (e) Arteriovenous fistula. At 'A' there is a fistula. This presents a low-resistance vascular bed. Flow to the fistula exhibits high-velocity low-pulsatility waveforms. (f) Renal artery stenosis. The pressure drop through the stenosis and distal vasodilatation produce a low-velocity damped-flow waveform. When compared with (e), velocities are substantially lower.*

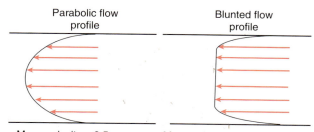

Parabolic flow profile — Mean velocity = 0.5 v_{max}

Blunted flow profile — Mean velocity = approx. v_{max}

Figure 3.13 *Flow profiles in laminar flow. Laminar flow describes flow in which layers of blood slide over adjacent layers with no mixing. The diagram shows a flow profile in fully developed flow when the profile becomes parabolic in cross-section (left). In entrance regions or as a result of rapid acceleration, the flow profile becomes more blunted (right). Both flow profiles can occur in laminar flow.*

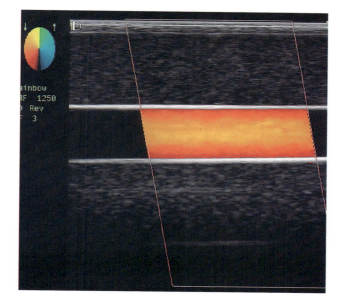

Figure 3.14 *Continuous laminar flow in a tube phantom. The orange hues show high velocities at the center of the lumen.*

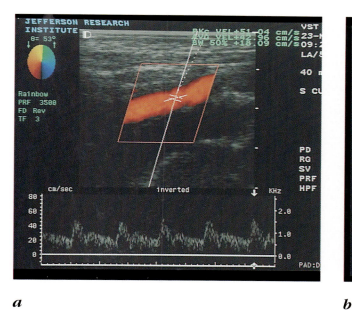

a

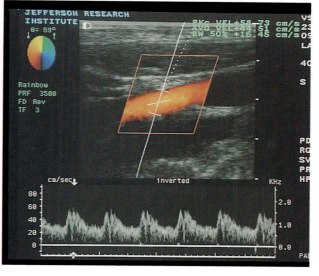

b

Figure 3.15 *Sampling within an artery. (a) If a small Doppler sample volume is placed in the center of the vessel, only the highest velocities are obtained. (b) If the sample volume is enlarged, low velocities near the wall contribute to the Doppler spectrum. The spectrum has a greater width than that in (a) and can be described as being spectrally broadened.*

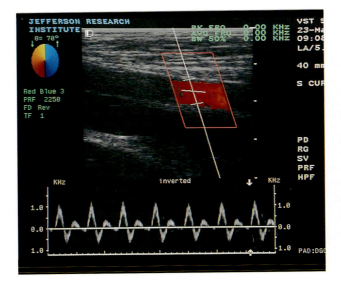

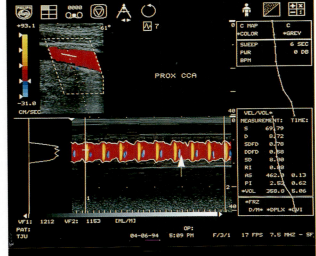

Figure 3.16 *Color flow image of a superficial femoral artery at peak systole. The color hue is uniform across the vessel. The sample volume insonates the entire vessel, yet the spectrum shows little spectral broadening.*

Figure 3.17 *Color M-mode of the origin of the common carotid artery. The M-mode displays a region of blue-coded flow concurrent with red-coded flow in the postsystolic phase (white arrow). The velocity vectors do not have uniform direction at this time.*

peripheral arteries at rest) have high accelerations and decelerations; flow profiles are more blunt during acceleration, producing more uniform color across the vessel diameter and showing Doppler spectra with little spectral broadening (Fig. 3.16).

The flow profile cannot always be assumed to be symmetrical. Curvature, bifurcations and confluences all produce secondary fluid flow which may extend along an artery or vein. The asymmetry may vary throughout the cardiac cycle (Fig. 3.17).

FLOW WITHIN BIFURCATIONS, CURVATURE, ARTERIOVENOUS FISTULAS AND ANEURYSMS

BIFURCATIONS

Flow at bifurcations is often complex, with the presence of a time-varying region of flow separation and strong secondary flows. Velocities are usually highest at the dividing wall, with flow separation likely at the opposite wall. The extent and duration of the region of separation is dependent on several factors, including the angle of bifurcation. These factors can make it difficult to measure velocity components accurately within the bifurcation region (Fig. 3.18). The waveform becomes more ordered distally due to the gradual damping of secondary flow.

CURVATURE

Curvature can cause skewing of the velocity profiles and, if severe enough to cause kinking, can give rise to narrowing. This sometimes occurs after vascular surgery if the course of the artery is tortuous (Fig. 3.19). In severe cases, accurate interpretation of the color image may be difficult and can produce errors in the measurement of flow velocity vectors.

ANEURYSMS AND PSEUDOANEURYSMS

Flow in aneurysms is typified by large secondary flows due to the sudden increase in cross-sectional area and increase in local static pressure. Swirling, multidirec-

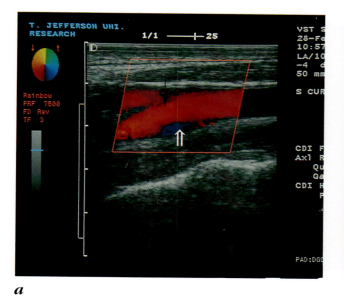

a

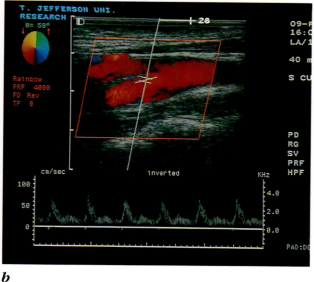

b

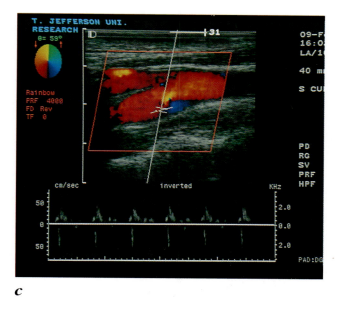

c

Figure 3.18 *Flow within a carotid bifurcation. (a) The color image shows high forward velocities at the dividing wall (solid arrow) with an area of flow separation in the carotid bulb (open arrow). (b) The spectral sample volume is placed near the dividing wall. The spectrum shows an ordered flow waveform throughout the cardiac cycle. (c) The spectral sample volume is placed in the area of flow separation. The time-varying pattern of flow is evident, with large fluctuations of velocity vector amplitude and direction.*

tional flow is often seen in the color image (Fig. 3.20). The Doppler spectrum may show disordered flow, depending on the position of the sample volume. Pseudoaneurysms also often show evidence of a swirling flow pattern (Fig. 3.21) which may be cyclic. The communicating tract leading to the pseudoaneurysm demonstrates forward flow in systole and complete reversal of flow in diastole (Fig. 3.22).

ATERIOVENOUS FISTULAS

Whether created intentionally or not, arteriovenous fistulas present a path of low resistance between an artery and vein. Doppler findings usually show a high-velocity low-pulsatility flow waveform in the artery leading to the fistula (Fig. 3.12e), with disturbed flow at the artery–vein junction (Fig. 3.23).

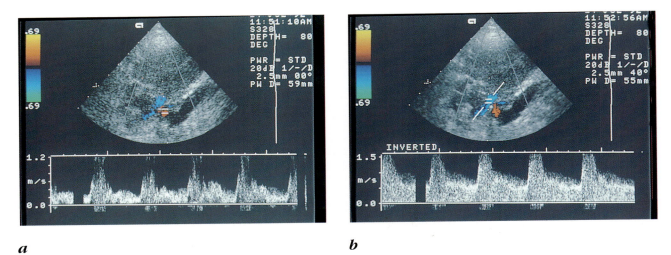

a   *b*

Figure 3.19 *Flow in a renal transplant artery. (a) Flow is towards the transducer. Peak velocity is approximately 100 cm/s. (b) Tight curvature causes elevated velocities to 160 cm/s. The direction of flow has changed by approximately 130° from that in (a) within a short distance.*

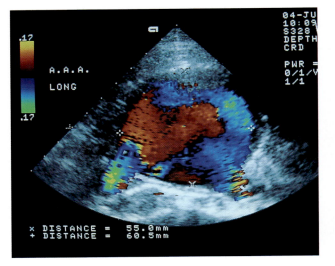

Figure 3.20 *Flow in an abdominal aortic aneurysm. Flow enters at the lower left of the image and exits lower right. The aneurysm contains swirling flows in the plane of measurement.*

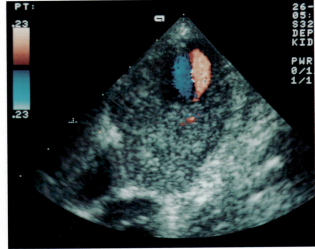

Figure 3.21 *Flow in a pseudoaneurysm. The color image shows half of the pseudoaneurysm with flow towards the transducer, and half away from it. The image results from a swirling flow within the volume.*

The turbulence at the fistula can lead to a large pressure drop as high-velocity flow is turned through 180° into the vein. Further along the vein, flow becomes ordered and may show arterial-like pulsations.

FLOW THROUGH STENOSES

Many practical and theoretical studies have been made of the flow through stenoses and the ability of

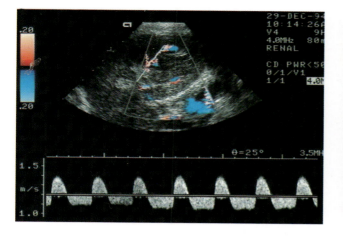

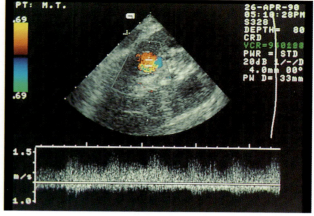

Figure 3.22 *Flow in a communicating tract supplying a pseudoaneurysm. The flow waveform shows forward and reversed flow as flow enters the pseudoaneurysm during systole and is ejected in diastole.*

Figure 3.23 *Flow at a fistula. The color image shows an area of intense color with many hues. The spectral display shows grossly disturbed flow.*

Doppler ultrasound to detect the presence and severity of a stenosis. Velocity changes through stenoses can lead to distal flow disturbances. If these are severe, turbulent losses will be added to the increased viscous resistance through the stenosis lumen and will result in a distal pressure loss and inadequate blood supply to downstream tissue. In the carotid arteries, it is thought that turbulent flow arising from stenoses may be a contributing factor in the formation of emboli. In the peripheral arteries, the pressure drop across a stenosis may limit the supply of blood to distal tissue. In the renal arteries, a pressure drop can lead to renal hypertension.

The effects of a stenosis can be measured by Doppler ultrasound either directly by examining velocity changes at the stenosis site or indirectly by measuring flow waveform changes downstream. By far the more reliable technique, if it is possible, is to examine changes at the site of stenosis.

The change in flow velocities occurring through a stenosis is shown diagrammatically in Fig. 3.24. The narrowing causes an increase in velocity through the stenosed lumen. The change in velocity vectors in the stenosis entrance region can lead to increased Doppler frequency shifts, depending on the direction of the flow vector and the velocity beam. Distally, the stenotic jet dissipates in the expansion region (Figs

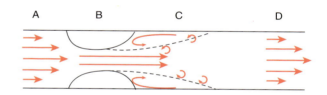

Figure 3.24 *Flow through a stenosis. Before stenosis (A), the flow velocity profile has lowest velocities near the wall, with high velocities in the center stream. Within the stenosis (B), a jet of high-velocity blood occurs due to the decreased lumen size. The flow profile becomes plug-like at this point. Distally (C), the jet dissipates and there is a post-stenotic region of disturbed flow. Vortices and flow separation (the region within the dotted lines) produce multidirectional velocity vectors. Distally (D), the flow reorganizes.*

3.24, 3.25 and 3.26). There may be a region of flow separation evident in the expansion region resulting from the increased cross-sectional area (Fig. 3.27). The recirculating flows in this region combine with

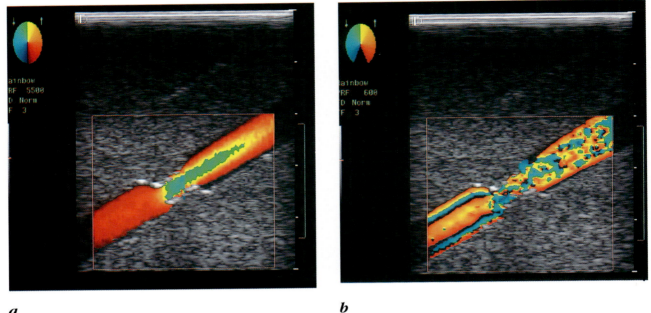

a   *b*

Figure 3.25 *Flow through a 50% diameter model narrowing. Color flow observations (flow is from left to right). (a) The color flow PRF is set so that the velocity jet is coded green (aliased). Distally, the jet dissipates and peak velocity gradually decreases downstream. (b) The color flow PRF is set low (notice the aliasing in the prestenotic laminar flow). This setting is more sensitive to subtle velocity vector variations. In the stenosis jet, there are many hues arising from the many velocity vectors caused by the entrance to the stenosis. Distally, flow is seen to contain a wide range of velocity vectors as the jet dissipates and causes local vortices.*

the vortex shedding of the stenotic jet to give velocity vectors with a range of amplitudes and directions. The Doppler ultrasound spectral display shows this as 'spectral broadening', although its extent is very dependent on the size and placement of the sample volume. In stenoses up to 50% diameter reduction, flow disturbances are not generally a reliable guide, because the Doppler characteristics associated with low level of turbulence (some spectral broadening and chaotic color flow image arising from multivector flow) can be artificially created by the user.

In theory, velocity measurement through a stenosis should provide an accurate measure of the degree of narrowing of the vessel. Continuity of flow means that the decrease in lumen size is accompanied by a corresponding rise in mean velocity in the vessel. Unfortunately, mean velocity is difficult to measure accurately with Doppler techniques. In addition, stenoses often occur near or at bifurcations, so that a comparison of proximal velocity with velocity within

the stenosis is limited by the multiple vascular beds which the proximal vessel supplies. Peak velocity does not change in proportion to the mean velocity rise. The flow profile through the stenosis becomes plug-like, so that a halving of area does not lead to twice the peak velocity (although mean velocity does increase by that much).

The characteristics of direct color flow and spectral Doppler investigation of stenoses are illustrated in in-vitro models of a stenosis (Figs 3.25, 3.26 and 3.27) and in in-vivo examples (Figs 3.28 and 3.29). A small degree of stenosis may not be manifested by velocity increases, depending on the vascular bed in which it occurs. Criteria for velocity increases have been obtained empirically and have been shown to be reliable in, for example, disease of the internal carotid artery. It may be that the only evidence obtained in some abdominal sites is a high velocity (Fig. 3.30); in such cases, there is no need to try to image the pre- or post-stenotic flow.

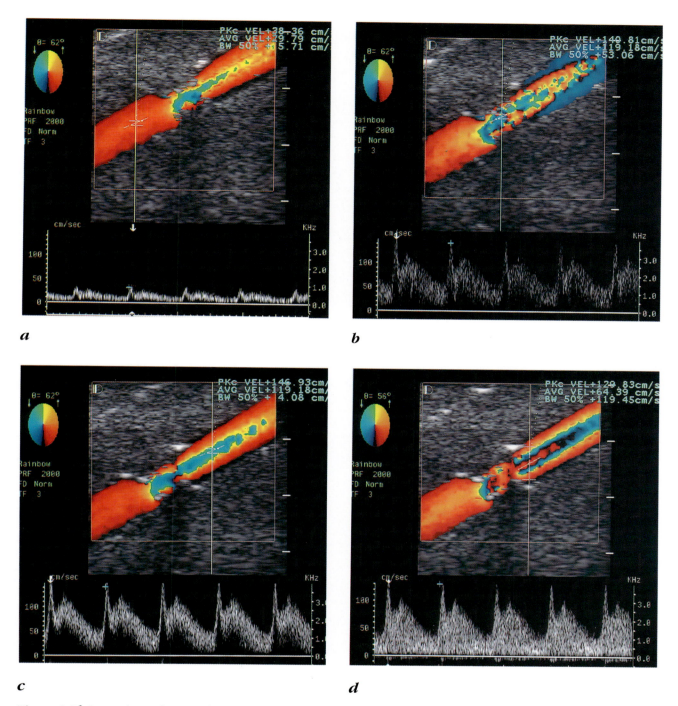

Figure 3.26 *Spectral Doppler in pulsatile flow in a model stenosis. (a) Prestenosis, peak velocity is 32 cm/s. (b) In the stenosis, measured peak velocity is 141 cm/s. The angle correction is based on the direction of the lumen and may not take account of the true velocity vectors in this model. (c) Post-stenosis in the center stream there is little spectral broadening. (d) With the sample volume expanded, there is spectral broadening caused by the multidirectional flow. There is some evidence of 'reversed-flow' components.*

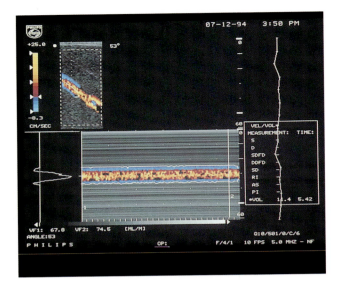

Figure 3.27 *Color M-mode of steady flow through a stenosis. Flow is from right to left. The flow profile (lower right) shows the reversed-flow component near the wall of the post-stenotic flow separation region.*

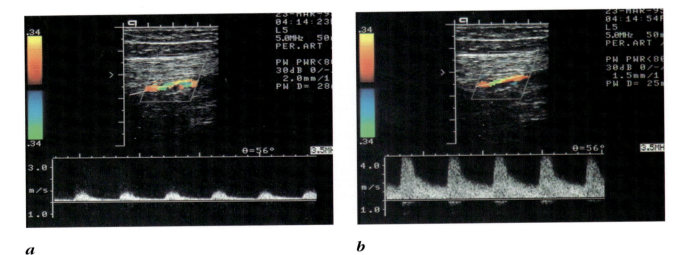

a   *b*

Figure 3.28 *In vivo stenosis, superficial femoral artery. (a) Prestenosis, the sample volume is placed in an area coded red. Measured peak velocity is under 1 m/s. (b) Within the stenosis, there is color aliasing. Measured peak velocity is over 5 m/s, indicating a severe reduction in cross-sectional area.*

If the narrowing is severe enough, the pressure loss through the stenosis causes damped flow distally (see Fig. 3.12f). The pressure drop can be exacerbated by increased bloodflow through the stenosis. The distal flow waveform may be affected by many factors, however, of which the stenosis is only one.

VENOUS FLOW

Compared with arterial flow, venous flow is characterized by lower velocities, pulsatility which depends on downstream pressure changes, and low-pressure vessels which are often readily compressed.

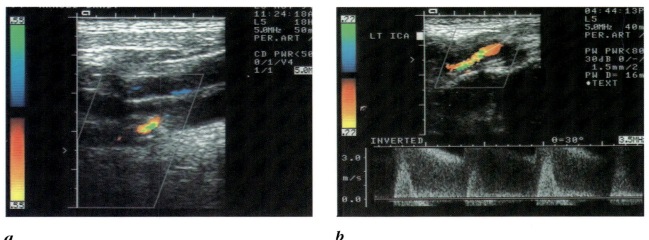

a   b

Figure 3.29 *In vivo stenoses, internal carotid artery. (a) The color PRF is set high. Only the stenotic jet registers on the image. The gray scale shows the presence of disease. (b) The color PRF is set high. There is aliasing in the artery. The sample volume is placed in the stenosis. The spectral display also shows aliasing, with measured peak velocities exceeding 5 m/s.*

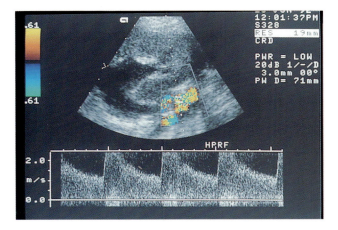

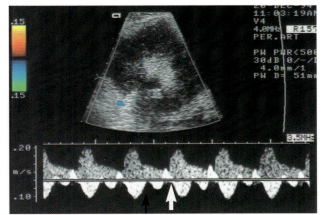

Figure 3.30 *Stenosis of a renal transplant artery. The color flow image of the anastomosis is confused with many velocity vectors present. The spectral Doppler sample volume is placed at the site of the anastomosis. No angle correction has been made; velocities must be at least as great as that measured. The waveform shows the characteristic renal artery shape but with velocities in the region of 2.5 m/s, indicative of a stenosis.*

Figure 3.31 *Arterial and venous flow waveforms. The image is of a renal transplant. The patient's venous pressure was high, which resulted in good transmission of the right atrial pressures down to the level of the renal veins. The arterial waveform shows the normal low-resistance forward flow. The venous waveform shows two periods of deceleration in every cardiac cycle. The reverse flow (white arrow), just prior to ventricular systole, is caused by the increased pressure of atrial systole. Deceleration is also caused by filling of the right atrium prior to opening of the tricuspid valve (black arrow).*

Because of the lower velocities, scanner settings for Doppler investigation of veins may have to be changed from those used for arterial flow. Typically, a lower pulse repetition frequency and more persistence are used to enhance the venous signals. The amount of pulsatility varies considerably, depending on the site being evaluated. Veins in the abdomen may exhibit velocity fluctuations due to pressure changes in the right atrium of the heart (Fig. 3.31). These may be further modulated by changes in pressure caused by respiration (Fig. 3.32). Further away from the heart (in the iliac veins, for instance) the respiratory changes dominate (Fig. 3.33). In the extremities, there may be little natural variation in velocity. Changes can be induced by asking the patient to cough or, in the exceptionally talented patient, having them perform a Valsalva maneuver. Flow may be augmented by squeezing a limb distally (Fig. 3.34).

The presence of naturally occurring changes in phase with breathing or the right heart is an indication that there is no major occlusion or thrombosis between the right heart and the site of measurement. Bilateral differences (e.g. a right femoral vein with fluctuations, and a left femoral vein with constant velocity) give cause for suspicion that one side has thrombus present (Fig. 3.35).

Venous reflux in legs is readily demonstrated by Doppler ultrasound. With the patient standing, a squeeze of the calf sends blood up towards the heart. If the venous valves are functioning adequately, release of the calf causes a slight backflow (as blood descends under gravity) which is quickly checked by closure of the valves (Fig. 3.36a). In cases of incompetent valves, blood flows back down the leg (Fig. 3.36b).

FURTHER READING

Bernstein EF, ed, *Vascular Diagnosis*, 4th edn (Mosby-Year Book: St Louis, 1993).

Burns PN, Haemodynamics. In: Taylor KJW, Burns PN, Wells PNT, *Clinical Applications of Doppler Ultrasound*, 2nd edn (Raven Press: New York, 1995) 35–54.

Carter SA, Hemodynamic considerations in peripheral and cerebrovascular diseases. In: Zwiebel WJ, *Introduction to Vascular Ultrasonography*, 3rd edn (WB Saunders: Philadelphia, 1992) 3–18.

Evans DH, McDicken WN, Skidmore R, Woodcock JP, *Doppler Ultrasound: Physics, Instrumentation and Clinical Applications* (Wiley: Chichester, 1989).

Strandness DE, Sumner DS, *Hemodynamics for Surgeons* (Grune and Stratton: New York, 1975).

Kopinski AM (ed), An overview of peripheral arterial disease and its diagnosis. *J Vasc Technol* (1994) **18**:225–322.

Cardullo PA (ed), Overview of venous disease and its diagnosis. *J Vasc Technol* (1988) **12**:77–123.

Zwiebel WJ, Spectrum analysis in Doppler vascular diagnosis. In: Zwiebel WJ, *Introduction to Vascular Ultrasonography*, 3rd edn (WB Saunders: Philadelphia, 1992) 45–66.

BACKGROUND

Caro GG, Pedley JG, Schroter RC, Seed WA, *The Mechanics of the Circulation* (OUP: New York, 1978).

Nichols WW, O'Rourke M, *McDonald's Blood Flow in Arteries*, 3rd edn (Edward Arnold: London, 1990).

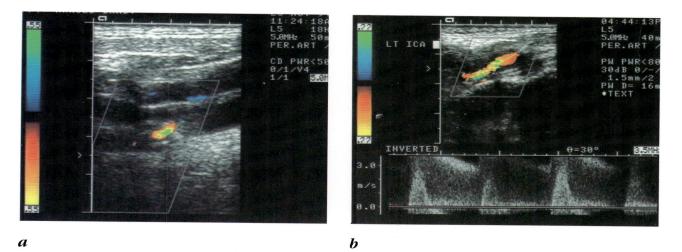

a **b**

Figure 3.29 *In vivo stenoses, internal carotid artery. (a) The color PRF is set high. Only the stenotic jet registers on the image. The gray scale shows the presence of disease. (b) The color PRF is set high. There is aliasing in the artery. The sample volume is placed in the stenosis. The spectral display also shows aliasing, with measured peak velocities exceeding 5 m/s.*

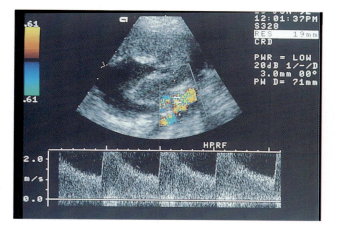

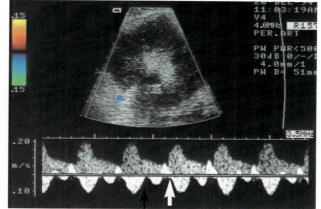

Figure 3.30 *Stenosis of a renal transplant artery. The color flow image of the anastomosis is confused with many velocity vectors present. The spectral Doppler sample volume is placed at the site of the anastomosis. No angle correction has been made; velocities must be at least as great as that measured. The waveform shows the characteristic renal artery shape but with velocities in the region of 2.5 m/s, indicative of a stenosis.*

Figure 3.31 *Arterial and venous flow waveforms. The image is of a renal transplant. The patient's venous pressure was high, which resulted in good transmission of the right atrial pressures down to the level of the renal veins. The arterial waveform shows the normal low-resistance forward flow. The venous waveform shows two periods of deceleration in every cardiac cycle. The reverse flow (white arrow), just prior to ventricular systole, is caused by the increased pressure of atrial systole. Deceleration is also caused by filling of the right atrium prior to opening of the tricuspid valve (black arrow).*

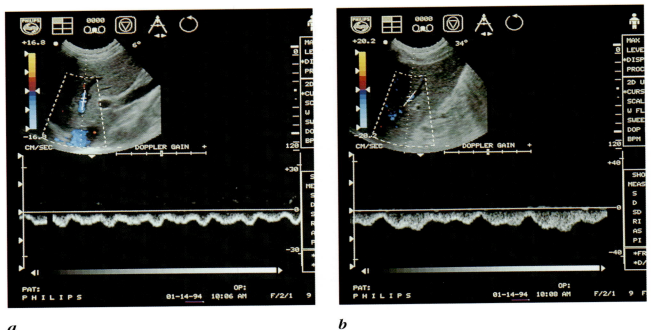

a
b

Figure 3.32 *Flow in a hepatic vein. (a) With the patient holding her breath, the venous waveform shows fluctuations from the right heart. (b) With the patient breathing normally, longer-period fluctuations also occur due to the changing pressure gradients in inspiration and expiration.*

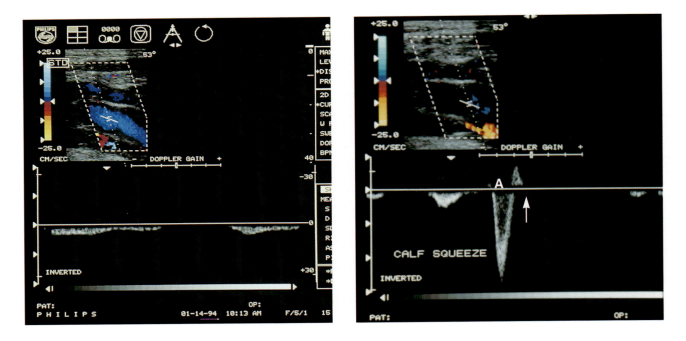

Figure 3.33 *Venous flow in the popliteal vein. There is no evidence of right heart fluctuations; some variation remains due to breathing.*

Figure 3.34 *Venous flow is augmented by a distal squeeze of the calf at A. There is a momentary reflux of blood which causes valve closure (arrow).*

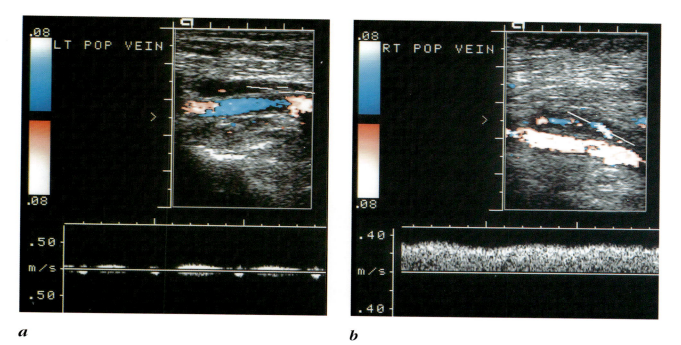

Figure 3.35 *Effects of thrombus on venous flow waveforms. (a) In the unaffected popliteal vein, velocities are low and show normal cyclic variation. (b) In the contralateral popliteal vein, velocities are high because of thrombus in the vein which reduces the lumen size. Velocity fluctuations arising from downstream pressure changes are less apparent.*

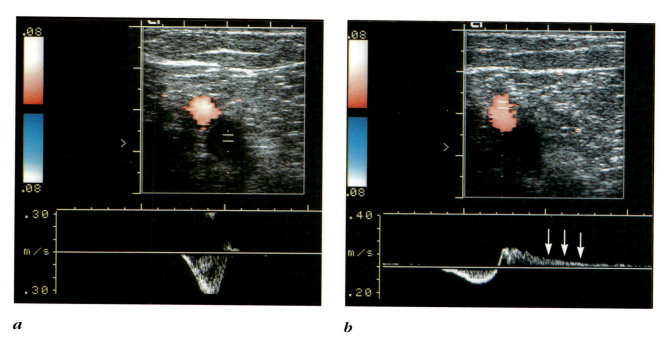

Figure 3.36 *Incompetent venous valves. (a) Normal valve function. The cursor is located in the femoral vein. Following a calf squeeze, during which blood travels towards the heart, the venous valve stops the return of blood back down the leg. Only very brief retrograde flow is seen on the sonogram. (b) Incompetent valve. The cursor is placed in the long saphenous vein in which there is an incompetent valve. Following a calf squeeze, blood returns back down the leg over several seconds (arrows).*

Because of the lower velocities, scanner settings for Doppler investigation of veins may have to be changed from those used for arterial flow. Typically, a lower pulse repetition frequency and more persistence are used to enhance the venous signals. The amount of pulsatility varies considerably, depending on the site being evaluated. Veins in the abdomen may exhibit velocity fluctuations due to pressure changes in the right atrium of the heart (Fig. 3.31). These may be further modulated by changes in pressure caused by respiration (Fig. 3.32). Further away from the heart (in the iliac veins, for instance) the respiratory changes dominate (Fig. 3.33). In the extremities, there may be little natural variation in velocity. Changes can be induced by asking the patient to cough or, in the exceptionally talented patient, having them perform a Valsalva maneuver. Flow may be augmented by squeezing a limb distally (Fig. 3.34).

The presence of naturally occurring changes in phase with breathing or the right heart is an indication that there is no major occlusion or thrombosis between the right heart and the site of measurement. Bilateral differences (e.g. a right femoral vein with fluctuations, and a left femoral vein with constant velocity) give cause for suspicion that one side has thrombus present (Fig. 3.35).

Venous reflux in legs is readily demonstrated by Doppler ultrasound. With the patient standing, a squeeze of the calf sends blood up towards the heart. If the venous valves are functioning adequately, release of the calf causes a slight backflow (as blood descends under gravity) which is quickly checked by closure of the valves (Fig. 3.36a). In cases of incompetent valves, blood flows back down the leg (Fig. 3.36b).

FURTHER READING

Bernstein EF, ed, *Vascular Diagnosis*, 4th edn (Mosby-Year Book: St Louis, 1993).

Burns PN, Haemodynamics. In: Taylor KJW, Burns PN, Wells PNT, *Clinical Applications of Doppler Ultrasound*, 2nd edn (Raven Press: New York, 1995) 35–54.

Carter SA, Hemodynamic considerations in peripheral and cerebrovascular diseases. In: Zwiebel WJ, *Introduction to Vascular Ultrasonography*, 3rd edn (WB Saunders: Philadelphia, 1992) 3–18.

Evans DH, McDicken WN, Skidmore R, Woodcock JP, *Doppler Ultrasound: Physics, Instrumentation and Clinical Applications* (Wiley: Chichester, 1989).

Strandness DE, Sumner DS, *Hemodynamics for Surgeons* (Grune and Stratton: New York, 1975).

Kopinski AM (ed), An overview of peripheral arterial disease and its diagnosis. *J Vasc Technol* (1994) **18**:225–322.

Cardullo PA (ed), Overview of venous disease and its diagnosis. *J Vasc Technol* (1988) **12**:77–123.

Zwiebel WJ, Spectrum analysis in Doppler vascular diagnosis. In: Zwiebel WJ, *Introduction to Vascular Ultrasonography*, 3rd edn (WB Saunders: Philadelphia, 1992) 45–66.

BACKGROUND

Caro GG, Pedley JG, Schroter RC, Seed WA, *The Mechanics of the Circulation* (OUP: New York, 1978).

Nichols WW, O'Rourke M, *McDonald's Blood Flow in Arteries*, 3rd edn (Edward Arnold: London, 1990).

Chapter 4 Abdominal applications of color flow imaging

Daniel A Merton and Barry B Goldberg

INTRODUCTION

The addition of color flow imaging (CFI) to conventional gray scale ultrasound has significantly increased the range and specificity of ultrasound diagnoses within the abdomen and retroperitoneum. As in other applications of Doppler flow analysis, CFI does not replace the more quantitative aspects of duplex Doppler with spectral analysis. However, because of the large areas under evaluation in this region of the body, examinations requiring bloodflow data can typically be done in a more time-efficient and thorough manner by utilizing CFI. Conversely, at times the qualitative nature of CFI is not a limiting factor because, often, only information regarding the presence and direction of bloodflow is necessary. For these applications CFI is the most efficient, non-invasive and cost-effective method of obtaining the necessary diagnostic information. When more specific bloodflow characterization is necessary, CFI plays an important role by providing a 'road map' guide for sample volume placement to acquire spectral Doppler waveforms.

As in all uses of ultrasound, prerequisites to achieving a proper diagnosis are a thorough knowledge of both the anatomy and physiology of the region under investigation, and equipment optimization techniques necessary for the specific application. While a complete discussion on abdominal anatomy and physiology is beyond the objectives of this book, specific applications dealt with here will demonstrate many of the most commonly encountered abnormalities detectable with abdominal CFI, as well as scanning techniques which will often facilitate successful diagnoses. Additionally, normal examples of CFI findings are included for comparison.

Technical limitations of CFI in the abdomen include the depth of vessels to be imaged and other attenuating factors such as intervening bowel. These limitations have proven to be a handicap, particularly

in the evaluation of flow in deeper vessels within the body and especially in the obese patient. A lack of flow on CFI may, for example, be due to an inadequate Doppler angle, or signal attenuation. Scanning techniques which provide more acute Doppler angles, such as approaching the vessel from a different plane and reducing the depth by using compression of the intervening tissue with the transducer, may reduce or eliminate some of these limitations. In the future the use of vascular ultrasound contrast agents will increase the flow signal-to-noise ratio and allow for more complete visualization of most vessels, including those at depths and angles encountered within the abdomen and retroperitoneum.

THE ABDOMINAL AORTA AND ITS BRANCHES

In most cases bloodflow in the abdominal aorta is easily visualized using CFI, along with its branches, particularly the celiac axis and superior mesenteric artery (Figs 4.1–4.3). Detection of flow in the renal arteries with CFI, because of their lateral location on the wall of the aorta, is often more difficult (Fig. 4.4). The inferior mesenteric artery, due to its small caliber, is typically more easily detected with the use of CFI than by gray scale imaging alone (Fig. 4.5). The proximal common iliac artery and distal external iliac vessels can usually be visualized with CFI; however, the mid-portions of the iliac arteries are often obscured by overlying gas-filled bowel (Figs 4.6 and 4.7).

Abnormalities in which CFI may provide additional information over that of gray scale imaging include demonstrating the extent of the functional lumen in cases of aneurysms, and detecting flow separations or other flow disruptions which occur in arterial aneurysms throughout the vascular system (Figs

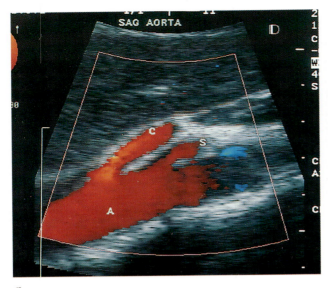

a

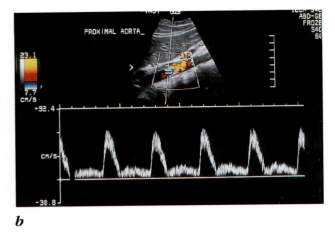

b

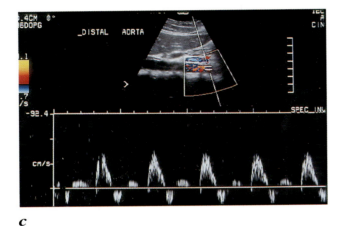

c

Figure 4.1 *Longitudinal CFI (a) of the abdominal aorta (A) and its two major ventral branches, the celiac axis (C) and superior mesenteric artery (S). In a different patient (b), pulsed Doppler spectral analysis of the proximal aorta (above the celiac axis) demonstrates a monophasic-continuous waveform due to the relatively low vascular resistance of flow to the visceral organs, whereas a waveform obtained from the distal aorta (c) demonstrates a triphasic spectral signal as a result of the higher resistance of flow to the pelvis and lower extremities. These differences in pulsatility can also be demonstrated using CFI with adequate temporal resolution (see Fig. 4.6).*

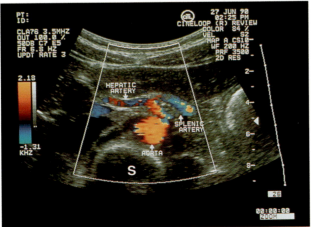

Figure 4.2 *Transverse CFI of the celic axis with its bifurcation into the common hepatic and splenic arteries. Flow direction in the hepatic artery is nearly perpendicular to the angle of insonation, resulting in ambiguous directional information. The left crus of the diaphram is visualized anterior to the aorta. By demonstrating no flow in this hypoechoic structure, CFI can help avoid mistaking it for a vessel. S, spine.*

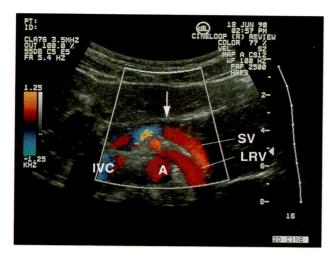

Figure 4.3 *Transverse CFI of the aorta at the level of the left renal vein (LRV) and splenic vein (SV). Flow in the SV changes direction in relation to the transducer, resulting in a red to blue transition (arrow). The superior mesenteric artery is seen in cross-section. IVC; inferior vena cava.*

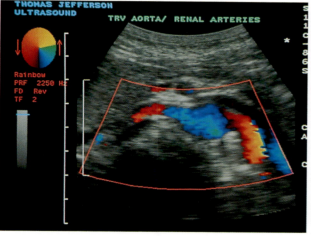

a

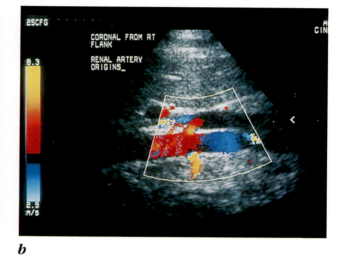

b

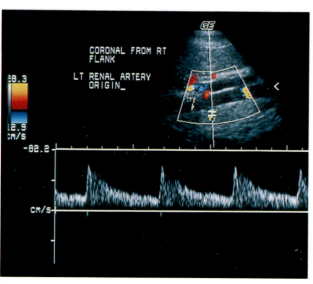

c

Figure 4.4 *The renal artery origins can be viewed from either a midline transverse view of the aorta (a) at the level of the renal artery origins approximately 1–2 cm inferior to Fig. 4.3, or a coronal view (b) obtained from the right costal margin. The coronal view can be especially useful to acquire pulsed Doppler spectral data (c) from the renal artery origins in patients being examined for suspected renal artery stenosis. This is an example of a normal renal artery waveform.*

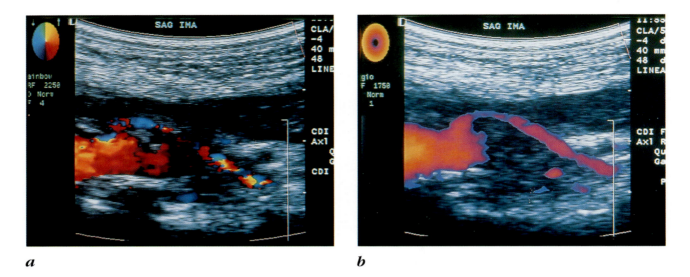

a   *b*

Figure 4.5 *Sagittal conventional color (a) and color amplitude (b) images of the distal aorta and inferior mesenteric artery (IMA). Note the improvement in flow continuity visualized with CAI and the lack of aliasing artifacts which are present in the conventional color flow image. This patient had mild stenosis of the IMA detected by pulsed spectral Doppler velocity estimation (not shown) and confirmed by X-ray angiography.*

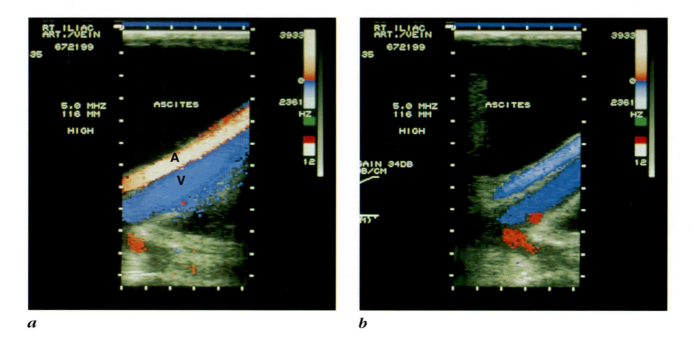

a   *b*

Figure 4.6 *CFI can demonstrate in real time the normal hemodynamics which occur over the cardiac cycle. In this case a longitudinal CFI of the right external iliac artery (A) and vein (V) at peak systole (a) indicates the flow direction in the artery is antegrade (color coded red), whereas the normal early diastolic flow reversal (in blue) is seen in (b). A marked amount of ascites within the abdomen and pelvis facilitates visualization of these structures.*

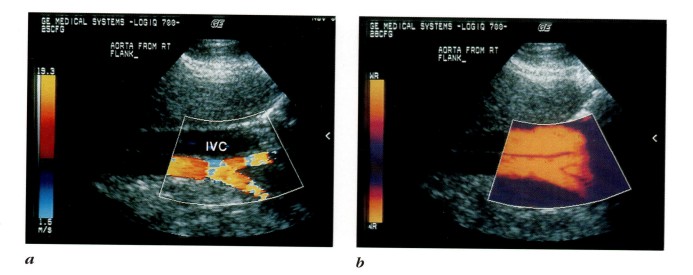

Figure 4.7 *Conventional (mean Doppler frequency shift) CFI of the distal aorta and bifurcation obtained from the patient's right flank (a) demonstrates good flow in the aorta and its terminal branches; however, to achieve this level of vessel filling requires such a low pulse repetition frequency that the image has significant aliasing artifacts. Also note the lack of flow information from the inferior vena cava (IVC). The same view obtained using the amplitude of the color Doppler signal or color amplitude imaging (CAI) (b), because of its non-directionality, increased signal-to-noise ratio and reduced angle dependence, demonstrates the flow in the aorta as well as that in the IVC.*

4.8–4.12). Additionally, in cases of aortic dissection, demonstration of flow within the true and false lumens can be demonstrated using CFI as well as in cases of intimal flaps where complete dissection has not occurred (Fig. 4.13). Temporal information, including differences in flow during systole and diastole, can be demonstrated so that CFI, often supplemented by pulsed spectral Doppler, is useful in understanding the physiology of normal and abnormal flow. To properly interpret the CFI information obtained from the abdominal aorta, the physiology of the regions supplied by this vessel must be understood and considered. The proximal aorta supplies blood to all of the visceral organs of the abdomen, including the kidneys, bowel and liver, which are relatively low-resistance vascular beds. Spectral Doppler waveforms obtained at this level of the aorta would be expected to contain a moderate level of diastolic flow, in contrast to the distal aorta which supplies the pelvis and lower extremities, which are higher-resistance vascular beds (Fig. 4.1). Spectral Doppler waveforms obtained from the distal aorta typically demonstrate a lack of diastolic flow,

often with a reversal of flow in early diastole. These temporal changes in flow can all be observed using properly adjusted CFI systems. In addition to confirming normal hemodynamics, CFI may provide additional information on disease processes which lead to changes in vascular resistance within organs.

CFI can facilitate detection of vascular stenoses within the abdomen by detecting a reduction in functional lumen size, increased flow velocities, and downstream turbulence (Figs 4.14 and 4.15). However, pulsed Doppler with spectral analysis is required to determine more accurately the severity of the stenosis. In cases of suspected vascular occlusion, CFI can demonstrate the lack of flow in the affected vessel segment, and may help to detect collateralization when present (Fig. 4.16). For patients having symptoms resulting from suspected bowel ischemia, such as post-prandial pain or unattempted weight loss, CFI can be used to localize stenoses of one or more of the the arteries supplying the bowel (Figs 4.17 and 4.18). These include the celiac axis, superior mesenteric artery and the smaller inferior mesenteric artery. The primary role of CFI in this application is

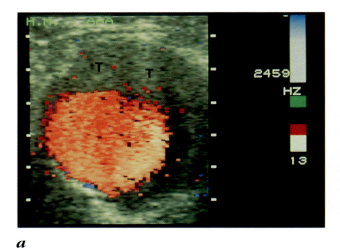

a

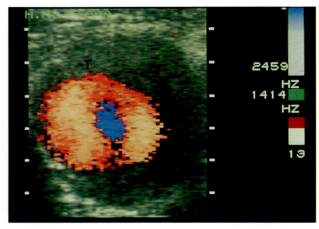

b

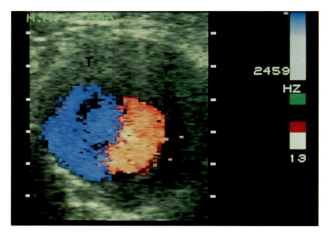

c

Figure 4.8 *Sequential transverse CFIs of an abdominal aortic aneurysm with intramural thrombus (T) obtained over different points of the cardiac cycle. A color flow image obtained at peak systole (a) demonstrates forward flow throughout the functional lumen. (b) An image obtained during early diastole with shades of blue representing a flow separation in the center of the lumen. At end diastole (c) helical flow is seen with half of the lumen color coded red and half color coded blue. CFI can help determine the functional lumen size and degree of intraluminal thrombus in aneurysms.*

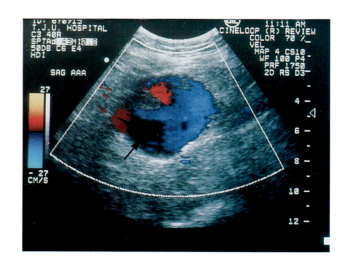

Figure 4.9 *Transverse CFI of a distal aortic aneurysm with a suspected area of thrombus extending from the right anterolateral wall (arrow). The lack of flow in this area supports the initial diagnosis of intraluminal thrombus suggested by gray scale imaging (not shown).*

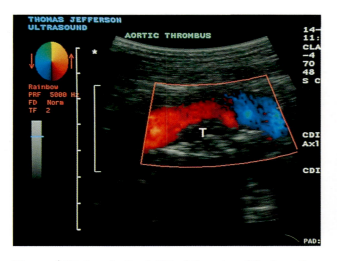

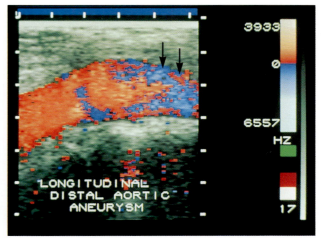

Figure 4.10 *Longitudinal CFI of thrombus (T) along the posterior wall of the abdominal aorta. In this patient with coagulopathy no aneurysm was identified.*

Figure 4.11 *Longitudinal CFI of a small distal aortic aneurysm in a 35-year-old female with pain following trauma from a lap restraint during a motor vehicle accident. A small area of flow separation is present due to the caliber increase at the level of the aneurysm. Ambiguous flow direction is demonstrated in the distal-most aorta (arrows) as a result of the poor Doppler angle.*

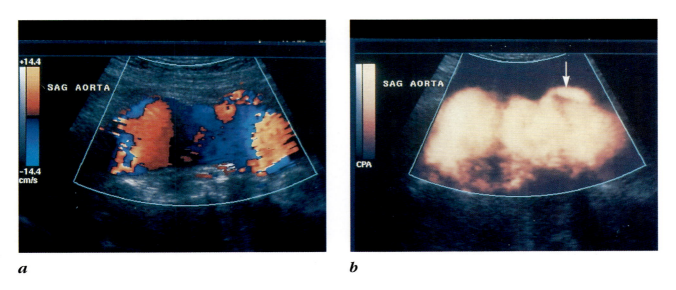

a

b

Figure 4.12 *Sagittal conventional color (a) and color amplitude (b) images of a distal aortic aneurysm. Note the flow turbulence (demonstrated as changes in flow direction) detected with the conventional color mode which cannot be demonstrated with CAI. However, CAI better demonstrates the location of the inferior mesenteric artery (arrow), but is more susceptible to artifacts related to transmitted vascular pulsations. This example demonstrates the complementary nature of the information obtained with the two different CFI modalities.*

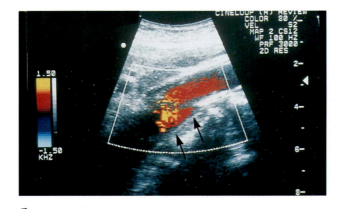

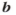

a

b

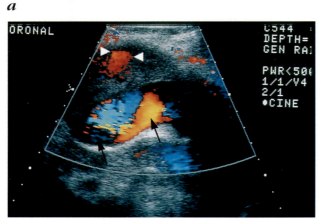

c

Figure 4.13 *Sequential longitudinal color flow images of an aortic dissection (arrows) during systole (a) with flow into the blind dissection pocket (color coded red), and diastole (b) with flow reversed in the dissection (color coded blue). CFI (c) demonstrates flow within the primary functional lumen (arrows) and the dissection (arrow heads) in a different patient with known chronic abdominal aortic dissection.*

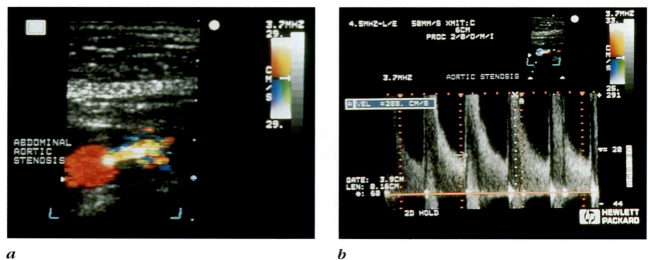

a

b

Figure 4.14 *This 45-year-old female was referred for ultrasound with bilateral lower extremity claudication. CFI of the mid-aorta (a) identified a focal area of functional lumen narrowing, with an increase in flow velocity, and downstream turbulence (note the use of a 'variance' color map) consistent with an aortic stenosis. Angle-corrected pulsed Doppler spectral analysis (b) confirms a high-velocity jet through the stenotic segment. Note the spectral aliasing with the peak systolic flow velocity greater than 291 cm/s.*

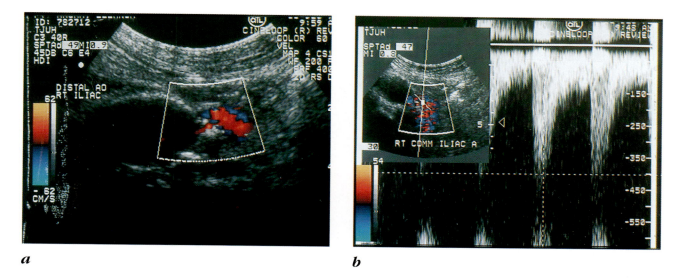

a   *b*

Figure 4.15 *CFI (a) demonstrates a stenosis at the origin of the left common iliac artery. A pulsed Doppler spectral wave form (b) obtained from the area of narrowing demonstrates typical spectral findings of high systolic frequency shifts, reduced pulsatility, and spectral broadening.*

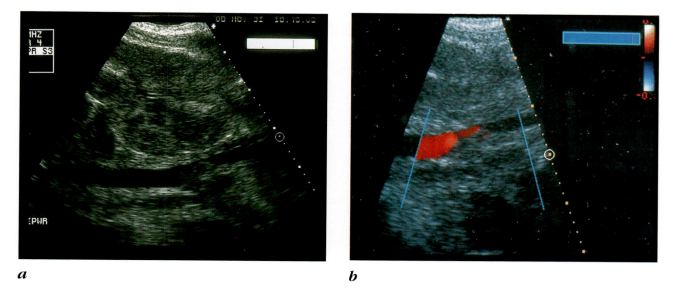

a   *b*

Figure 4.16 *After removal of an umbilical artery catheter a physical examination revealed reduced pulses in this premature neonate's right lower extremity. A pulsed spectral Doppler examination of the right leg (not shown) detected reduced flow velocity and signal amplitude from the right femoral artery when compared to the left. A coronal gray scale image (a) of the common iliac arteries suggested thrombosis within the right iliac artery with extension through the aortic bifurcation into the left iliac artery. CFI (b) confirmed complete occlusion of the right iliac artery and partial functional lumen narrowing on the left iliac artery. CFI also detected multiple pelvic collateral vessels which provided flow to the right leg. Serial ultrasound examinations were used in this case to non-invasively monitor resolution of the thrombus.*

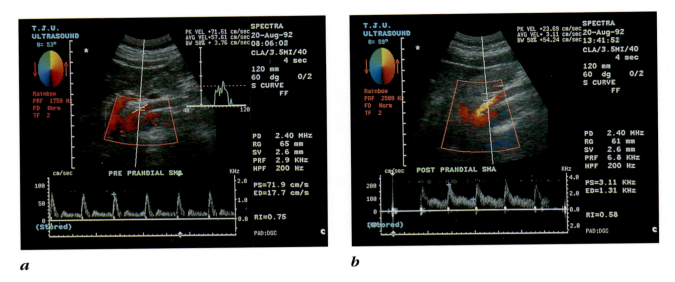

a   *b*

Figure 4.17 *The normal physiologic response to a meal is demonstrated in these color flow images with spectral analysis of the superior mesenteric artery (SMA) pre- (a) and post- (b) prandially. The preprandial spectral wave form has reversed or absent early diastolic flow and low end-diastolic flow indicative of increased downstream resistance. After a meal, peripheral resistance of flow to the bowel decreases resulting in a loss of the early diastolic flow reversal, an increase in end-diastolic flow, and a reduction in the resistive index (RI).*

to act as a guide to direct placement of a pulsed Doppler sample volume at the point of maximum functional lumen narrowing and acquire velocity information via spectral analysis. Comparing flow velocity estimations obtained proximal and distal to the stenotic area to that of the stenotic segment will determine if there is a hemodynamically significant stenosis by using established criteria. In cases of occlusion to one or more of the vessels feeding the bowel it is common to have collateralization of flow through communicating vasculature which can be detected with CFI. After therapeutic angioplasty or surgical reconstruction, CFI with Doppler spectral analysis can be used to monitor for re-stenosis, possibly identifying hemodynamically significant stenoses prior to the onset of the patient's symptoms, when interventional radiographic measures are still a treatment option.

CFI can assist in the identification of normal vascular anatomic variations when present, such as a replaced right hepatic artery, duplication of the renal arteries, or a common origin of the celiac and

superior mesenteric arteries (Figs 4.19–4.23). Detection of stenoses or aneurysmal dilatation of these vessels can also be seen. The use of various patient positions and probe compression maneuvers may help to displace overlying bowel when it presents problems in visualization of abdominal and retroperitoneal structures.

THE INFERIOR VENA CAVA AND ITS BRANCHES

The hepatic portion of the inferior vena cava (IVC) can usually be visualized deep to the liver, passing through the diaphragm and into the right atrium of the heart. The middle to distal portions of the IVC may be obscured by overlying gas-filled bowel. Compression of the overlying tissues, placing the patient in a left lateral decubitus position and using

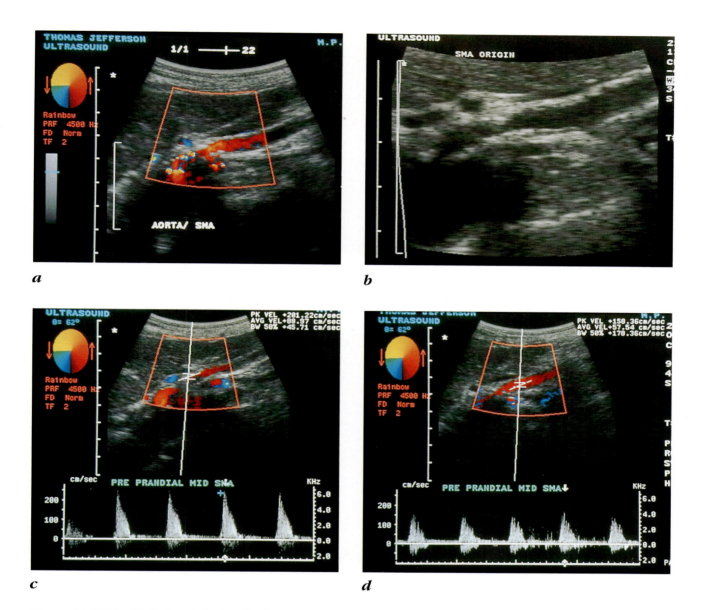

Figure 4.18 *This elderly female had a chief complaint of mid-abdominal pain after eating, and progressive weight loss over several months time. Longitudinal color flow images of the tortuous aorta (a) at the level of the superior mesenteric artery (SMA) demonstrates a focal narrowing of the SMA lumen with aliasing at that level, and an increase in vessel diameter downstream from the suspected stenosis. A magnified gray scale image (b) of the area better delineates the intimal thickening and atherosclerotic changes within this vessel segment, and helps localize the point of maximum narrowing for Doppler sample volume placement. A spectral Doppler velocity estimate (c) of 239 cm/s at the narrowed segment was nearly 6 times the velocity of the aorta at this level. Distal to this point (d) spectral Doppler demonstrated a reduction in velocity with spectral broadening and turbulence. These findings suggest a stenosis of the SMA. A subsequent X-ray angiographic examination identified an 80% stenosis of the SMA at the location first identified with CFI ultrasound. Successful balloon angioplasty of this vessel segment resolved the patient's symptoms. CFI can also be used to non-invasively monitor for re-stenosis in patients who have had prior therapeutic angioplasty.*

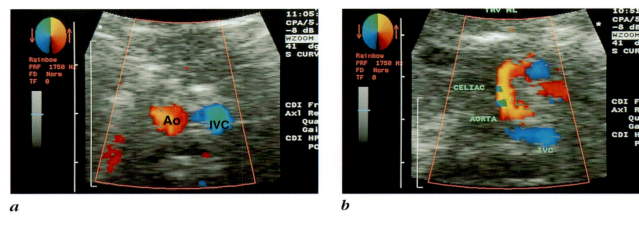

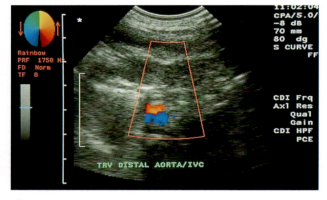

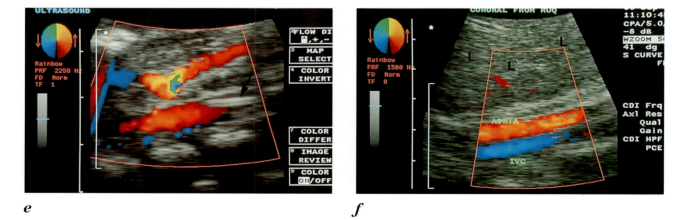

Figure 4.19 *CFIs of a neonate with a left-sided inferior vena cava (IVC), a normal anatomic variation. Transverse view (a) of the proximal aorta (Ao). Transverse view (b) at the level of the celiac axis. Transverse view (c) at the level of the renal artery origins. Note the location of the IVC posterior to the left renal artery (LRA). RRA, right renal artery. Transverse view (d) at the level of the IVC and aortic bifurcations. Longitudinal view (e) of a single ventral branch giving rise to both the celiac axis and superior mesenteric arteries, another anatomic variation identified in this newborn. Note the presence of an umbilical artery catheter in the distal aorta (arrow). Coronal view (f) from the right upper quadrant demonstrating the proximal abdominal aorta to the right of the IVC. L, liver.*

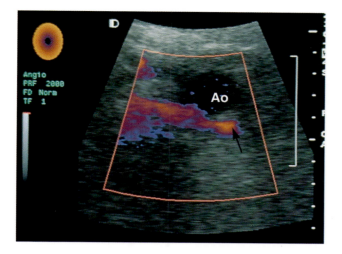

Figure 4.20 *Transverse color amplitude image of the aorta (Ao) obtained in diastole in a patient with a known retro-aortic left renal vein (arrow), a normal anatomic variant.*

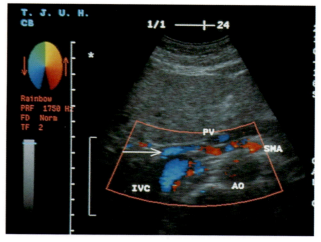

Figure 4.21 *Transverse CFI of the origin of a replaced right hepatic artery arising from the superior mesenteric artery (SMA). This anatomic variant is seen in approximately 14% of the population, and can be identified by its course posterior to the main portal vein (arrow). The more typical location of the hepatic artery is anterior to the portal vein. IVC; inferior vena cava; AO, aorta; PV, main portal vein.*

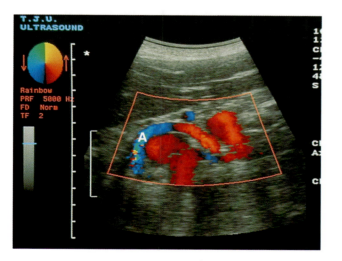

Figure 4.22 *Longitudinal image obtained to the left of the abdominal aorta with a tortuous unidentified artery (A) visualized. CFI allows rapid detection of flow in unsuspected vascular structures such as this, and may aid in determining their relationship to adjacent organs or vessels. Spectral Doppler analysis may be necessary to characterize flow in these structures more accurately.*

the Valsalva maneuver can often result in improvement in CFI visualization of flow in these portions of the IVC. Visualization of flow in the IVC is best demonstrated after the release of the Valsalva maneuver, when there is increased flow of blood back to the patient's chest with a reduction in intrathoracic pressure (Fig. 4.24). Another beneficial technique which can also improve CFI visualization of flow in the IVC requires elevation of the lower extremities, with or without manual compression of the muscles in the leg, which typically produces an augmentation of flow from the lower extremities.

Gray scale ultrasound is often used to identify the location of IVC filters including documenting their proper position inferior to the renal veins. Using CFI it is possible to demonstrate both the functional lumen and filling defects due to intralumenal thrombus. Extension of tumor thrombus into the IVC via the renal or hepatic veins can also be seen (Figs 4.25 and 4.26). Bloodflow in the hepatic veins is typically well visualized using CFI (Fig. 4.27). When not readily detected, however, hepatic vein flow can be elicited by using the Valsalva maneuver as mentioned above. Bloodflow in the renal veins can be detected

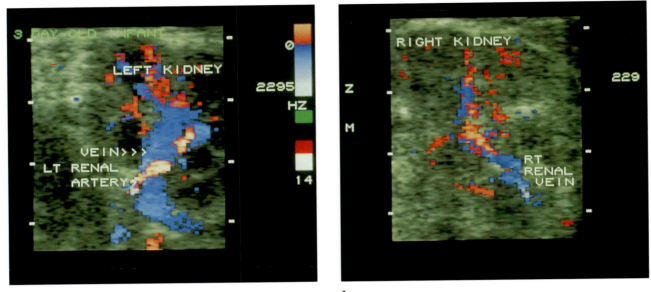

a

b

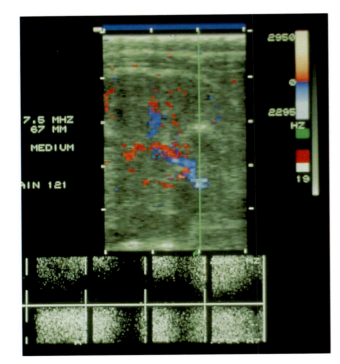

c

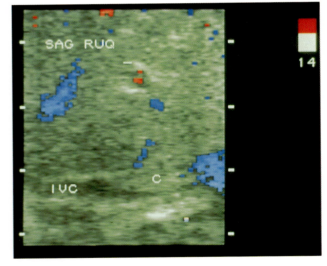

d

Figure 4.26 *Transverse CFI image (a) demonstrates normal flow through the left renal vein of a newborn. CFI of the right kidney (b) demonstrated a relative decrease in renal vein lumen diameter with spectral Doppler findings (c) of increased flow velocity (note aliasing) and a lack of normal phasicity. These combined findings are consistent with renal vein thrombosis which resulted from dehydration. CFI (d) of the IVC detects extension of the echogenic clot (c) into the IVC. Ultrasound with CFI was used in this case to serially monitor the resolution of the thrombosis in this infant. A 6-month follow-up examination (not shown) detected atrophy of this infant's right kidney.*

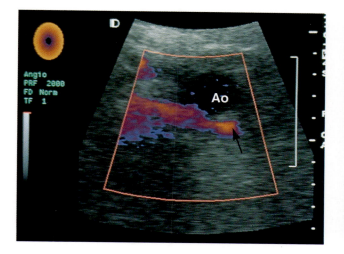

Figure 4.20 *Transverse color amplitude image of the aorta (Ao) obtained in diastole in a patient with a known retro-aortic left renal vein (arrow), a normal anatomic variant.*

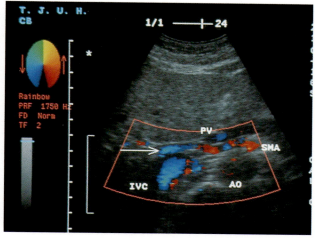

Figure 4.21 *Transverse CFI of the origin of a replaced right hepatic artery arising from the superior mesenteric artery (SMA). This anatomic variant is seen in approximately 14% of the population, and can be identified by its course posterior to the main portal vein (arrow). The more typical location of the hepatic artery is anterior to the portal vein. IVC; inferior vena cava; AO, aorta; PV, main portal vein.*

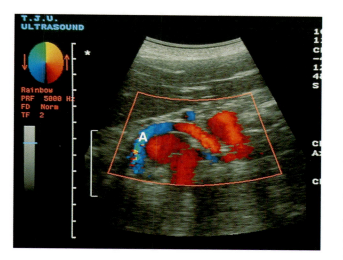

Figure 4.22 *Longitudinal image obtained to the left of the abdominal aorta with a tortuous unidentified artery (A) visualized. CFI allows rapid detection of flow in unsuspected vascular structures such as this, and may aid in determining their relationship to adjacent organs or vessels. Spectral Doppler analysis may be necessary to characterize flow in these structures more accurately.*

the Valsalva maneuver can often result in improvement in CFI visualization of flow in these portions of the IVC. Visualization of flow in the IVC is best demonstrated after the release of the Valsalva maneuver, when there is increased flow of blood back to the patient's chest with a reduction in intrathoracic pressure (Fig. 4.24). Another beneficial technique which can also improve CFI visualization of flow in the IVC requires elevation of the lower extremities, with or without manual compression of the muscles in the leg, which typically produces an augmentation of flow from the lower extremities.

Gray scale ultrasound is often used to identify the location of IVC filters including documenting their proper position inferior to the renal veins. Using CFI it is possible to demonstrate both the functional lumen and filling defects due to intralumenal thrombus. Extension of tumor thrombus into the IVC via the renal or hepatic veins can also be seen (Figs 4.25 and 4.26). Bloodflow in the hepatic veins is typically well visualized using CFI (Fig. 4.27). When not readily detected, however, hepatic vein flow can be elicited by using the Valsalva maneuver as mentioned above. Bloodflow in the renal veins can be detected

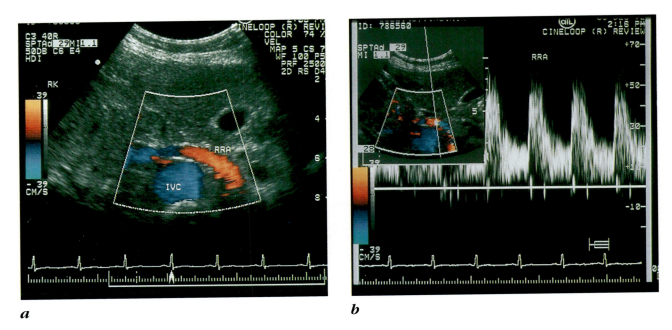

a

b

Figure 4.23 *Another normal anatomical variation is seen in this transverse color flow image (a) of the right renal artery (RRA) anterior to the inferior vena cava (IVC). Spectral analysis of this vessel (b) demonstrates a typical renal artery wave form with forward flow throughout the cardiac cycle.*

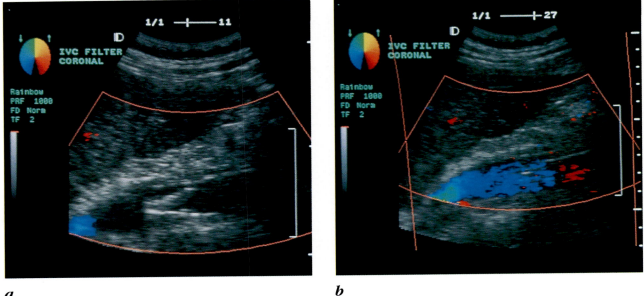

a

b

Figure 4.24 *Longitudinal CFI of the inferior vena cava (IVC) with a Greenfield filter obtained (a) during and (b) after Valsalva. During Valsalva, bloodflow to the chest is reduced and the IVC distends, allowing for better gray scale visualization of the presence and location of the filter device, while blood flow through the IVC and filter is better demonstrated after exhalation. When evaluating flow in the veins of the abdomen it is important to consider the effects of the breathing instructions given to the patient, and to use them advantageously to evaluate both anatomic structure and physiologic events.*

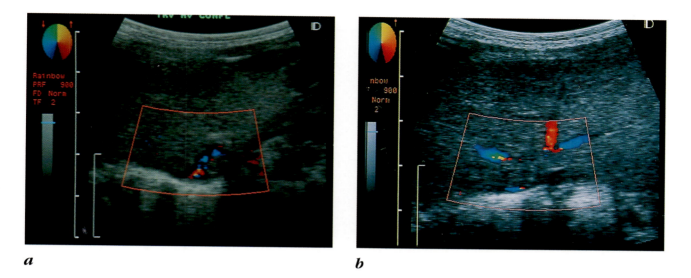

a   *b*

Figure 4.25 *Transverse CFI (a) of a non-occlusive IVC thrombus (arrow) at the hepatic vein confluence in a premature infant. This thrombus was incidentally detected during a routine echocardiographic examination. A color flow image obtained slightly inferior to the hepatic vein confluence (b) demonstrates patency of the hepatic veins with mild reflux (in red) noted in one, a normal finding.*

with CFI by insonating the vessels from either a coronal or axial scan plane angled from the patient's flank toward the IVC on the right to identify flow in the shorter right renal vein, or in a transverse plane using an anterior approach where the longer left renal vein can usually be visualized crossing anterior to the aorta and posterior to the superior mesenteric artery. The location of the left renal vein can also be used as a landmark to help identify the location of the origin and proximal portion of the left renal artery. Other IVC branches are more difficult to image, although with changes in patient position and transducer compression in the lower abdomen and pelvis it is often possible to visualize portions of the right and left iliac veins. Normal anatomic variants of the IVC or its branches can often be more easily identified and better delineated with the help of CFI.

HEPATIC APPLICATIONS

The portal venous system, including the intra- and extrahepatic circulations, is one of the abdominal regions most commonly evaluated with CFI. The effects of portal hypertension include reversed (hepatofugal) portal vein flow, the formation of portosystemic varices and collateral vessels, and portal vein thrombosis—all of which can be diagnosed using CFI. Often the first imaging study requested in patients suspected of having portal hypertension is an ultrasound examination to determine the liver and spleen size, and to evaluate the hemodynamics of the portal venous system. In this capacity the qualitative nature of CFI is usually not a limiting factor, because only the presence and direction of flow is necessary. However, for documentation purposes or to better characterize portal blood-flow, Doppler spectral analysis will often be included in the examination. In patients with known portal hypertension, serial ultrasounds with CFI can help monitor their condition and assist in clinical management decisions.

The primary tributaries of the main portal vein include the splenic and superior mesenteric veins. Bloodflow in the splenic vein can usually be detected from its exit from the spleen in a coronal or axial scan of the left upper quadrant, and again as it courses posterior to the pancreas using an anterior approach in a transverse plane (Fig. 4.28a and b). The portal vein confluence of the superior mesenteric vein and splenic vein is usually visualized as a region of focal enlargement posterior to the pancreatic neck.

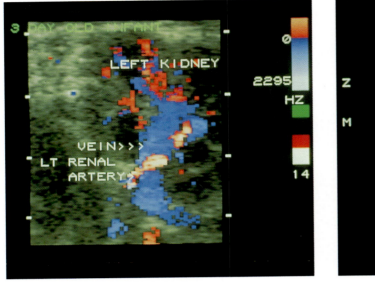

a

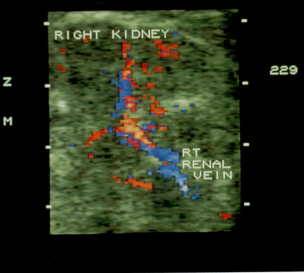

b

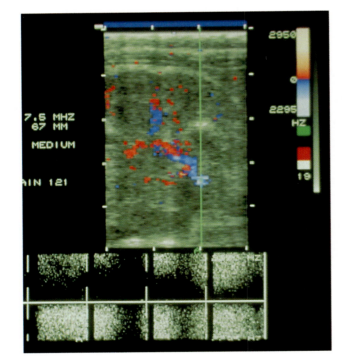

c

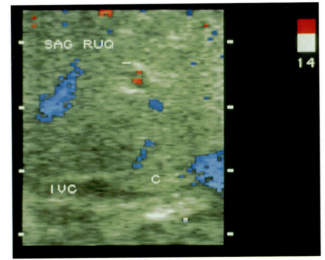

d

Figure 4.26 *Transverse CFI image (a) demonstrates normal flow through the left renal vein of a newborn. CFI of the right kidney (b) demonstrated a relative decrease in renal vein lumen diameter with spectral Doppler findings (c) of increased flow velocity (note aliasing) and a lack of normal phasicity. These combined findings are consistent with renal vein thrombosis which resulted from dehydration. CFI (d) of the IVC detects extension of the echogenic clot (c) into the IVC. Ultrasound with CFI was used in this case to serially monitor the resolution of the thrombosis in this infant. A 6-month follow-up examination (not shown) detected atrophy of this infant's right kidney.*

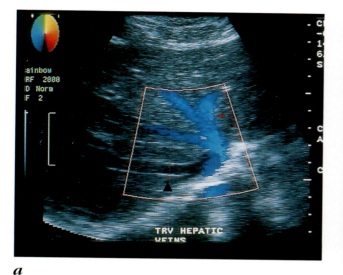

a

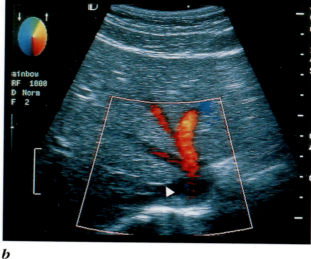

b

c

Figure 4.27 *Transverse color flow images of the hepatic vein confluence obtained during right atrial diastole (a) and systole (b). Note the normal reflux of blood (displayed in red) into the hepatic veins during atrial systole. The lack of flow in the right hepatic vein (arrow head) is a result of the poor Doppler angle. Spectral Doppler (c) can be used to demonstrate these temporal changes of flow. The arrow indicates the normal reversed flow component seen with CFI in (b).*

Using the confluence as a landmark, the superior mesenteric vein can be visualized by imaging in a sagittal plane and directing the CFI beam inferiorly to acquire a sufficient Doppler angle to flow (Fig. 4.28c). The extrahepatic main portal vein is best identified by positioning the transducer to obtain an oblique plane from the patient's left hip to right shoulder (Fig. 4.29). By again using a variety of probe maneuvers to acquire an adequate Doppler angle, flow can usually be detected from this segment of the portal vein. Care must be taken by the investigator to acquire unambiguous CFI information on the direction of flow throughout the portal system. At times indirect indications of flow direction, such as the direction of flow in vessel branches, may reduce the likelihood of an incorrect diagnosis.

Partial or complete thrombosis of the portal system may result from a variety of causes, including sepsis,

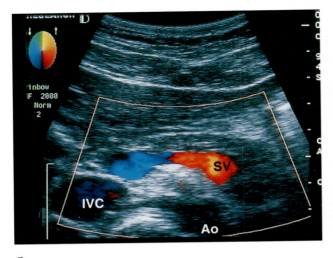

a

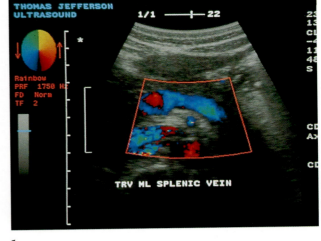

b

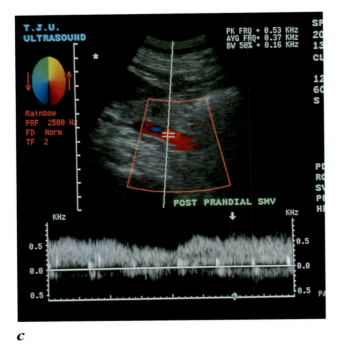

c

Figure 4.28 *The CFI examination of the portal venous system often begins with the evaluation of the two major vessels delivering blood to the liver; the splenic vein (SV) and superior mesenteric vein (SMV)—to document the presence and direction of flow. A transverse color flow image of a normal splenic vein (a) demonstrates flow directed toward the main portal vein (hepatopedal), color coded red where flow is directed toward the transducer, and blue as it courses into the portal vein confluence. (Ao, aorta; IVC, inferior vena cava.) A similar image (b) in a patient with portal hypertension indicates flow directed toward the spleen (hepatofugal). The reversed flow in the splenic vein is an indirect indication of the presence of portosystemic collaterals, the location of which should be determined during the CFI examination. The SMV is best identified in a sagittal projection (c) deep to the pancreas (P) using the portal vein confluence as an anatomic landmark. The degree of flow through the SMV will be reduced if a patient has been fasting for a long period of time, making detection of flow in the SMV more difficult. Postprandially, however, flow is usually not difficult to detect in the SMV, with a spectral Doppler waveform demonstrating normal mild temporal variations of flow.*

pancreatitis and venous stasis. Thrombosis may involve a small segment of the portal vein, an individual branch vessel, or, less commonly, the entire portal system (Fig. 4.30). Additionally, tumor invasion of the portal or hepatic veins occurs in as many as one-third of patients diagnosed with primary hepatic malignancies, and these tumors may obstruct flow in the hepatic vasculature (Fig. 4.31). In cases of venous invasion by hepatic malignancies, spectral Doppler signals obtained from areas with flow identified with CFI may demonstrate arterial flow resulting from tumor neovascularity. Using proper technique

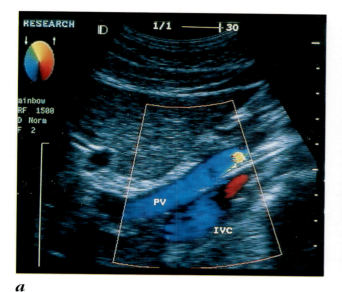

Figure 4.29 *In this patient an oblique color flow image (a) displays blood flow in the main portal vein (PV) in blue because of its flow direction away from the transducer (IVC; inferior vena cava). Pulsed Doppler spectral analysis of this vessel (b) demonstrates the normal mild variations of flow. In a patient with severe tricuspid valve regurgitation (c), pulsed Doppler of the portal vein demonstrates a biphasic spectral signal as a result of increased resistance to flow into the liver.*

and parameter adjustments, portal vein thrombosis can be detected with CFI (Figs 4.32 and 4.33). Complete thrombosis will be suggested by the total absence of flow in a portal vein segment, whereas partial thrombosis is typically identified with CFI as a reduction in the size of the portal vein's functional lumen by a filling defect representing intraluminal thrombus which, in the acute stage, may be anechoic on gray scale imaging. In the chronic stage, recanalized flow through thrombosed portal veins presents, on CFI, as small channels of flow through typically echogenic clot. In cases of main portal vein occlu-

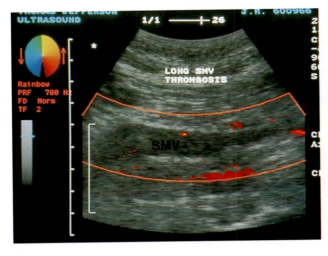

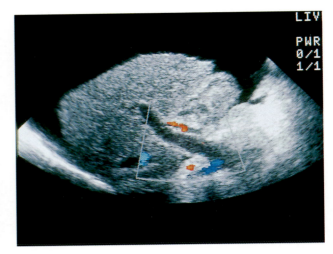

a

b

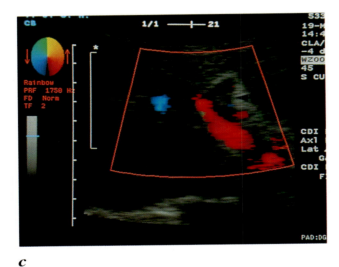

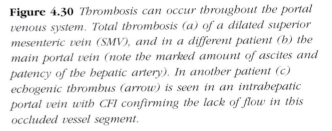

Figure 4.30 *Thrombosis can occur throughout the portal venous system. Total thrombosis (a) of a dilated superior mesenteric vein (SMV), and in a different patient (b) the main portal vein (note the marked amount of ascites and patency of the hepatic artery). In another patient (c) echogenic thrombus (arrow) is seen in an intrahepatic portal vein with CFI confirming the lack of flow in this occluded vessel segment.*

c

sion, small portal venulae (venea comitantes) may dilate, resulting in cavernous transformation of the portal vein (Fig. 4.34). This is most often evident in the region of the porta hepatis.

Within the liver the main portal vein branches into right and left portal veins which, in turn, branch into anterior and posterior right and medial and lateral left portal veins. The vessels within the liver are important identifiable landmarks used to demarcate the segmental anatomy of the liver. The direction of flow in the intrahepatic portal veins can be compared to the direction of flow in the adjacent hepatic arteries (Fig. 4.35). Normally, flow in the two vessels should be in the same direction (hepatopedal). However, in cases of hepatofugal flow the two vessels will have flow in opposite directions (Fig. 4.36). This can be demonstrated either with CFI alone or by obtaining a spectral Doppler tracing by using a large (10 mm) sample volume positioned so as to acquire flow information simultaneously from the two vessels. The

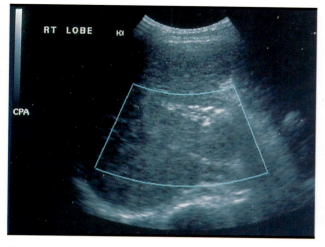

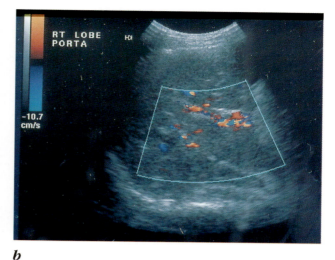

a

b

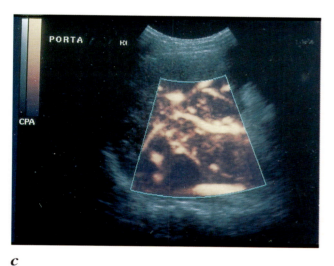

c

Figure 4.31 *Primary hepatic malignancies may infiltrate vessels within the liver. Here a patient with a poorly defined mass in the right lobe of the liver is found with gray scale imaging (a) to have echogenic material presumed to be thrombus within the right and main portal veins. CFI (b) detected scattered flow signals within the portal veins. While this may represent recanalized flow through the thrombus, pulsed spectral Doppler guided by the CFI signals (not shown) demonstrated an arterial waveform. This is an example of hepatocellular carcinoma (HCC) with tumor invasion into the portal venous system. CAI (c) better demonstrated the increased vascularity in the region of the porta hepatis and continuity of small arterial branches coursing from the hepatic artery into the tumor thrombus. In this case CFI facilitated a correct diagnosis by demonstrating vessels within what was initially thought to be benign thrombus in the portal vein, thereby identifying the presence of an infiltrative neoplasm (i.e. HCC).*

latter technique can be a useful method to document, via hard copy format, hepatofugal flow when present.

The presence of portal venous varices and collaterals can be demonstrated using CFI (Figs 4.34, 4.37–4.39). The most common locations include the splenic hilum, porta hepatis, and around the stomach and gastroesophageal junction. Reversed portal vein flow due to increased intrahepatic pressure can also result in patent paraumbilical veins (Fig. 4.37). When hepatopedal flow is detected in the main and left portal veins, but hepatofugal flow is found in the right portal vein, a patent paraumbilical vein should be suspected. In these instances the hepatopedal flow in the main portal vein is directed out of the liver by way of the dilated paraumbilical veins that often anastomose with systemic pelvic veins, forming portosystemic collaterals. In patients with portal hypertension, flow reversals may be total or partial and can change even during the course of a single

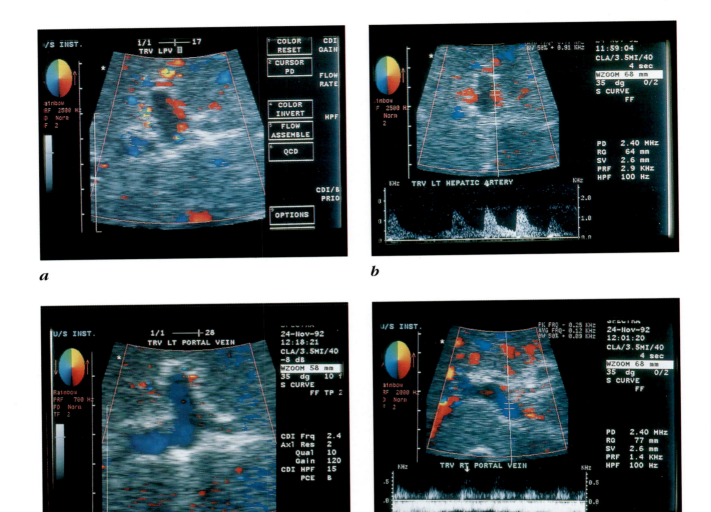

Figure 4.32 *CFI is commonly used to establish the presence and direction of flow within the portal venous system in patients suspected of having portal hypertension. However, the color flow system parameters will directly influence the lowest detectable flow velocities. In this transverse color flow image (a) of the umbilical portion of the left portal vein using a pulse repetition frequency (PRF) of 2500 Hz, the absence of flow in the vein is suggested while flow is identified in the adjacent hepatic artery. A pulsed Doppler spectral waveform (b) confirms the arterial nature of flow from the left hepatic artery. With a color PRF of 700 Hz, however, (c) flow directed away from the transducer (i.e. out of the liver) is detected in this portal vein segment. A Doppler waveform obtained from the right portal vein (d) confirms hepatofugal flow and provides an indirect indication of the presence of portosystemic collateral vessels.*

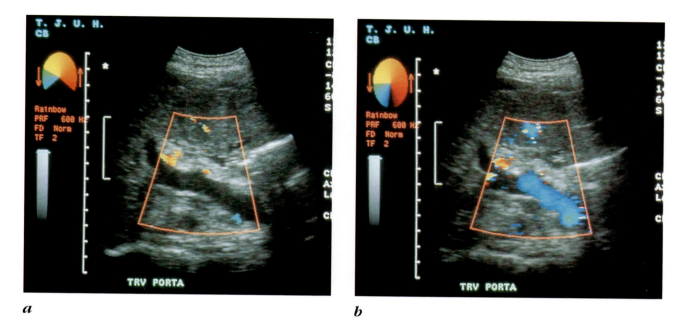

Figure 4.33 *In addition to a low pulse repetition frequency (PRF), a low color wall filter should be used to detect the low-velocity flow often encountered in cases of PHT. In this example using a 100 Hz wall filter (a), CFI indicates no flow in the portal vein; however, by reducing the wall filter to 25 Hz (b), hepatofugal flow is visualized. The presence and direction of flow in the portal system is important for clinical management when considering surgical intervention in patients with PHT. The wall filter level is indicated by the black wedge on the color wheel.*

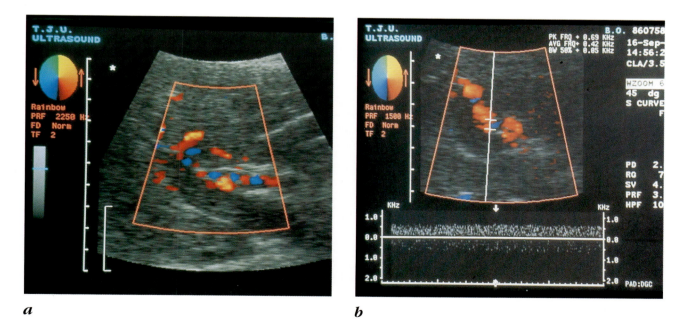

Figure 4.34 *In this magnified color flow image of the porta hepatis (a), flow in the portal vein is not seen. Instead, multiple small vessels surround an echogenic area. This finding is typical of cavernous transformation of the portal vein, the result of portal vein thrombosis and dilatation of small periportal veins (venea comitans). The portal vein is occluded with echogenic thrombus suggestive of a chronic process. Pulsed Doppler spectral analysis (b) provides confirmation of venous flow in these vessels.*

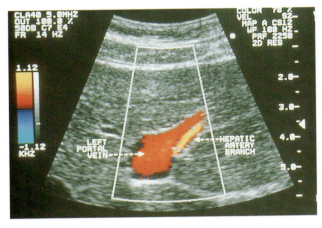

a

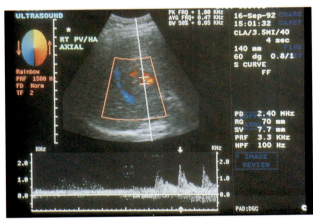

c

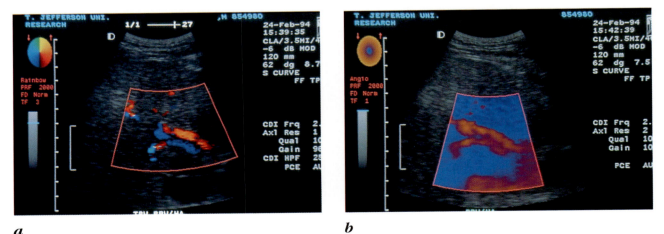

b

Figure 4.35 *The flow direction in an intrahepatic portal vein can be quickly determined by comparing it to the direction of flow in the adjacent hepatic artery branch. Normally, flow in the portal vein should be in the same direction as in the hepatic artery. CFI is an ideal method of demonstrating normal (hepatopedal) flow within the left (a) and right (b) portal veins and hepatic arteries in different patients. A pulsed Doppler spectral display acquired with a large sample volume (c) can also be used to demonstrate this, and provides a good means of documenting the direction of flow in the intrahepatic portal system.*

a   *b*

Figure 4.36 *Conventional color (a) and color amplitude (b) images of the portal vein and hepatic artery in a patient with hepatofugal portal vein flow. Using the conventional CFI mode, the reversed flow in the portal vein is readily apparent when compared to the flow direction in the adjacent hepatic artery. However, owing to its non-directional nature, CAI cannot provide information on flow direction. This example demonstrates why CAI is not well suited for examinations requiring flow-directional information.*

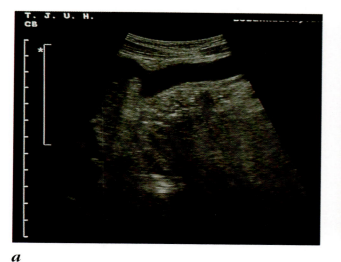

a

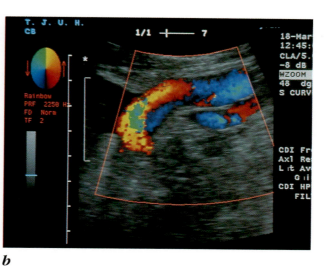

b

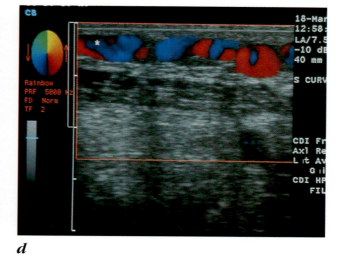

c

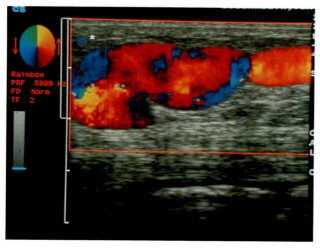

d

e

Figure 4.37 *A sagittal gray scale image (a) of the inferior tip of the left lobe of the liver in a patient with known PHT demonstrates a tubular structure extending from the left lobe towards the anterior abdominal wall. CFI (b) detected flow within this structure with flow directed out of the liver—findings consistent with a patent paraumbilical vein. CFI facilitates mapping of the course of this vessel, which continued inferiorly (c) toward the umbilicus. Using a higher frequency transducer to image the subcutaneous tissues adjacent to the umbilicus demonstrated a typical color flow pattern of varices (d and e). These vessels continued into the patient's left lower quadrant, presumably collateralizing with systemic veins of the pelvis.*

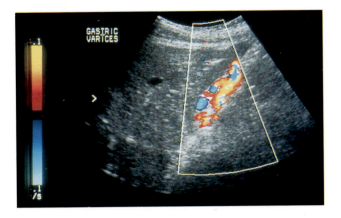

Figure 4.38 *CFI of gastric varices in a patient with known PHT. CFI facilitates detection of flow in these unsuspected abnormal vessels.*

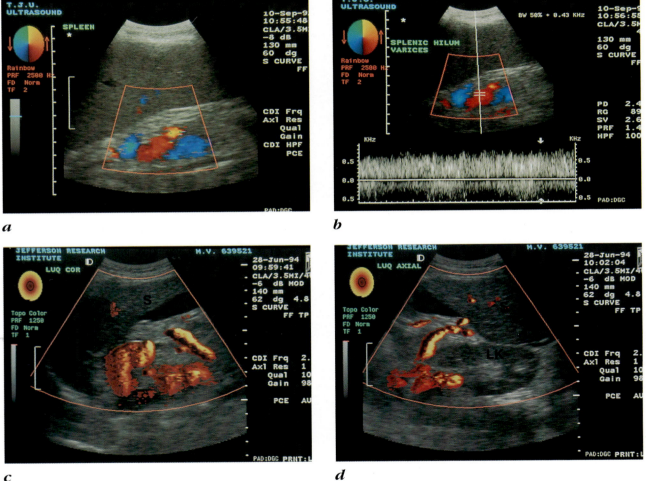

a

b

c

d

Figure 4.39 *Coronal color flow image of the spleen (a) demonstrating multiple vessels within the splenic hilum in a patient with known cirrhosis consistent with the diagnosis of splenic vein varices. Pulsed Doppler spectral analysis (b) better characterizes the venous nature of these vessels. The swirling flow in varices results in flow displayed above and below the spectral baseline. In a different patient with known PHT a coronal color amplitude scan (c) detected multiple varices in the splenic hilum. Further examination of this area (d) identified communication of these portal system varices with the left renal vein. Note the ascites medial to the spleen. LK, left kidney; S, spleen.*

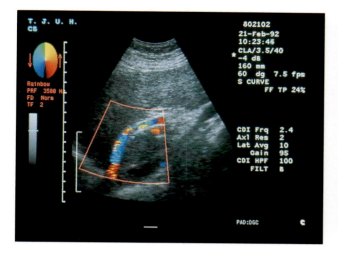

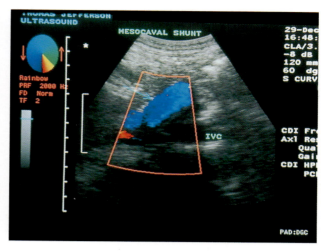

Figure 4.40 *Longitudinal view of the liver shows an angiographically placed transjugular intrahepatic portosystemic shunt (TIPS) connecting the portal vein (red) with the hepatic vein. This shunt diverts flow from the portal circulation into the systemic circulation via the hepatic vein. The echogenic walls of the metallic stent are well visualized. CFI can reliably demonstrate flow through TIPS, non-invasively confirming shunt patency.*

Figure 4.41 *Longitudinal view of a surgically placed mesocaval shunt (arrow) diverting blood from the mesenteric vein to the inferior vena cava (IVC) in a patient with PHT. CFI facilitates detection of flow through surgically created portosystemic shunts, which are often difficult to visualize with gray scale imaging alone.*

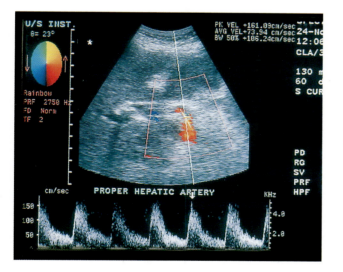

Figure 4.42 *CFI is used to locate the proximal portion of the hepatic artery allowing for quantitative Doppler spectral analysis, which demonstrates a normal waveform from this vessel.*

day due to variations in pressure within the portal system.

CFI can be a useful addition to the gray scale and pulsed spectral Doppler evaluation of portosystemic shunts (Figs 4.40 and 4.41). A recently developed angiographic technique used to relieve portal pressure in patients with portal hypertension is to place, via a jugular vein access site, a vascular stent between the portal venous and hepatic venous systems within the liver. This procedure is known as a transjugular intrahepatic porto-systemic shunt (TIPS). CFI can be used to document patency of TIPS shunts and determine if there is a narrowing of the functional lumen. CFI can also determine the direction of flow through the TIPS; however, because of the depth of the shunt it is often necessary to utilize a low CFI pulse repetition frequency, which may result in aliasing of the color flow signal. In these cases a spectral Doppler signal may be necessary to accurately determine bloodflow direction through the TIPS. Other portosystemic shunts, either developing spontaneously or surgically created, can usually be evaluated more thoroughly and with less technical difficulty by using CFI rather than by gray scale

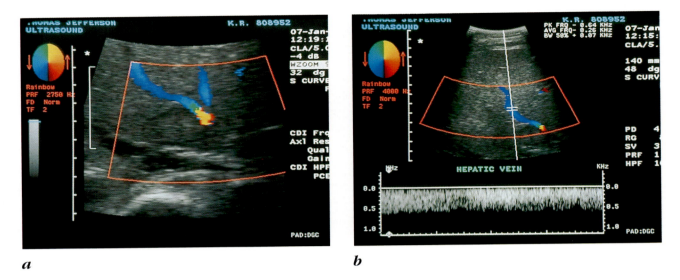

a   *b*

Figure 4.43 *A magnified transverse view of the middle hepatic vein (a) in a patient with liver metastases. A focal lesion is causing a mechanical obstruction of flow through the hepatic vein. Note the color aliasing at the site of luminal narrowing. A pulsed Doppler spectral display (b) of flow proximal to the level of obstruction demonstrates a lack of normal pulsatility in the hepatic vein consistent with partial obstruction of flow through this vessel.*

ultrasound with spectral Doppler analysis alone. The most common is a Warren or splenorenal shunt (between the splenic vein and left renal vein), or between the mesenteric vein and IVC (mesocaval shunt). In both of these two types of shunts, their variable location deep within the abdomen and presence of overlying bowel can present problems in ultrasonic imaging. However, several reports indicate that the ability to adequately evaluate flow in these shunts is improved with the use of CFI. When the actual shunt is not well visualized, information obtained with CFI, such as the direction of flow in the portal vein or its branches, can provide useful indirect information on the likelihood of a shunt's patency. Hepatofugal main portal vein flow in a patient with a mesocaval shunt, for example, indicates probable shunt patency due to the portal flow taking the path of least resistance through the shunt.

The common hepatic artery normally arises from the celiac trunk and courses laterally to the right to divide into the gastroduodenal artery and the proper hepatic artery (Fig. 4.42). The gastroduodenal artery courses over the pancreatic head to divide rapidly into multiple smaller branches which are variable in course and number and supply the proximal portion of the pancreas and duodenum. The proper hepatic artery can usually be identified in its normal position just anterior and medial to the main portal vein. Bloodflow in the intrahepatic hepatic artery branches can be detected within the right and left lobes of the liver adjacent to the larger portal veins. At times it may be difficult to identify the more peripherally located intrahepatic arteries. This is particularly true in obese patients when there is significant attenuation of signal, or in liver transplant recipients in the acute stage with limited acoustic access due to surgical dressings. One approach which may be helpful is to examine the region immediately adjacent to the portal triads with a low CFI pulse repetition frequency and high color priority and gain settings. A large pulsed Doppler sample volume placed over to the portal triads may also prove useful in detecting and characterizing flow in the adjacent hepatic artery. A normal waveform obtained from a hepatic artery has forward flow throughout diastole, with a reduction or loss of diastolic flow indicating increased peripheral resistance.

Bloodflow at the level of the confluence of the hepatic veins with the IVC is usually not difficult to

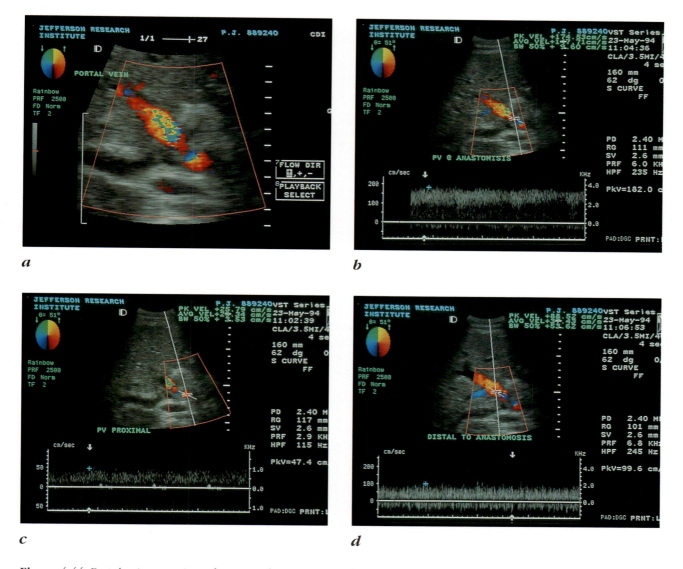

Figure 4.44 *Portal vein stenosis at the surgical anastomosis of a patient with a transplanted liver. CFI (a) demonstrates a focal narrowing of the functional lumen and guides for sample volume placement to obtain flow velocities from the stenotic segment (b) of 182 cm/s. Spectral Doppler of the proximal (c) and distal (d) segments estimated the velocities to be 47 cm/s and 100 cm/s respectively. Turbulence (identified as flow above and below the baseline) is detected from the distal segment and supports a diagnosis of a hemodynamically significant stenosis.*

detect with CFI (see Fig. 4.27). The spectral Doppler waveforms obtained from the hepatic veins at this location typically have a high level of pulsatility as a result of their close proximity to the right heart. During right atrial diastole, bloodflows from the hepatic veins and IVC towards the heart, whereas during right atrial systole it is normal to have some reflux of blood back into the IVC and hepatic veins. Hepatic vein dilatation and increased reflux of flow may result from congestive heart failure, among other cardiac causes. These events can be depicted using a CFI system with an adequately high level of temporal

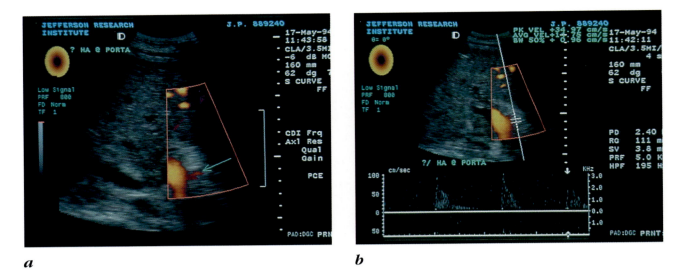

Figure 4.45 *In this patient who recently received a liver transplant, flow in the hepatic artery was not detected using conventional (mean Doppler frequency shift) CFI. However, flow in the hepatic artery was detected using CAI (a), which then enabled confirmation of the arterial signal (b) with spectral Doppler analysis. (Note the lack of flow in diastole—a non-specific finding.) The high temporal averaging and color persistence of the amplitude mode may be beneficial when evaluating flow in highly pulsatile vessels. Displaying flow for a longer period of time allows the operator to identify the location of the origin of flow signals and guide for more definitive spectral analysis.*

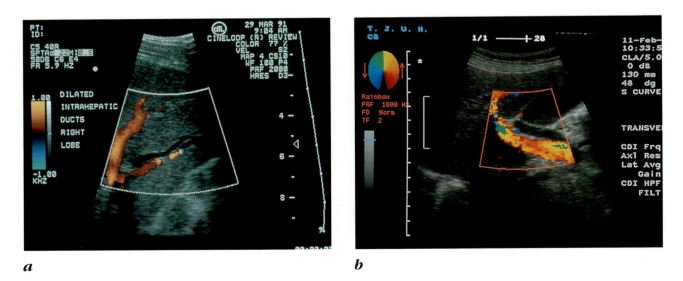

Figure 4.46 *CFI can help differentiate vascular structures from those of non-vascular origins. Here, the intrahepatic portal veins are shown in color (a) with the adjacent bile ducts displayed without flow. In a different patient (b) the tubular structure adjacent to the portal vein represents a dilated common bile duct posterior to the gallbladder which contains sludge.*

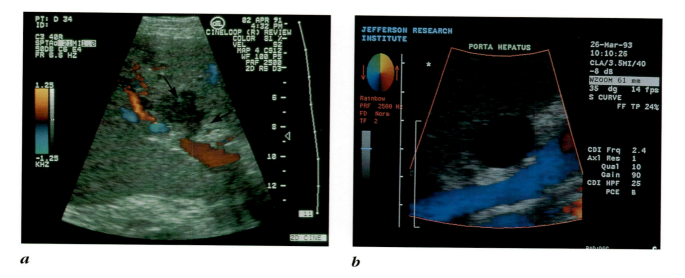

Figure 4.47 *A complex area within the liver (arrows) following blunt abdominal trauma is shown by CFI to contain no flow (a). This was later determined to represent an area of intrahepatic hemorrhage. In a patient with a recent liver transplant (b) CFI demonstrates good flow through the portal vein anastomosis but no flow in an adjacent fluid collection.*

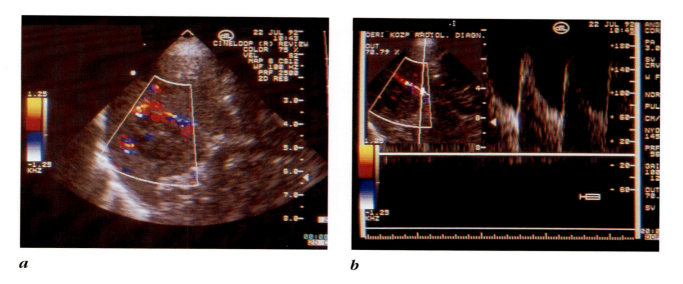

Figure 4.48 *CFI of a hepatocellular carcinoma (a) detects increased vascularity at the tumor periphery with angle-corrected pulsed Doppler spectral analysis (b) demonstrating the increased velocity (i.e. systolic velocity >150 cm/s) and low pulsatility of flow in these tumor vessels. Courtesy of Z. Harkanyi.*

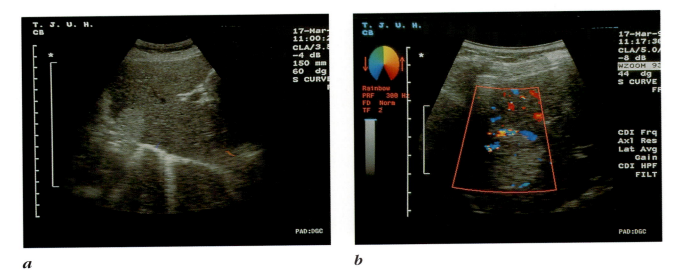

a   b

Figure 4.49 *Longitudinal view of the right lobe of the liver (a) demonstrates a well-circumscribed, uniformly echogenic mass near the dome of the diaphragm highly suggestive of a hemangioma. CFI of this region (b) shows flow within the normal parenchyma of the liver and around the edge of the mass but no flow within the mass. While not pathognomonic, the lack of flow is probably due to the very slow flow of blood within hemangiomas.*

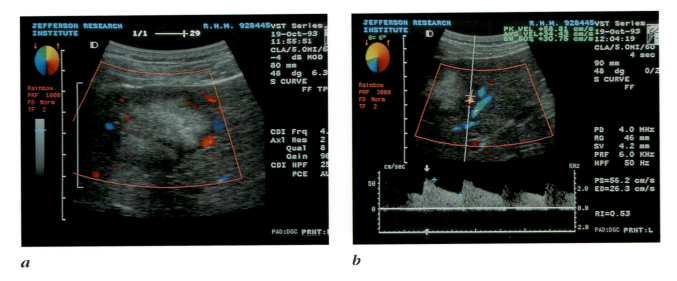

a   b

Figure 4.50 *Transverse CFI of a large liver metastasis (a) in a patient with known gastric cancer. A spectral Doppler waveform obtained from the tumor periphery (b) detects an elevated peak velocity and increased diastolic flow yielding a low resistive index (RI) of 0.53 consistent with tumor-feeding vessels.*

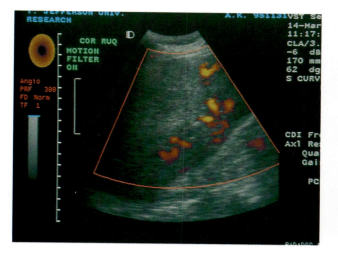

Figure 4.51 *A longitudinal color amplitude image of a liver metastasis in a patient with a history of colorectal cancer and chemotherapy over the course of 1 year. The relative hypovascularity of the tumor is well demonstrated using this color flow mode, which detects flow in the normal liver parenchyma around the tumor.*

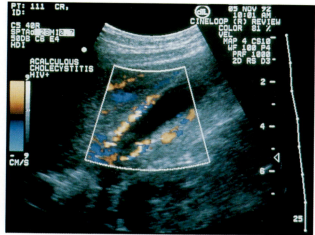

Figure 4.52 *This patient presented with gallstones and acute right upper quadrant pain. Murphy's sign was positive. A longitudinal color flow image of the gallbladder demonstrates increased vascularity. It is normal to see some flow in the anterior division of the cystic artery in the proximal quarter to third of the gallbladder, but flow more distally and on the posterior wall usually indicates the presence of inflammatory hyperemia due to acute cholecystitis. Inflammatory hyperemia may be absent very early or very late in the course of acute cholecystitis and is absent in chronic cholecystitis unless there is superimposed acute cholecystitis. Courtesy of T. Stavros.*

resolution. The lack of bloodflow in the hepatic veins on CFI indicates complete thrombosis of one or more of the hepatic veins or Budd–Chiari syndrome (Fig. 4.43). Thrombosis of the hepatic veins may be complete or partial and involve one or more of the veins and IVC. Flow in previously thrombosed but recanalized hepatic veins can be detected using CFI. Chronic processes may lead to the development of fibrous webs which may or may not significantly obstruct flow from the liver.

The liver transplant recipient is also a candidate for CFI evaluation, both before and after transplantation. Prior to transplantation, documentation of patency of the intra- and extrahepatic vasculature, and determining the presence and location of collateral vessels, is important. Both during and after liver transplantation the integrity of the vascular anasto-

moses, especially of the important hepatic artery, can be accomplished portably in the acute post-transplantation stage using ultrasound with CFI (Figs 4.44 and 4.45). Here again, serial CFI examinations can provide information on the status of the transplanted liver in the least traumatic, and most non-invasive and cost-effective, manner.

Other indications for performing CFI of the liver include identifying non-vascular structures such as dilated bile ducts, diagnosing vascular malformations, and characterizing hepatic lesions and determining their effect on surrounding structures such as compression of normal vessels (Figs 4.34, 4.46 and 4.47). In some cases, flow in hepatic tumor vessels can be detected with CFI. This is particularly true with primary hepatic malignancies (Figs 4.31 and 4.48). Metastatic lesions in the liver tend to have less vascu-

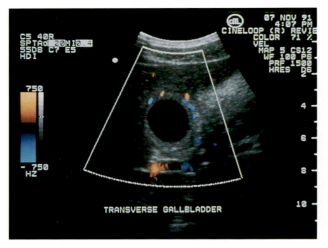

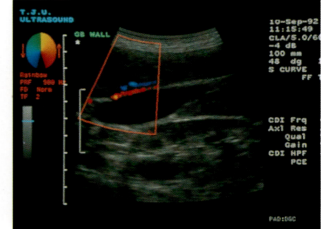

Figure 4.53 *This patient presented with gallstones and acute right upper quadrant pain. A transverse color flow image of the gallbladder detects flow within multiple small branches of the cystic artery in its anterior wall. The CFI detection of flow within multiple small branches usually indicates the presence of inflammatory hyperemia due to acute cholecystitis. Courtesy of T. Stavros.*

Figure 4.54 *CFI of a normal gallbladder. The use of a 5.0-MHz transducer with a 4.0 MHz color Doppler frequency facilitates detection of flow in this normal cystic artery branch.*

larity and the slow flow known to occur in hemangiomas is typically difficult to detect with currently available CFI systems (Figs 4.43, 4.49–4.51). CFI has also been beneficial in detecting increased size and flow of vessels of the gallbladder wall in cases of acute cholecystitis (Figs 4.52 and 4.53). However, the CFI information alone does not constitute a diagnosis of gallbladder disease, as normal gallbladder wall flow may be detected with CFI (Fig. 4.54). Communications may develop between the portal and hepatic venous systems, either congenital or traumatic, as well as communications between a hepatic artery and portal or hepatic vein (arteriovenous malformation) (Fig. 4.55). The use of CFI in conjunction with Doppler spectral analysis for the evaluation of suspected hepatic vascular communications will facilitate more time-efficient and accurate diagnoses.

RENAL APPLICATIONS

In the past few years Doppler ultrasound evaluation of renal bloodflow has increasingly been utilized as a screening device for patients with suspected renovascular hypertension. This is due, in part, to significant improvements in CFI technology and new scanning techniques and protocols used to derive a diagnosis. The demonstration of intrarenal vascularity using CFI is normally not difficult (Fig. 4.56); however, adequate detection of flow in the main renal arteries and veins is heavily dependent on equipment sensitivity, operator experience and the patient's body habitus and cooperation. The performance of an ultrasound examination for suspected renovascular hypertension is labor-intensive and requires the proper equipment and significant operator dedication to reach a satisfactory level of sensitivity. It is not unusual to devote an hour or more using low-frequency (i.e. 2.0 MHz) transducers designed for deep abdominal applications to obtain a diagnosis. The variety of pathologic processes that may result in a renal artery stenosis, such as atherosclerosis or fibromuscular hyperplasia, also add to the complexity of this examination.

There are two ultrasound imaging protocols currently being applied to diagnose renovascular hypertension. The historic approach requires a

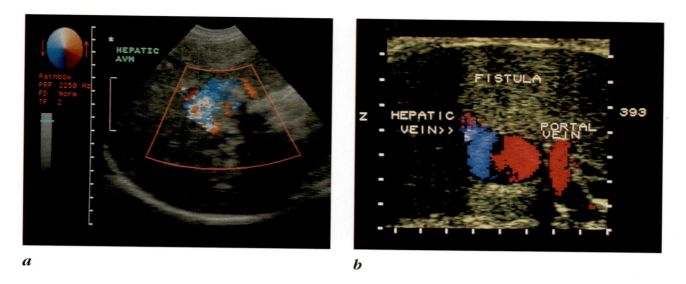

Figure 4.55 *(a) CFI of a congenital arteriovenous malformation (AVM) of the liver. (b) CFI of an iatrogenic portal vein – hepatic vein fistula and pseudoaneurysm which resulted from the inadvertent puncture of the two vessels during an interventional biliary catheterization procedure. The flow within the pseudoaneurysm is color coded red on the right and blue on the left (with red indicating flow towards the transducer) because of the counter-clockwise direction of bloodflow within this vascular abnormality. This finding was incidentally detected in a patient with a liver transplant, and did not require surgical intervention.*

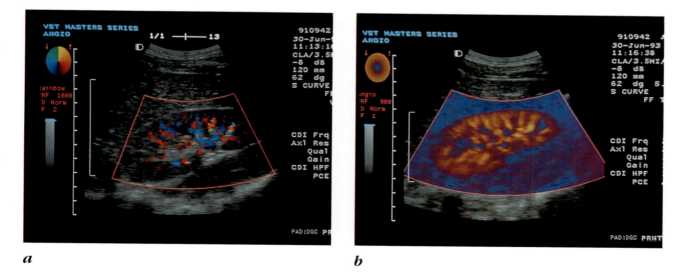

Figure 4.56 *Longitudinal conventional color (a) and color amplitude (b) images of a normal right kidney. The color amplitude mode appears to improve visualization of bloodflow in the renal cortex and may be useful for the detection of regional differences of flow in abdominal and retroperitoneal organs.*

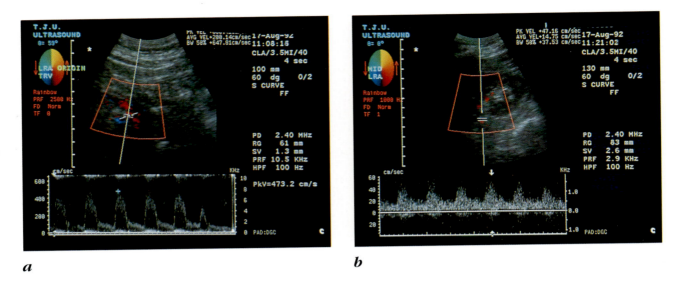

a *b*

Figure 4.57 *CFI can significantly aid in the evaluation of the renal arteries in patients suspected of having renovascular hypertension. Primarily used as a screening device prior to angiography, CFI with pulsed Doppler spectral analysis of the renal arteries can detect stenoses by identifying focal increases in velocities, and downstream flow disturbances. Dilatation of the vessel distal to the stenosis may also be identified. Here (a) a velocity estimate obtained at the origin of the left renal artery detects a flow velocity of 473 cm/s, which was more than four times the velocity of the aorta at this level (not shown). Using a left-flank approach of the middle to distal portion of the renal artery (b), flow disturbances are identified with Doppler spectral analysis. These combined findings suggest a hemodynamically significant stenosis. A subsequent X-ray angiogram confirmed an 80% stenosis in this location. Following balloon angioplasty the patient's blood pressure dramatically decreased to within the normal range. Ultrasound with CFI can also be used to non-invasively monitor for re-stenosis following surgical reconstruction or therapeutic angiographic procedures.*

thorough CFI evaluation of the entire main renal artery on each side (Fig. 4.57). CFI is then used to guide for sample volume placement to perform Doppler spectral analysis and determine the peak systolic velocities from selected segments of the renal arteries. This information is then compared to the peak systolic velocity of the aorta at the level of the renal artery origins. A ratio of the peak systolic velocity detected in the renal vessel over the peak systolic velocity in the aorta of greater than or equal to 3.5 indicates a stenosis of greater than 60% on the affected side. Other indirect indications of a stenosis, such as the presence of flow disturbances or vessel dilatation downstream from a suspected area of stenosis, also raise the likelihood of the presence of a hemodynamically significant lesion. This technique sounds much simpler than it actually is when

practiced in the clinical setting, for it is fraught with pitfalls and technical limitations, some of which have been discussed. Other limiting factors include the inability to adequately visualize the complete course of each of the renal arteries or to detect duplicate or accessory renal arteries. Identification of the presence and location of accessory renal vessels and, more importantly, stenoses which may be present within these typically smaller vessels is facilitated by the use of CFI (Fig. 4.58). The benefit of this technique in diagnosing renal artery stenosis is in its ability to identify the exact site of functional lumen narrowing.

The second more recently developed protocol used to diagnose renovascular hypertension with CFI involves the evaluation of flow in the segmental renal arteries of each kidney. In this case CFI-guided spectral Doppler waveforms are obtained from the

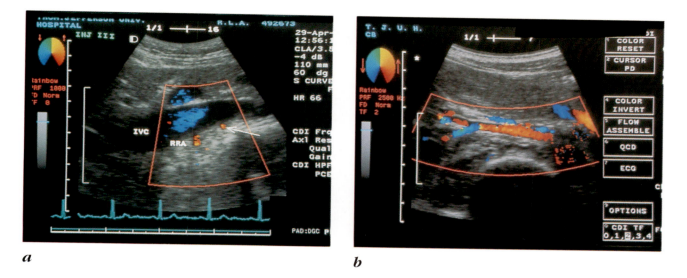

Figure 4.58 *Significant anatomic variations occur in the blood vessels supplying the kidneys, and CFI can facilitate the identification of these normal variations when present. On this longitudinal image (a) of the inferior vena cava (IVC) the main right renal artery (RRA) is seen with an accessory renal artery identified inferiorly (arrow). In a different patient (b) a transverse color flow image identifies branching of the main right renal artery proximal to the renal hilum.*

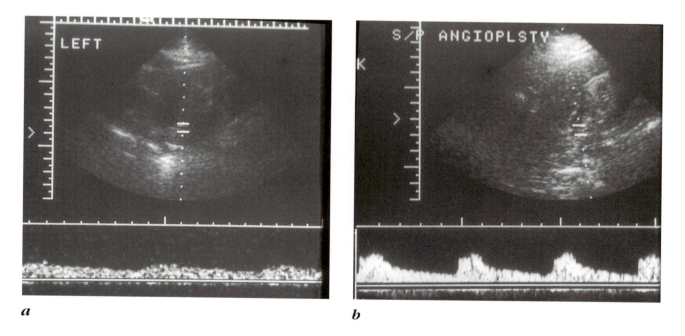

Figure 4.59 *Pulsed Doppler spectral waveforms obtained from the left renal artery at the hilum before (a) and after (b) percutaneous transluminal angioplasty for left renal artery stenosis. Note the reduced velocity, increased systolic rise time, and loss of the early systolic compliance peak on the pre-angioplasty waveform compared to the post-angioplasty waveforms. This patient's blood pressure returned to normal a short time after the angioplasty procedure.*

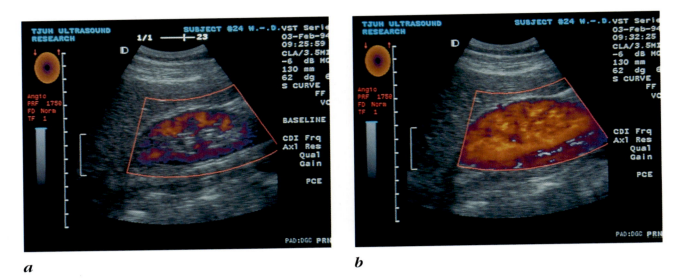

a　　　　　　　　　　　　　　　　　　　　　　　　*b*

Figure 4.60 *These images provide an example of the ability of vascular ultrasound contrast agents to improve our ability to detect bloodflow. In this case CAI was used to evaluate flow in the kidney of a normal volunteer during the FDA phase I trial of Echogen™ (Sonus Pharmaceuticals, Bothell, WA). Both the pre-injection (a) and post-injection (b) images were obtained using identical color flow parameters. The improvement in flow information is a result of the increase in reflective properties of the blood following the administration of contrast.*

upper-, middle-, and lower-pole segmental arteries. From this spectral Doppler information a number of quantifying parameters, including the time to systolic rise, the acceleration index and the peak systolic velocities, are measured. What is sought here are the downstream effects of a more proximal renal artery stenosis (Fig. 4.59). The theoretical benefits of performing this examination are that it can be used on a much greater portion of the population, it can detect stenoses of duplicate renal arteries if present, and it is typically less labor- and time-intensive than the complete CFI evaluation of both main renal arteries. The limitations are that this technique does not localize the exact site of a stenosis. However, used as a screening tool, if the ultrasound examination indicates that there is a strong likelihood of a renal artery stenosis, the patient typically will have a more definitive angiogram with or without therapeutic angioplasty.

Each of the two protocols described above obviously have their own strengths and weaknesses. The choice of which one to use can, at times, be determined on an individual basis depending on the operator's expertise, equipment and time available, and the patient's body habitus. The use of vascular ultrasound contrast agents to enhance both color and spectral Doppler flow signals, which is discussed in Chapter 8, has the potential to improve considerably the ability of ultrasound to detect a variety of vascular abnormalities, including renal artery stenosis (Fig. 4.60).

In addition to evaluating the patient suspected of having renovascular hypertension, CFI is useful in a variety of other renal applications. CFI can provide information on the relative vascularity of a suspected renal tumor, or aid in determining whether a region suspected on gray scale ultrasound to be abnormal has regionally different vascularity, as well as detecting the effect a tumor has on other surrounding structures (Figs 4.61–4.64). CFI can also help delineate focal areas of renal infarction by demonstrating a lack of flow in one region of the kidney, or to confirm renal artery occlusion which results in no arterial flow detected from within the main renal artery (Figs 4.65–4.66). Owing to the highly vascular nature of kidneys, color displays using the amplitude of the

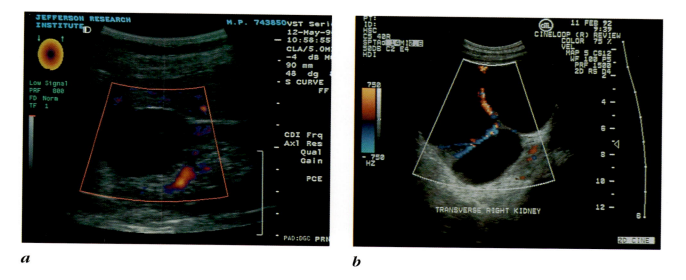

Figure 4.64 *This patient was referred to our laboratory for an ultrasound-guided diagnostic aspiration of a renal cyst which was found with gray scale to contain septations. CAI (a) optimized for low flow sensitivity detected no flow in the abnormal area. This was proven to represent a benign renal cyst. In a different patient, CFI (b) demonstrates flow within the walls of a multiseptated cystic renal tumor.*

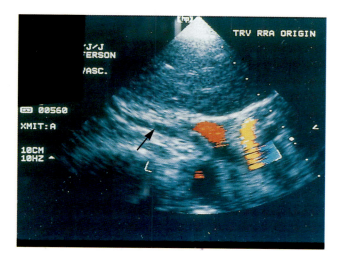

Figure 4.65 *Transverse CFI of an angiographically proven right renal artery (arrow) occlusion. Note the low-level echoes seen within the vessel lumen. Bloodflow is identified in the IVC located anterior to the renal artery.*

differentiate between a vascular aneurysm or simple cyst. Increased pulsatility of bloodflow in the kidneys which results from obstructive hydronephrosis can be demonstrated using CFI; however, the added benefit of displaying the flow dynamics over time with Doppler spectral analysis is probably better suited for this or similar applications. Dilated veins in the renal hilum may mimic hydronephrosis (Fig. 4.68). CFI can be used to demonstrate the presence of flow in these vessels and help avoid a false-positive diagnosis of ureteral obstruction. Renal vein thrombosis (partial or complete) resulting from primary renal tumor invasion or other causes can also be detected using CFI (Fig. 4.26).

CFI evaluation of the urinary bladder can demonstrate both normal and abnormal ureteric jets (Fig. 4.69). Additionally, with CFI bloodflow within tumors of the urinary bladder wall and, at times, tumor invasion into the bladder wall from adjacent neoplasms can be detected (Fig. 4.70).

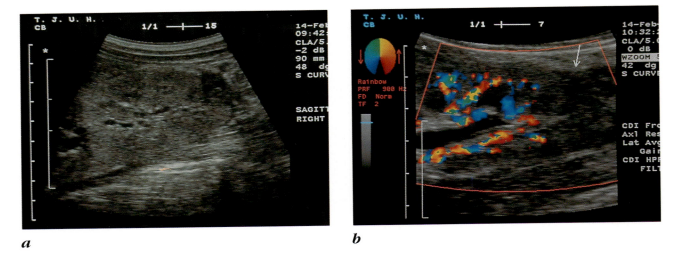

Figure 4.66 *Longitudinal gray scale image (a) of the right kidney demonstrates a wedge-shaped area of decreased echogenicity in the lower pole. With CFI (b) this area (arrow) had no detectable bloodflow, consistent with a lower-pole renal infarction.*

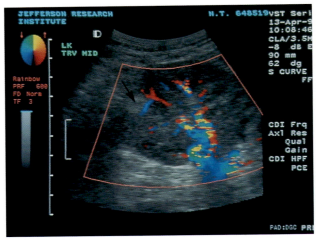

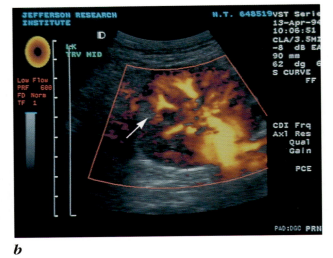

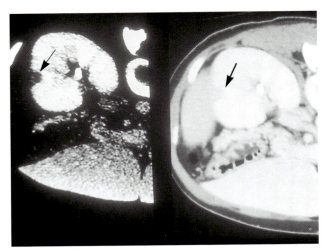

Figure 4.67 *This patient had multiple areas of increased echogenicity within both kidneys identified with gray scale ultrasound. With conventional CFI (a) much of the renal cortex, including these areas, was void of flow. However, better flow information was obtained using CAI (b), which demonstrated flow in the normal appearing portions of the cortex and the lack of flow in these echogenic areas (arrow). A subsequent CT examination (c) confirmed multiple renal infarcts in this patient. Note: the CT images have been rotated to correlate with the ultrasound plane of section. In this case renal infarctions as small as 1.0 cm were diagnosed using CAI.*

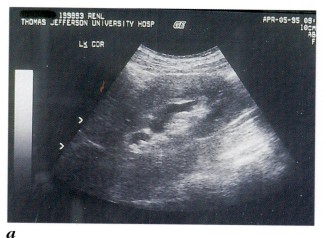

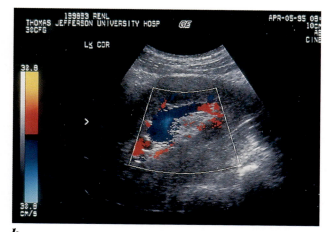

a

b

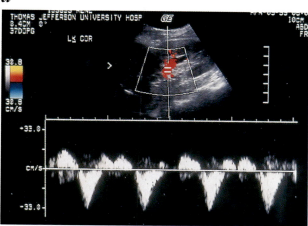

c

Figure 4.68 *This patient presented with microscopic hematuria. A gray scale image of the left kidney (a) suggested dilatation of the renal collecting system. However, using CFI (b) it was determined that the fluid-filled spaces in the renal sinus actually represented dilated renal veins, probably due to the patient's known tricuspid valve regurgitation. A spectral Doppler waveform (c) confirmed the highly pulsatile biphasic nature of the flow in these veins. In this case an incorrect diagnosis was avoided by including CFI during the initial examination.*

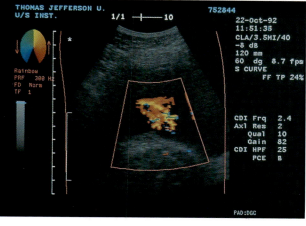

a

b

Fig 4.69 *This patient was referred to ultrasound with right flank pain after passing a renal calculus. CFI of the urinary bladder demonstrated bilateral ureteric jets, however, flow was much more conspicuous and at a higher velocity from the left ureteral orifice (a) than from the right (b). This was a consistent finding which was thought to be the result of inflammation and/or spasm of the right ureter.*

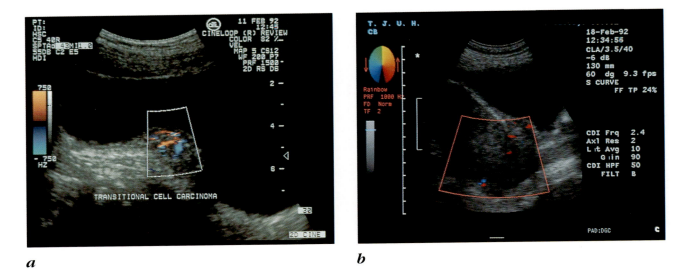

a   *b*

Figure 4.70 *CFI (a) of a moderately distended urinary bladder demonstrates a solid mass which has abnormal vascularity arising from the posterior wall mucosa. This lesion represents a transitional cell carcinoma of the urinary bladder. In a different patient with known uterine cervical cancer a longitudinal CFI (b) demonstrates elevation of the posterior bladder wall by an abnormally thickened cervix and a poorly demarcated boundary between the uterus and bladder wall. Bloodflow was detected from small vessels within this abnormal area. These findings suggest a diagnosis of direct invasion of the bladder wall by the cervical cancer. A subsequent MRI examination confirmed bladder wall invasion.*

RENAL TRANSPLANTS

CFI has proven useful for the evaluation of a number of abnormalities associated with transplanted kidneys. This results, in part, from their superficial location which allows use of higher-frequency transducers, a lack of movement, known major vessel anatomy, and the highly vascular nature of kidneys, providing dramatic color displays of bloodflow (Figs 4.71 and 4.72). CFI permits rapid qualitative assessment of flow in the transplanted kidney, thereby confirming patency of the main renal artery and vein (Figs 4.73 and 4.74). More quantitative information, when necessary, can be obtained with pulsed spectral Doppler (Fig. 4.75). A variety of indices have been used to identify normal flow in the transplanted kidney. The most common of these is the resistive index (RI). An RI of 0.5–0.7 is considered normal, and an RI of 0.9 or greater is abnormal. An RI of 0.7–0.9 is indeterminate; however, serial studies may demonstrate changes in flow over time which can be quantified and determined using RI. When placed in the clinical context these serial evaluations may provide

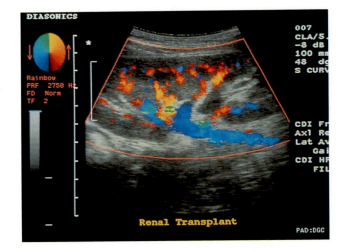

Figure 4.71 *Owing to the relatively superficial location of transplanted kidneys in the iliac fossa, CFI with pulsed Doppler spectral analysis can be used to assess both flow through the surgical vascular anastomoses and intrarenal flow patterns in cases of suspected organ rejection. Here a longitudinal color flow image of a renal transplant shows normal bloodflow distribution within the kidney and patency of the renal vein.*

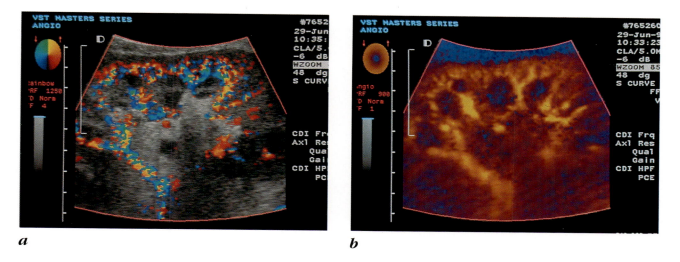

a

b

Figure 4.72 *Conventional color (a) and color amplitude (b) images of a renal transplant using similar color flow parameters. Note the severe color aliasing on the conventional color image and the improvement in cortical bloodflow information obtained with the color amplitude mode. CAI is ideally suited for the qualitative assessment of flow in renal transplants.*

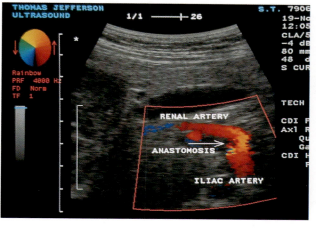

a

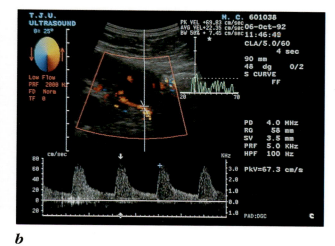

b

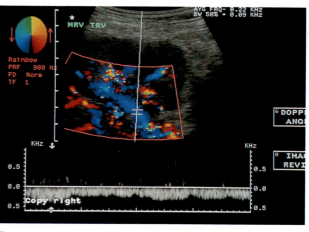

c

Figure 4.73 *CFI can facilitate the evaluation of bloodflow through the anastomotic sites of both the renal artery and renal vein. Pulsed spectral Doppler should be utilized to exclude hemodynamically significant stenoses.*

A transverse color flow image (a) of the donor renal artery anastomosis with the native iliac artery in a patient after recent renal transplantation demonstrates good flow with no evidence of stenosis. In a different patient (b) CFI detects flow in the main renal artery, with pulsed spectral Doppler demonstrating a normal waveform. CFI (c) guides for pulse Doppler sample volume placement to demonstrate normal flow in the main renal vein. In the acute stage the ultrasound evaluation of a renal transplant should include assessment of both the main renal artery and vein to confirm patency of the surgical anastomoses of these vessels.

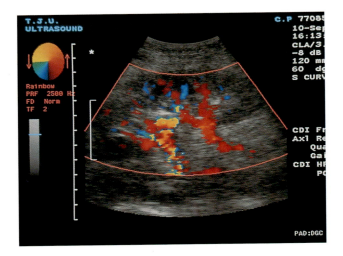

Figure 4.74 *CFI demonstrates paired renal arteries entering the hilum of a transplanted kidney. In this case, because of the lack of intrarenal vascular communications, both arteries of the donor kidney were anastomosed to the patient's iliac artery, and were evaluated during the ultrasound examination.*

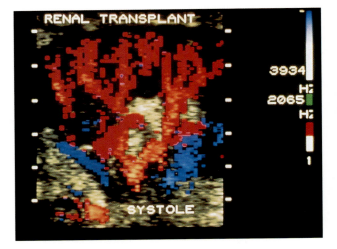

a

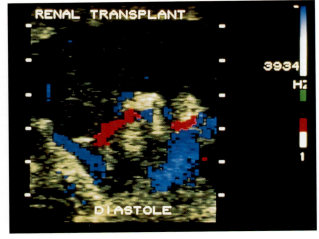

b

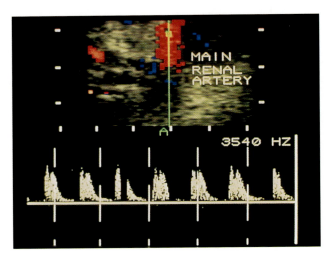

c

Figure 4.75 *CFI can demonstrate temporal changes of flow in real time. In this longitudinal view of a renal transplant during systole (a), bloodflow is detected within the renal parenchyma; however, in diastole (b) no flow is visualized. A pulsed Doppler spectral waveform (c) of the main renal artery confirmed a total absence of diastolic flow. Although this is an abnormal finding it is non-specific, possibly representing acute tubular necrosis, organ rejection, or other complications.*

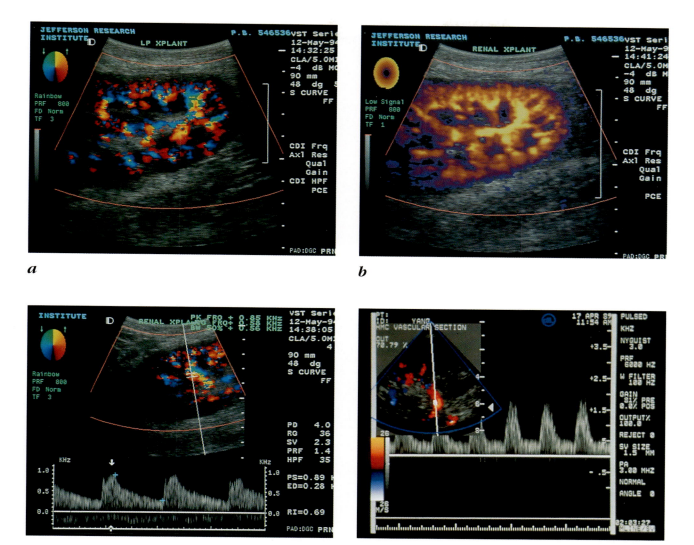

Figure 4.76 *Longitudinal conventional color (a) and color amplitude (b) images of the lower pole of a renal transplant in a patient with a slight rise in his creatinine. Pulsed Doppler spectral analysis of a segmental renal artery (c) demonstrates good flow with a normal resistive index (RI) of 0.69. Although normal on ultrasound the patient had a subsequent needle biopsy which detected mild acute cellular rejection which responded to medical therapy. In a patient with known acute tubular necrosis (d), a pulsed spectral Doppler waveform obtained from the main renal artery appears within normal limits, with an RI of approximately 0.70. These two cases demonstrate Doppler ultrasound's inability to reliably detect some complications of renal transplants, and emphasize the importance of placing the ultrasound findings in the context of other diagnostic tests and clinical observations.*

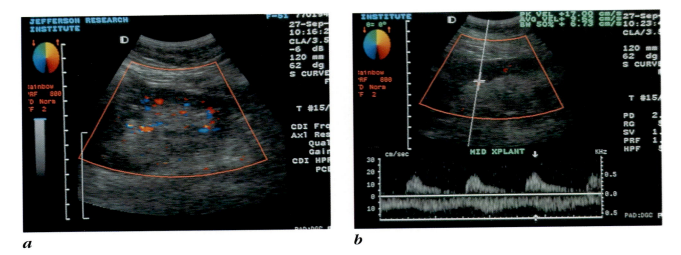

Figure 4.77 *Longitudinal CFI (a) of an abnormal renal transplant with decreased visualization of bloodflow. A spectral Doppler waveform obtained from an interlobar vessel (b) indicates increased resistance with a lack of end-diastolic flow (RI = 1.0). This kidney was subsequently biopsied, which determined the presence of chronic tubulointerstitial nephritis and acute tubular necrosis. In this case the qualitative information obtained with CFI suggested an abnormality; however, spectral Doppler analysis was necessary to better quantitate the abnormal flow. If serial ultrasound examinations are performed, the quantitative nature of the data obtained with spectral Doppler is also more comparable than that obtained by CFI alonee.*

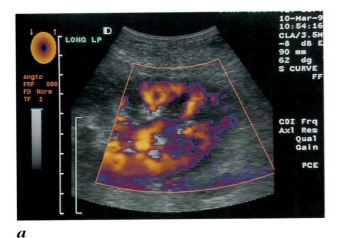

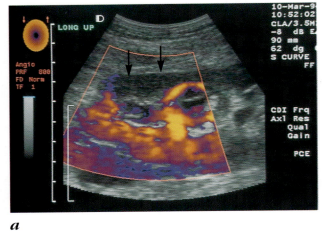

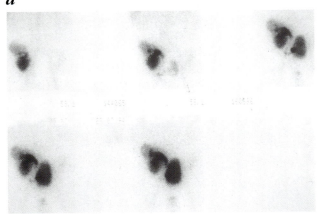

Figure 4.78 *Longitudinal color amplitude images of a renal transplant lower (a) and upper (b) poles using identical color parameters. Compared to the lower pole, in the upper pole there is an area (arrows) with no flow detected consistent with an area of renal ischemia. A nuclear medicine examination (c) was consistent with reduced perfusion in the upper pole region, but was less specific in delineating the ischemic area than was ultrasound. Multiple follow-up ultrasound examinations confirmed the lack of flow in this area.*

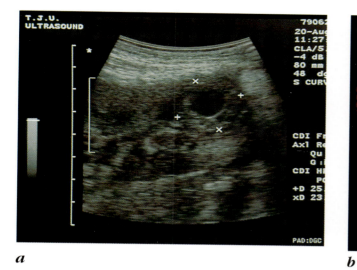

a

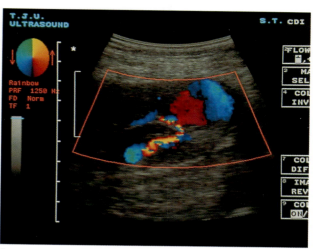

b

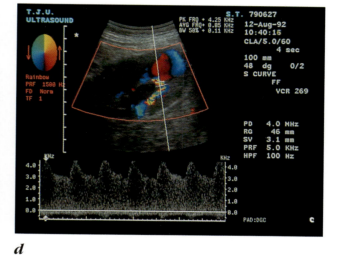

c

d

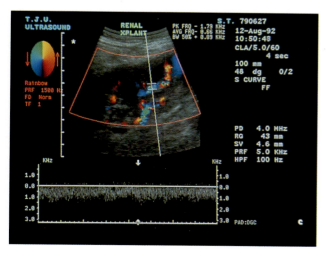

e

Figure 4.79 *CFI can detect vascular abnormalities following invasive procedures such as tissue biopsies of abdominal organs. This longitudinal gray scale image of a renal transplant (a) shows a complex cystic area in the lower pole (cursors), the site of a previous percutaneous biopsy. CFI of that region (b) demonstrated a whirling flow pattern within this mass. Pulsed spectral Doppler of this area (c) demonstrated bidirectional flow. Further spectral Doppler evaluation of this area detected a communicating tract with flow into the lesion in systole and reversed flow in diastole, consistent with a pseudoaneurysm. Doppler spectral analysis of an adjacent vessel with abnormal flow patterns on CFI (d) detected unusually high diastolic flow indicating low peripheral resistance. Spectral analysis of an adjacent vein (e) detected flow which was pulsatile with the cardiac cycle. These findings are consistent with a concomitant arteriovenous fistula. These injuries were the result of inadvertent puncture of intrarenal vessels during the biopsy procedure.*

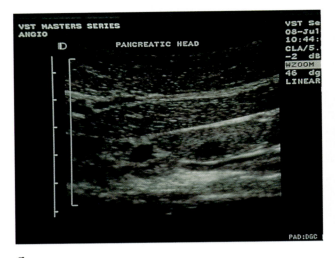

a

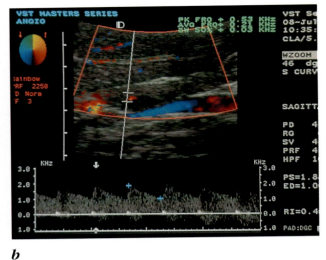

b

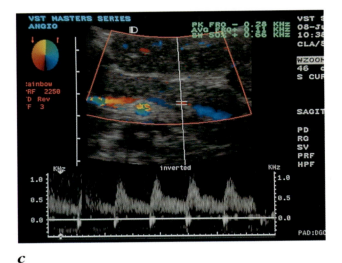

c

Figure 4.80 *A focal area of decreased echogenicity is seen on this sagittal gray scale image (a) of the pancreatic head. A CFI-guided pulsed Doppler spectral waveform (b) obtained from the periphery of this area indicates increased flow and decreased resistance, when compared to (c), a normal-appearing portion of the same gland. This was later determined to represent focal pancreatitis.*

additional information on the status of the transplanted kidney (Figs 4.76 and 4.77). The vascular anastomoses of the renal artery and vein may be the site of an obstruction of bloodflow to or from the kidney. An obstruction to the flow out of the kidney usually results in an increase in the pulsatility (or an increase in RI) of arterial waveforms obtained from the kidney and a reduction or loss of flow in the renal veins. This is in contrast to an arterial stenosis which, if severe enough, results in a reduction in pulsatility (or a decrease in RI) downstream from the stenotic segment.

As with native kidneys, focal regions of renal ischemia in the transplanted organ can be identified with CFI (Fig. 4.78). CAI appears to have the potential to better demonstrate regional differences in flow in organs in general, and the qualities of renal transplants discussed above are particularly relevant to using this new flow imaging modality for this application. After a needle biopsy of renal transplants, CFI may facilitate detection of abnormal vascular communications which result from inadvertent puncture of intrarenal vessels (Fig. 4.79). Ultrasound with CFI can be used to safely monitor these vascular abnormali-

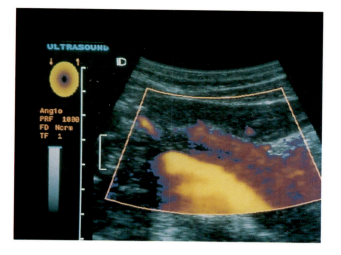

Figure 4.81 *Acute and chronic pancreatitis with hemorrhagic necrosis of the pancreatic head. This patient presented with acute right upper quadrant and epigastric pain. The gallbladder was sludge-filled, but did not have stones or evidence of hyperemia. The common bile duct was mildly dilated. The pancreas appeared abnormal. There was a pseudocyst in the pancreatic head, multiple pancreatic calcifications, and the pancreatic duct was severely dilated and 'beaded' in appearance. A color amplitude image of the pancreas demonstrates a diffuse parenchymal blush in the body and tail, which have increased bloodflow. There is no perfusion detected by this modality in an area of the pancreatic head larger than the size of the pseudocyst. High-bolus, thin-cut CT scan confirmed the lack of pancreatic blush in this area surrounding the pseudocyst. Courtesy of T. Stavros.*

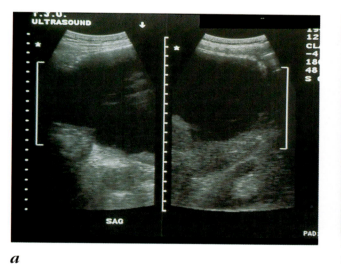

a

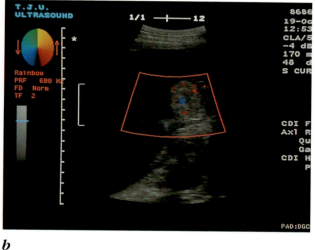

b

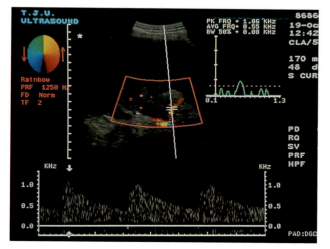

c

Figure 4.82 *Longitudinal gray scale image (a) of a predominantly cystic mass located in the region of the tail of the pancreas with a solid nodule on the wall. (Note: two images are placed side by side to demonstrate the extensive size of this mass, which measured approximately 18 cm.) CFI (b) demonstrated flow within the solid nodules and guided for pulsed Doppler sample volume placement. A spectral Doppler waveform (c) obtained from these vessels revealed low-resistance flow with a high amount of diastolic flow suggestive of a malignant tumor. This was surgically proven to represent a cystic adenocarcinoma of the pancreatic tail.*

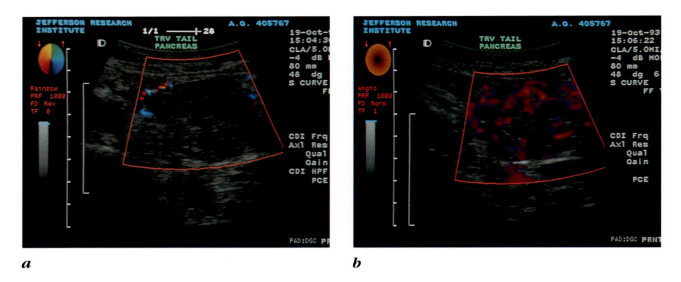

a *b*

Figure 4.83 *Transverse conventional color (a) and color amplitude (b) images of a mass involving the pancreatic tail. Note the increased visualization of the intratumoral vessels seen on the color amplitude image. This was proven to represent a microcystic adenoma.*

ties, and may help determine whether surgical intervention is indicated.

THE RETROPERITONEUM AND OTHER ABDOMINAL APPLICATIONS

Abnormalities within the pancreas that can be demonstrated with CFI are usually confined to distortion of vessels by tumors. However, inflammation resulting in increased flow can also be demonstrated (Figs 4.80 and 4.81). In general, pancreatic tumors tend to be hypovascular and thus have sparse vascularity. On occasion, however, hypervascular tumors may be detected (Figs 4.82 and 4.83). The relative vascularity of pancreatic tumors can be determined with CFI, with some indication of the malignant potential obtained with the information provided by CFI-guided spectral Doppler analysis of tumor vessels shown by increased diastolic (and on occasion systolic) flow related to the lower resistance in tumor vessels. Although this spectral Doppler pattern has been seen in other malignant tumors, it is not specific, since similar patterns have been seen with some benign tumors and in regions of inflammation. Pancreatic enzymes within pseudocysts may cause erosion of adjacent blood vessel walls, resulting in the development of a pseudoaneurysm or other abnormal vascular communications. CFI can help identify the affected vessel(s) and demonstrate flow in both the communicating tract and within the pseudoaneurysm (Fig. 4.84). This information can help in planning the interventional measures needed to correct these abnormalities. Recipients of pancreatic transplants are also candidates for CFI examinations. The transplanted gland derives its blood supply from the donor celiac and superior mesenteric arteries anastomosed to the recipient's iliac artery, and the donor portal vein is anastomosed to the iliac vein. Owing to their superficial location, these can often be adequately evaluated with CFI with spectral Doppler analysis to confirm patency of the vascular anastomoses and exclude graft ischemia.

CFI may be used to detect intratumoral vascularity and to determine the source of tumors of the abdomen and retroperitoneum, including the adrenal gland, by demonstrating the origin of a tumor's blood supply (Figs 4.85–4.88). However, the

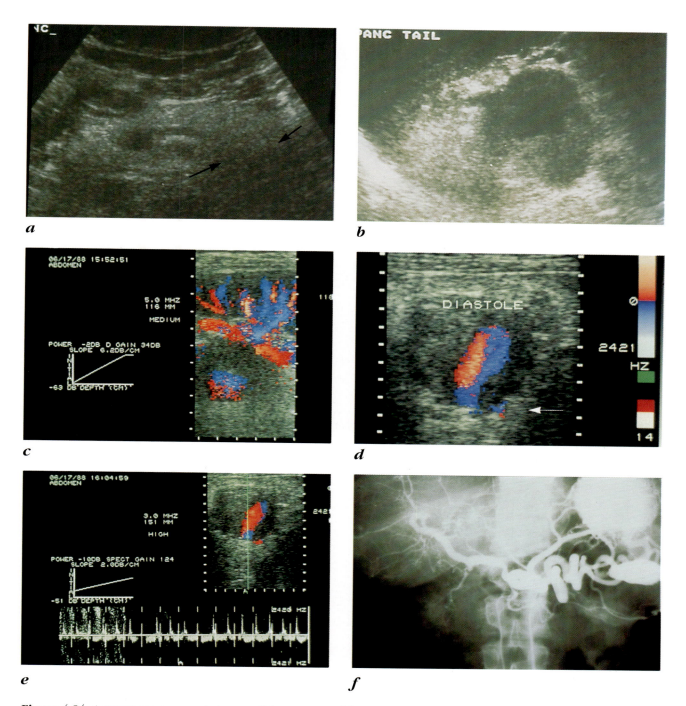

Figure 4.84 *A transverse gray scale image of the pancreas (a) in a patient with a history of pancreatitis demonstrates a normal pancreatic head and body, although there is evidence of a vague hypoechoic mass in the region of the pancreatic tail (arrows). This region was better visualized by a coronal scan from the left upper quadrant (b) which confirmed the presence of a complex mass. CFI of this area (c) demonstrated bloodflow in the spleen as well as flow within the center of the mass. Close examination of this area (d) detected a small vascular tract (arrow) with flow entering into the central area. Pulsed spectral Doppler obtained from this tract (e) revealed a waveform with forward systolic flow and diastolic flow reversal consistent with the diagnosis of a pseudoaneurysm. A subsequent angiogram (f) confirmed the presence of a pseudoaneurysm arising from the splenic artery, the result of partial destruction of the vessel wall by pancreatic enzymes contained within a pseudocyst.*

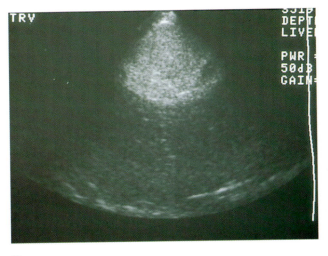

a

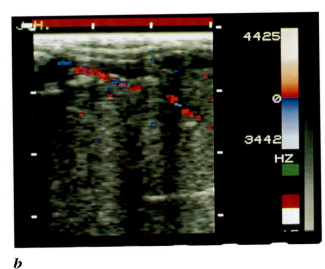

b

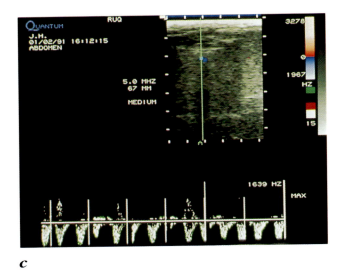

c

Figure 4.85 *By identifying the origin of the blood supply to tumors CFI may, in some cases, assist in determining (or excluding) the abdominal tumor's host organ. This gray scale image (a) demonstrates an echogenic mass anterior to the liver in an 18 month-old infant. Using CFI, no vascular communications were detected between the liver and this mass. However, using a high-resolution (7.5 MHz) transducer (b) small tumor-feeding vessels arising from the intercostal arteries were identified. Pulsed Doppler with spectral analysis of these vessels (c) demonstrated high resistance to flow. This mass was surgically confirmed to represent an extraperitoneal lipoblastoma arising from the anterior abdominal wall. At surgery, portions of the ribs were resected with this benign mass to maintain the integrity of the tumor capsule. The preoperative ultrasound results were especially helpful in the surgical management of this infant.*

exact source of the vascularity may be difficult to delineate due to the deep location and small size of the neovascular vessels. Enlarged lymph nodes resulting from inflammatory processes often show increased vascularity which can be detected with CFI (Fig. 4.89). If the adenopathy is due to tumor infiltration there may be distortion of the normal vascular architecture, whereas enlargement of nodes caused by inflammation tends to maintain the normal architecture. CFI can also detect compres-

sion of surrounding vessels, primarily veins, which results from lymphadenopathy or other abdominal masses (Figs 4.90 and 4.91).

As previously discussed, both normal and abnormal vascularity of abdominal organs can be depicted using CFI. CAI especially appears to be well suited for this application, by demonstrating differences in organ vascularity which result from tumor invasion, subcapsular hematomas, or other causes (Figs 4.92–4.94).

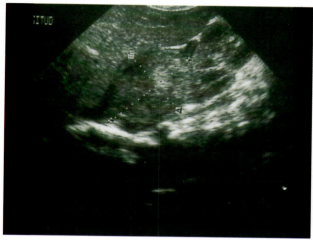

a

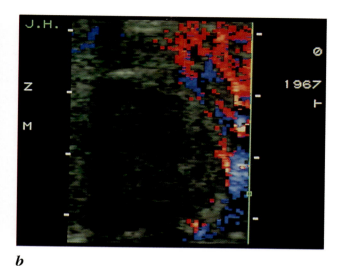

b

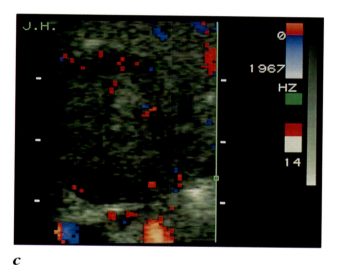

c

Figure 4.86 *This 3-month-old male infant was referred to our ultrasound laboratory after an outside gray scale ultrasound examination (a) detected a mass superior but immediately adjacent to the right kidney. While good flow was demonstrated in the right kidney, CFI (b) was unable to detect any vascular communications between the kidney and what appeared to be a hypovascular lesion in the region of the right adrenal gland. CFI of the mass (c) detected some intratumoral vessels. This was later confirmed to represent a neuroblastoma involving the right adrenal gland. In this case CFI helped to rule out a renal mass, which increased the confidence level of the ultrasound diagnosis of an adrenal tumor.*

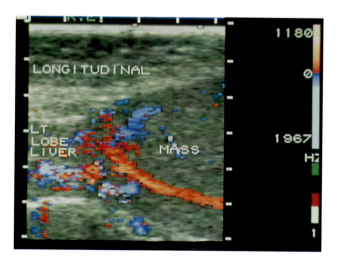

Figure 4.87 *This longitudinal color flow image of the inferior tip of the left lobe of the liver demonstrates continuity of flow from the liver into a large solid mass. By demonstrating this continuity, CFI provides information as to the host organ from which this mass is originating. This hypervascular lesion later was proven to represent multinodular hyperplasia. CFI can also be used during biopsy procedures to direct the approach so as to avoid both the major tumor vessels and areas of necrosis if present.*

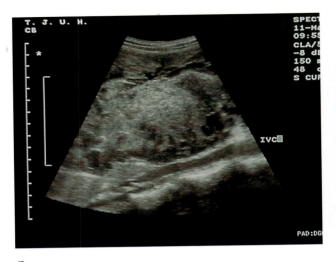

a

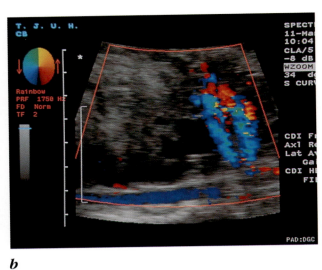

b

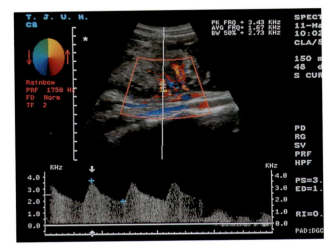

c

Figure 4.88 *Longitudinal gray scale image (a) of a large, predominantly solid mass anterior to the IVC. CFI (b) identifies the location of the major vessels within the mass and guides for sample volume placement to obtain a pulsed Doppler spectral waveform (c) which demonstrates a low-resistance, high-diastolic flow pattern. This was proven to represent metastatic spread from a known ovarian carcinoma (i.e. pseudotumor peritonei).*

GASTROINTESTINAL APPLICATIONS

Tumors of the bowel, including the stomach, may have increased and/or distorted vascularity which can be detected with CFI; however, tumors undergoing necrosis may not show any significant blood-flow (Fig. 4.95). Endorectal ultrasound, most commonly utilized to assess the prostate gland, can also be used to evaluate the rectal wall in patients with abnormalities that are detected during digital rectal examinations. Portions of the bowel with inflammation will usually demonstrate wall thickening with an increase in vascularity which can be detected with CFI. This has been seen in cases of acute appendicitis, Crohn's disease, and other inflammatory bowel processes (Figs 4.96–4.99). With the high level of flow sensitivity in currently available CFI systems, including the use of CAI, even the normal bowel walls may demonstrate some vascularity. Thus, the presence of vascularity alone does not indicate inflammation. The CFI information should be put into context with the patient's symptoms before a diagnosis is suggested.

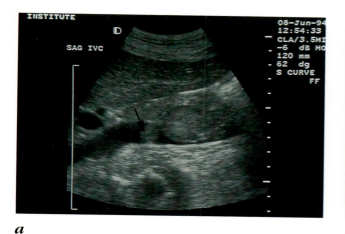

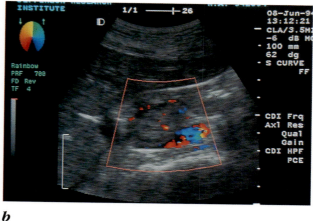

a

b

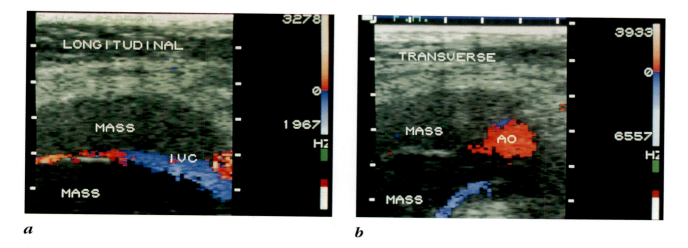

c

Figure 4.89 *Longitudinal gray scale image (a) of the IVC with compression by a solid anteriorly located mass and echogenic thrombus (arrow) within the IVC. CFI (b) demonstrates flow both within and along the periphery of the lesion, with pulsed Doppler spectral analysis (c) demonstrating a monophasic continuous signal. This patient had a history of a right nephrectomy for renal cell carcinoma. The solid mass represents a lymph node with tumor infiltration; however, it was unknown whether the thrombus within the IVC represented benign thrombus due to hemostasis or tumor extension from the primary cancer.*

a

b

Figure 4.90 *CFI is useful for detecting and demonstrating the effects of abdominal masses on adjacent structures such as blood vessels. In this case longitudinal (a) and transverse (b) color flow images demonstrate a mass surrounding the great vessels. This massive tumor is causing compression of a portion of the inferior vena cava (IVC), and surrounds the abdominal aorta (AO) both anteriorly and posteriorly. This was a mass of confluent lymphomatous nodes.*

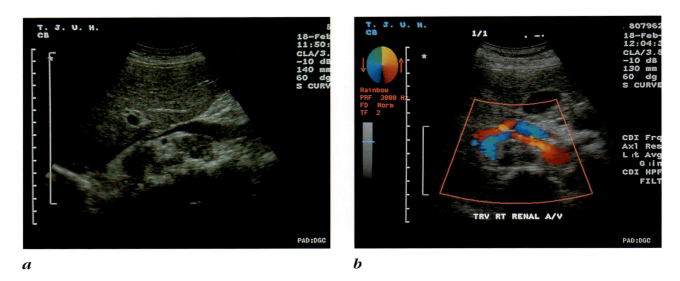

a   *b*

Figure 4.91 *In a patient with known uterine cervical carcinoma (see Fig. 4.70b) a sagittal gray scale image (a) demonstrates elevation of the IVC by enlarged lymph nodes surrounding the right renal artery. A transverse CFI of this area (b) confirms patency of the renal artery and vein. Note the change in color assignment as the flow in the two renal vessels changes in relation to the Doppler angle of insonation.*

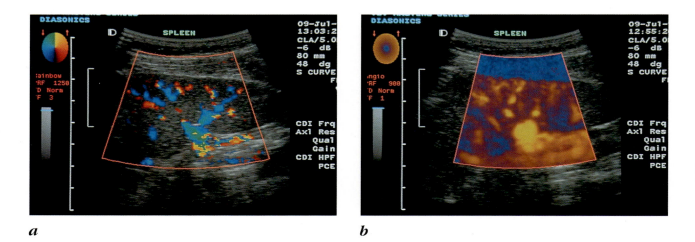

a   *b*

Figure 4.92 *CFI of a normal spleen using conventional color (a) and color amplitude (b) imaging. Note the better display of bloodflow out to the splenic capsule on the color amplitude image.*

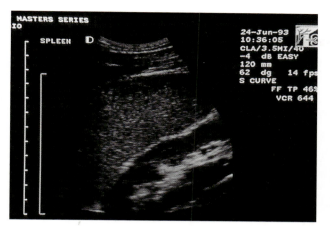

a

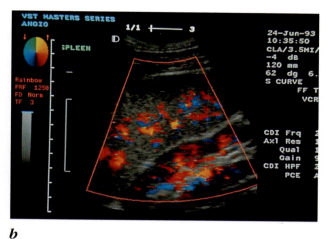

b

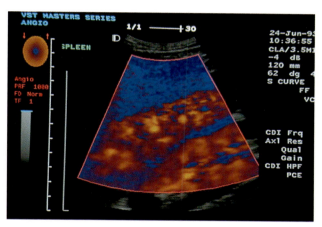

c

Figure 4.93 *A gray scale evaluation of the spleen (a) in a patient with recent abdominal trauma detected a region of reduced echogenicity at the splenic periphery. Conventional color (b) and color amplitude (c) imaging of the spleen demonstrated good flow in the left kidney (LK) and portions of the spleen, but no flow in this hypoechoic region. This area represented a post-traumatic subcapsular splenic hematoma.*

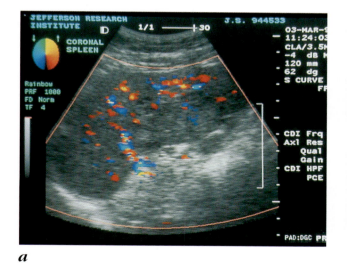

a

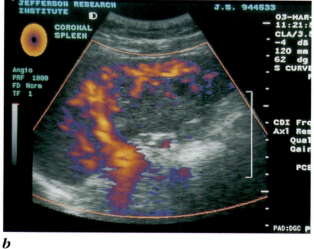

b

Figure 4.94 *CFI of the spleen in a patient with known metastases from ovarian cancer using conventional color (a) and color amplitude (b) modes with similar color flow parameters. Note the improved vessel continuity and better delineation of areas with and without flow on the color amplitude image. CAI appears to better demonstrate regional differences of flow in abdominal organs.*

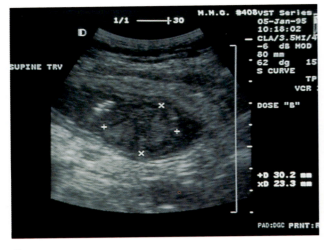

a

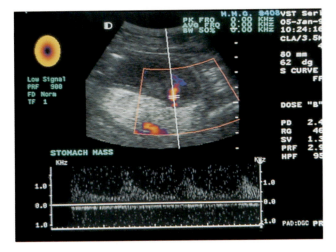

c

Figure 4.95 *Using gray scale ultrasound (a) a solid mass measuring 3.0 × 2.3 cm was detected within the stomach of this patient. CAI (b) detected a small feeding vessel and guided for sample volume placement (c) to obtain spectral Doppler waveforms. This mass was later determined to represent a primary gastric cancer.*

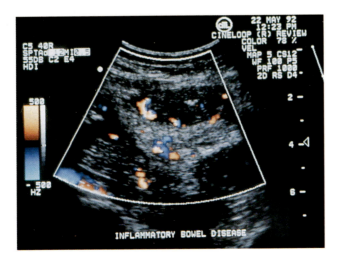

Figure 4.96 *This patient presented for sonography with acute right lower quadrant pain ruling out appendicitis. A normal-sized appendix was demonstrable. However, a loop of distal ileum was abnormally thickened due to a combination of edema and spasm, the small bowel mesentery was edematous, and both the bowel and mesentery showed evidence of increased bloodflow on CFI. This represents active Crohn's ileitis where bowel wall thickening, mesenteric edema and inflammatory hyperemia are usually extreme. During periods of inactivity these changes resolve. Courtesy of T. Stavros.*

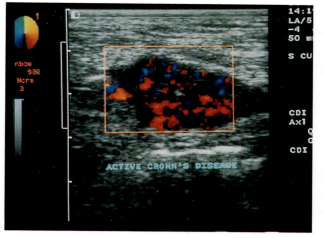

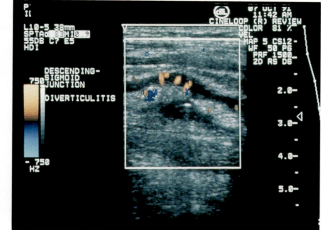

Figure 4.97 *Active Crohn's colitis. This patient had a long history of Crohn's disease and had had multiple segmental small bowel and colon resections in the past. She presented with pelvic pain. CFI detected a markedly thickened sigmoid apex with marked inflammatory hyperemia, indicating a new area of active disease. This represented a 'skip area' of involvement because the proximal sigmoid and descending colon appeared sonographically normal. Courtesy of T. Stavros.*

Figure 4.98 *Acute diverticulitis. This patient presented with left pelvic and lower quadrant pain. Sonography was requested to exclude a left ovarian etiology for pain. The patient's pelvic organs were sonographically normal. CFI of the area of maximum pain with a high-resolution probe demonstrated abnormal thickening of the proximal sigmoid wall and edema of the mesocolon. Centered within the edematous mesocolon deep to the bowel is a small fluid collection with an air bubble which represented a small diverticular abscess. These findings were confirmed by a CT scan. Abnormalities resolved over several weeks of antibiotic treatment. Courtesy of T. Stavros.*

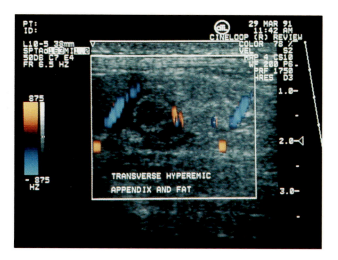

Figure 4.99 *Acute appendicitis. This patient presented with acute right lower quadrant pain. CFI demonstrated enlargement of the appendix, edema of the mesoappendix (medial to the appendix on this transverse view), and markedly increased bloodflow in the middle and outer layers of the appendiceal wall and within the mesoappendix. Bloodflow is usually not demonstrable within the normal appendix. Some flow may be seen within the normal mesoappendix, but normal spectral Doppler arterial waveforms will show a high-resistance pattern and venous waveforms will show respiratory phasicity. In cases of appendicitis, arterial waveforms will have a low-resistance pattern (i.e. increased diastolic flow) and venous flow is usually continuous, with decreased or absent respiratory variations. Venous waveforms frequently also show transmitted arterial pulsations. Even when the appendiceal mucosa is gangrenous, there is usually hyperemia within the mesoappendix. Courtesy of T. Stavros.*

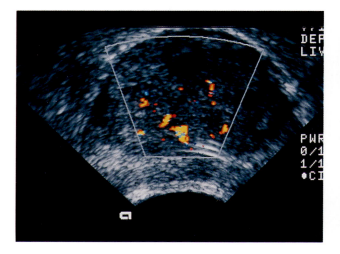

Figure 4.100 *Using the endorectal approach CFI demonstrated increased bloodflow throughout the prostate of this patient, especially within the peripheral zone. In this case the color flow information assisted in the selection of a site for transrectal needle biopsy. The pathology diagnosis was prostatitis.*

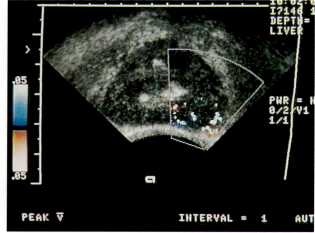

Figure 4.101 *CFI of prostate cancer. This lesion appeard vaguely hypoechoic and poorly delineated on gray scale imaging. However, CFI detected a focal area of increased vascularity within the peripheral zone of this patient who had an elevated prostate specific antigen level. A subsequent needle biopsy of this area confirmed a diagnosis of prostate cancer. Courtesy of A. Alexander.*

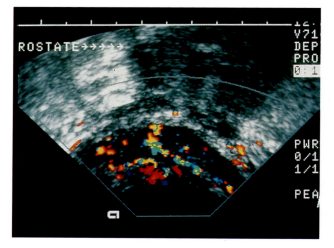

Figure 4.102 *Transverse color flow image of rectal wall cancer obtained using a dedicated endorectal probe. Ultrasound with CFI demonstrates the location of multiple vessels within the hypoechoic tumor and confirms this mass as extraprostatic in origin. Courtesy of A. Alexander.*

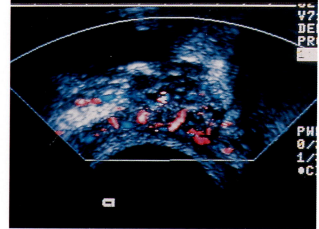

Figure 4.103 *This patient who presented with a palpable rectal mass detected during a routine clinical examimination had undergone prior prostatectomy for prostate cancer. Endorectal ultrasound with CFI detected a hypoechoic mass with increased vascularity anterior to the rectum. This area was later surgically confirmed to represent recurrence of prostate cancer with invasion into the perirectal tissues. Courtesy of A. Alexander.*

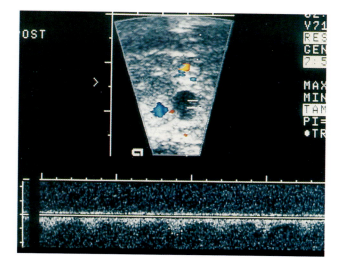

Figure 4.104 *Endorectal CFI detected flow within this small well-marginated hypoechoic mass located in the perirectal space. Guided by the color flow information, pulsed Doppler spectral analysis detected both arterial and venous bloodflow. This represents a perirectal lymph node in a patient with known rectal wall carcinoma. Courtesy of A. Alexander.*

PROSTATE APPLICATIONS

At present there is some controversy regarding the benefits of endorectal CFI for diagnosing abnormalities of the prostate gland. Various reports have described the ability of CFIs to detect increased bloodflow in cases of inflammation resulting from prostatitis, and to identify abnormal bloodflow in prostatic tumors, both benign (benign prostatic hypertrophy) and malignant (Figs 4.100 and 4.101). However, there exists considerable overlap in the CFI appearance of prostatic abnormalities, particularly that of hypervascular neoplasms and focal areas of prostatitis. Of interest are some reports of cases of unsuspected prostatic malignancies which were not detected using either the digital rectal examination or conventional endorectal gray scale imaging. In these cases tissue biopsies were performed solely guided by the CFI information, and resulted in the detection of an otherwise inconspicuous cancer. The bloodflow information obtained with CFI during ultrasound evaluation of the prostate is commonly viewed as a secondary diagnostic sign. When the CFI findings are used in the proper context of the physical examination, laboratory results (prostate-specific-antigen levels) and a gray scale examination, they may assist in the selection of a biopsy site, or may raise one's diagnostic confidence level and improve the overall utility of ultrasound imaging of this gland.

Endorectal ultrasound can also be used to evaluate patients with suspected rectal wall masses. In these cases CFI can provide information regarding the source of bloodflow to and relative internal and external vascularity of a mass. This information may help to determine the etiology of the lesion (Figs 4.102–4.104).

INTRAOPERATIVE APPLICATIONS

Owing primarily to its safety, portability, and flexibility, ultrasound has gained widespread acceptance in the operating room. The addition of CFI to gray scale imaging has the ability to greatly expand the diagnostic applications of intraoperative ultrasound. Unlike transcutaneous ultrasound, the intraoperative technique does not suffer from the attenuating effects of bone, intervening bowel, muscles, subcutaneous tissues, and skin. Therefore, higher frequency transducers can be utilized which improve flow sensitivity and provide better spatial resolution. As in other areas of ultrasound, a prerequisite for performing a thorough intraoperative examination is the ability to gain acoustical access to the structures which need to be evaluated. Factors such as the presence of adhesions or a small surgical incision may impose limitations on intraoperative ultrasound visualization of structures. The use of specialized intraoperative

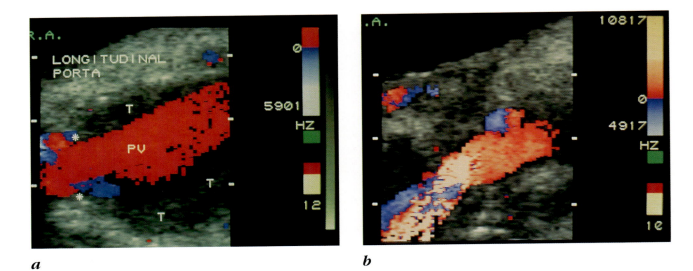

a   *b*

Figure 4.105 *Intraoperative CFI (a) of the anastomosis (*) between the native and donor portal vein (PV) in a patient receiving a liver transplant. Note the flow separations at the anastomosis indicated by the blue color coding. T, native portal vein thrombosis. Although CFI confirmed patency of the anastomosis, in a different view (b), there appeared to be some increase in flow velocity through the anastomosis. Angle-corrected pulsed Doppler with spectral analysis (not shown) indicated some elevation of flow velocity in this location, but not enough to warrant repair. The apparent increase in velocity demonstrated with CFI was, in part, related to the direction of flow in relation to the ultrasound beam. Quantitative spectral Doppler should be used in conjunction with CFI to determine the hemodynamic significance of suspected stenoses.*

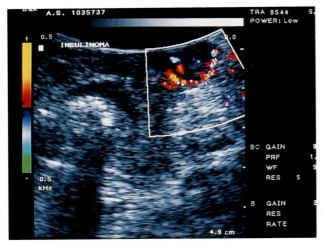

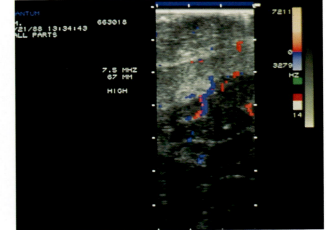

Figure 4.106 *Intraoperative CFI demonstrates the highly vascular nature of a hypoechoic pancreatic insulinoma. In this case CFI also assisted in the localization of the pancreatic duct and determined its relationship to the tumor, thereby assisting in the resection of the mass without injury to the duct. Intraoperative ultrasound was also used to exclude the presence of additional pancreatic masses in this patient.*

Figure 4.107 *Intraoperative CFI of a meningioma. Gray scale ultrasound was used to identify the margins of the tumor and helped determine the surgical approach to resection. CFI demonstrated the hypovascular nature of the brightly echogenic lesion, and localized the major feeding vessels, further assisting the resection.*

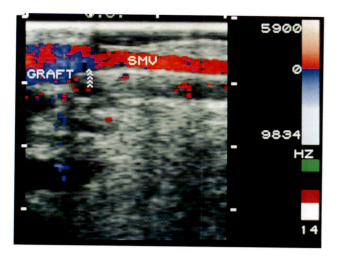

Figure 4.108 *Intraoperative CFI confirms patency of the anastomosis (arrow heads) between a mesocaval shunt (graft) and the superior mesenteric vein (SMV) in a patient with portal hypertension. A small amount of sterile saline placed in the surgical space facilitates adequate imaging of this graft by allowing the structures of interest to be positioned away from the transducer's 'main bang' (near field) and within the focal area of this transducer.*

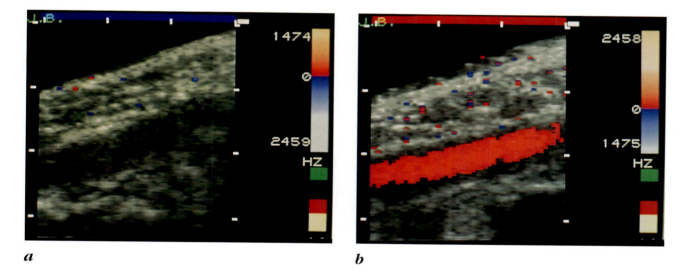

a   *b*

Figure 4.109 *Intraoperative CFI of a femoral artery to femoral artery graft. Initially (a), transcutaneous intraoperative CFI was used to confirm total occlusion of the graft prior to the planned thrombectomy. After the surgery (b) intraoperative CFI confirmed patency of this graft segment, and guided pulsed Doppler spectral analysis to better quantitate the flow through the various graft segments (not shown).*

probes can reduce some of these limitations. The results of pre-operative imaging studies are often used to focus the intraoperative ultrasound examination on a particular area of interest. However, intraoperative abdominal ultrasound (either open or via laparoscopy) is gaining popularity as a screening method for the detection of metastatic disease and cancer staging.

In patients receiving organ transplants, the vascular anastomoses can be evaluated with CFI to ensure functional lumen patency or to detect the presence of flow reducing lesions prior to closing the abdomen. This potentially obviates the need for intraoperative angiography or additional corrective procedures (Fig. 4.105). In cases of tumor resections, CFI may help determine the relative vascularity of a

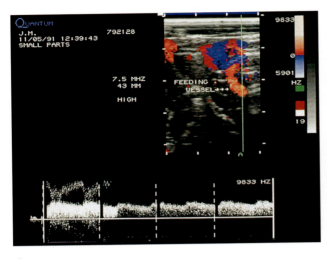

a

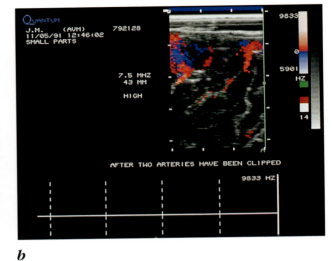

b

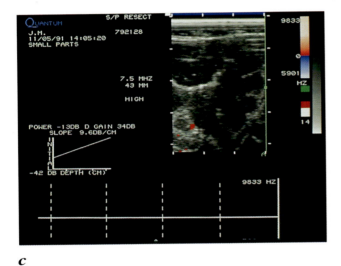

c

Figure 4.110 *Intraoperative CFI demonstrates the effects of afferent vessel ligation prior to resection of a cranial arteriovenous malformation (AVM). After craniotomy and prior to removal of the dura mater CFI (a) identifies the location and guides for spectral Doppler analysis of a major AVM feeding artery. After ligation of two of the feeding arteries (b), CFI demonstrates a reduction in flow within the AVM. After resection (c), CFI confirms total excision of the AVM and demonstrates the resultant cavity.*

lesion and ascertain its spatial relationship to both vascular and non-vascular stuctures (Figs 4.106 and 4.107). CFI used in this way can assist in planning the surgical approach.

Other intraoperative applications of CFI include the assessment of flow through vascular reconstructions and grafts within the abdomen, extracranial circulation, and periphery (Figs 4.108 and 4.109). CFI can confirm patency or occlusion of reconstructions or grafts and potentially detect abnormalities related to residual disease, competent valves, and technical complications such as intimal flaps, arterial kinks, strictures, or thrombi intraoperatively so that they can be corrected prior to completion of the surgical procedure.

Intraoperative CFI has also been used successfully to more accurately determine the location of arteriovenous fistulae (AVF) in situ. CFI can be quite

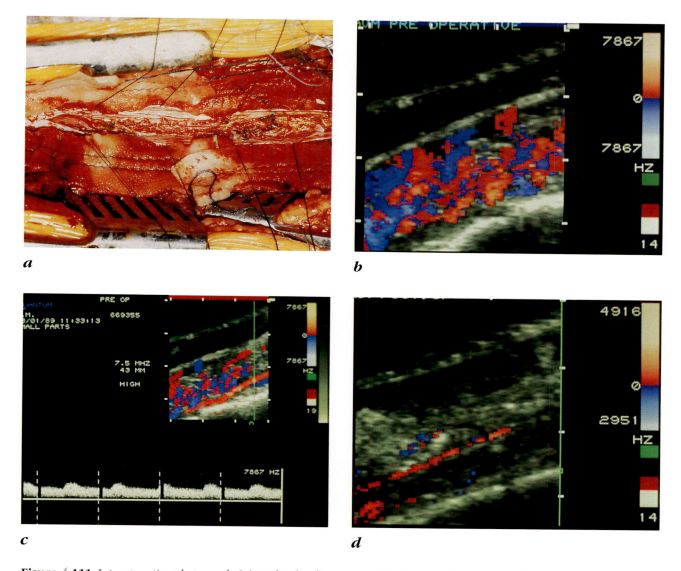

Figure 4.111 *Intraoperative photograph (a) and color flow image (b) of an arteriovenous malformation (AVM) of the spinal cord obtained in situ. Intraoperative CFI facilitated localization of the major afferent artery, which was confirmed by the reduced pulsatility identified with spectral Doppler analysis (c). After resection (d), CFI identified normal vascularity to the cord and no residual AVM, findings that were confirmed on a postoperative angiogram.*

useful, particularly in neurosurgical procedures, to identify the location of the afferent and efferent vessels of an AVF, which can vary in number, course and location, and to demonstrate the hemodynamic effects of surgical manipulations (Fig. 4.110). The addition of CFI for this application may minimize surgical exploration, reduce the time required to perform the resection, and potentially avoid catastrophic complications which may result from the

premature ligation of a major draining vein. CFI-guided pulsed Doppler with spectral analysis should be used to differentiate normal arteries from those feeding the AVF (Fig. 4.111). Typically, AVF vessels will have increased flow velocities (especially the diastolic component) and a lower pulsatility than arteries supplying normal territories. Hematomas which result from previous rupture of an AVF can be differentiated from vascular spaces using CFI and,

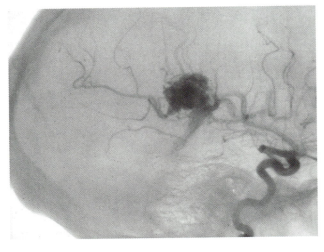

a

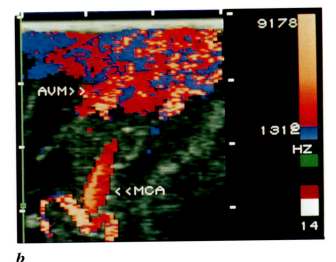

b

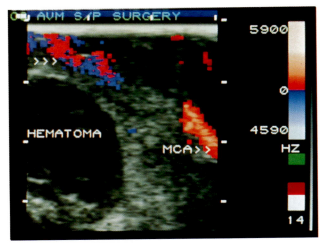

c

Figure 4.112 *Preoperative angiogram (a) and intraoperative CFI (b) of an intracranial arteriovenous malformation (AVM). Image (b) was obtained after craniotomy, prior to removal of the dura mater. In this case the major arterial feeding vessels were branches from the middle cerebral artery (MCA) located deep to the AVM, and not directly visualized. CFI assisted in the surgical approach to these afferent vessels prior to AVM resection. After resection (c), CFI identified the location of a known hematoma which resulted from prior rupture of AVM vessels and caused the patient's original episode of unconsciousness. (This episode was the first indication of an abnormality in this patient.) Prior to closure, CFI-guided evacuation of the hematoma and detected a small residual area of abnormal vascular communication (arrow heads). This was believed to represent a small residual component of the AVM and was, therefore, resected. A postoperative arteriogram confirmed total resection of the AVM.*

when necessary, can be evacuated under ultrasound guidance. Following AVF resection and prior to surgical closure, CFI can again be utilized to detect the presence of small residual abnormal vascular communications, thereby improving the effectiveness of the surgery and reducing the likelihood of, or eliminating the need for, additional procedures to correct recurrent abnormalities (Fig. 4.112). CFI can be used during surgical resection of vascular aneurysms to assist in the localization of the abnormality and guide the surgical approach. After surgical correction CFI

can help to confirm patency of the previously affected vessel (Fig. 4.113).

Many procedures previously performed using open surgery, such as cholecystectomies and various gynecologic procedures, are now being performed via laparoscopy. Dedicated laparoscopic ultrasound probes that are composed of a semi-steerable high frequency transducer on the end of a shaft are currently available with CFI capabilities. These specialized probes can be introduced through a standard laparoscopic trocar and used for a variety of applica-

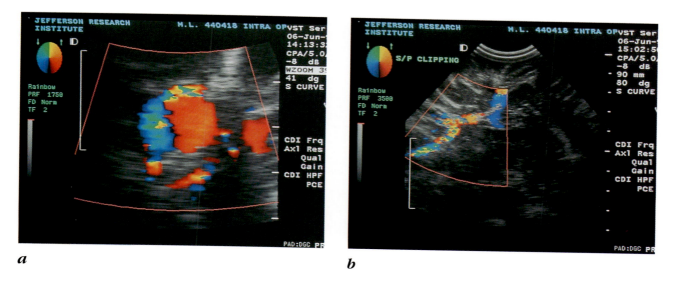

Figure 4.113 *Magnified color flow image of an anerurysm of an intracranial artery. CFI identifies the swirling flow pattern within the aneurysm and the location of the neck of the aneurysm relative to the native vessel. After surgical correction (b), CFI confirmed patency of flow and identified a slight kink in the previously affected vessel.*

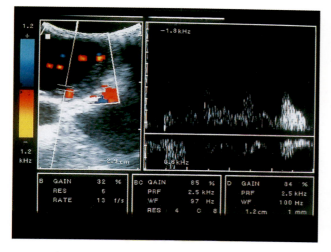

Figure 4.114 *Thoracoscopic CFI using a laparoscopic ultrasound probe identifies the location of vessels within the solid component of a complex (i.e. cystic and solid) mediastinal mass. CFI-guided pulsed Doppler spectral analysis of this vessel demonstrated arterial flow. This information helped in the selection of a site for tissue biopsy by confirming the neovascularity within this area of the mass. This was proven to represent a benign mesothelial cyst. Color artifacts are present within the cystic area of this tumor.*

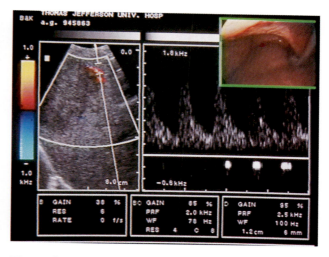

Figure 4.115 *Laparoscopic CFI identifies a vessel at the periphery of a large metastatic liver tumor in a patient with known colon cancer. Guided by the color flow information, a pulsed Doppler spectral wave form demonstrates arterial flow in this vessel. Note that the ultrasound image and the laproscopic view (top right, provided as a picture-in-a-picture) are on the same monitor. This feature provides information on the spatial location of the probe within the abdominal cavity to the individual performing the ultrasound examination, and facilitates the scanning procedure.*

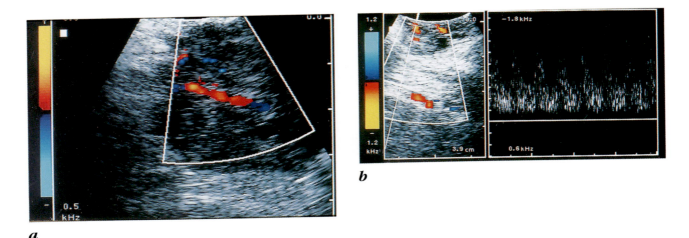

Figure 4.116 *Laparoscopic CFI (a) identifies an intratumoral vessel in a large pelvic mass that was later proven to represent ovarian carcinoma. In a different patient (b) laparoscopic ultrasound was used to minimize exploration of the pelvis in a patient with severe pelvic adhesions. In this case CFI-guided for spectral Doppler analysis confirmed abnormal flow in this pelvic mass. (Note the high diastolic flow component.) This mass was later proven to represent ovarian carcinoma.*

tions within the thorax, abdomen and pelvis (Figs 4.114–4.116). The addition of both gray scale and CFI can be useful during these procedures to provide a means of assessing structures which are not seen by laparoscopic visualization. During a cholecystectomy, for example, CFI can help identify the location of the common bile duct and determine the nature of other tubular stuctures within the porta hepatis to differenti- ate bile ducts from adjacent vessels (Fig. 4.117). At times it may be necessary to perform pulsed Doppler with spectral analysis to better characterize bloodflow (e.g. to differentiate arteries from veins). Laparoscopic ultrasound, both with and without CFI, has also proven useful to guide intraoperative needle biopsies, to determine the location of vessels both within and adjacent to tumors, and to minimize exploration in patients with severe adhesions.

Diagnostic ultrasound plays an important role during the cryosurgical ablation of tumors. In these cases, CFI can be useful to determine the location of adjacent vessels, or to detect abnormal vascularity in lesions that are not well visualized with gray scale imaging alone. With ultrasound guidance the thera- peutic probes can be correctly positioned to provide optimal freezing and destruction of a lesion, while sparing normal tissue and avoiding damage to adjacent structures.

Finally, intraoperative CFI can be used as a screen- ing device to identify situations where intraoperative angiography is indicated. With continued refinements in technology, including improvements in transducer configurations and higher resolution imaging, the use of intraoperative ultrasound with CFI is expected to expand to meet the needs of surgeons and reduce the complication rates of current and future surgical procedures.

CONCLUSION

CFI has proven useful in the evaluation of a wide range of abnormalities within the abdomen and retroperitoneum. Its uses include detection of blood- flow in normal and abnormal vessels, and the quali- tative analysis of focal areas of increased or decreased parenchymal flow. The detection of arterial stenoses, especially of the renal arteries, is an important application of CFI, especially in patients who are not candidates for diagnostic angiography. CFI can also aid in the evaluation of patients with portal hypertension, being used for the detection of portal vein thromboses and varices, and the evalua-

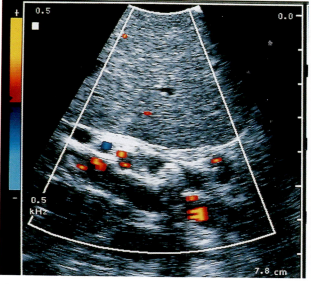

a

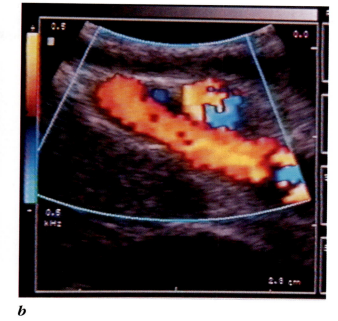

b

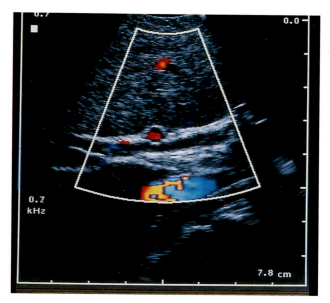

c

Figure 4.117 *Laparoscopic CFI is useful for differentiating vascular from non-vascular structures and demonstrating their spatial relationships within the porta hepatis during cholecystectomies. In this case (a) an unsuspected common bile duct stone (identified as a bright reflector with acoustic shadowing) was detected in a patient with known gallbladder stones. In a different case (b), laparoscopic CFI confirms this tubular structure to represent a normal caliber bile duct. Adequate near field resolution is critical for intraoperative examinations of this type. In a third case (c) laparoscopic CFI identifies a normal variation of the anatomy near the porta hepatis, with the bile duct situated between the portal vein posteriorly and the hepatic artery anteriorly.*

tion of flow through portosystemic shunts. Detecting bloodflow in tumor vessels can be accomplished non-invasively using CFI, which also can help identify the host organ of a tumor in cases where this is not readily apparent. Surgical procedures, both open and laparoscopic, can often be performed in a more timely fashion while obtaining a higher rate of success with the addition of gray scale and color flow imaging. The future introduction of vascular ultrasound contrast agents, which enhance the amplitude of both color and spectral Doppler signals and improve flow detectability, will undoubtedly increase the utilization of CFI for diagnosing a variety of abnormalities throughout the body.

FURTHER READING

TEXTBOOKS

Merritt CRB (ed.), *Doppler Color Imaging*, Clinics in Diagnostic Ultrasound **27** (Churchill Livingstone: New York, 1992).

Goldberg BB (ed.), *Textbook of Abdominal Ultrasound* (Williams & Wilkins: Baltimore, 1993).

Hagen-Ansert SL (ed.), *Textbook of Diagnostic Ultrasonography*, 4th edn (Mosby-Year Book: St. Louis, 1995).

GREAT VESSEL APPLICATIONS

Bluth EI, Murphey SM, Hollier LH, Sullivan MA. Color flow Doppler in the evaluation of aortic aneurysms, *Int Angiol* (1990) **9**:8–10.

Harris DD, Ruckle H, Gaskill DM et al, Intraoperative ultrasound: determination of the presence and extent of vena caval tumor thrombus, *Urology* (1994) **44**:189–93.

Iliceto S, Nanda NC, Rizzon P et al, Color Doppler evaluation of aortic dissection, *Circulation* (1987) **75**:748–55.

Stringer DA, Krysl J, Manson D et al, The value of Doppler sonography in the detection of major vessel thrombosis in the neonatal abdomen, *Pediatr Radiol* (1990) **21**:30–3.

Uno A, Ishida H, Naganuma H et al, Color Doppler findings in small abdominal aneurysms, *Abdominal Imaging* (1994) **19**:410–12.

Zwiebel WJ, Aortic and iliac aneurysms, *Seminars in Ultrasound, CT, MR* (1992) **13**:53–68.

HEPATIC APPLICATIONS

Abu-Yousef MM, Normal and respiratory variations of the hepatic and portal venous duplex Doppler waveforms with simultaneous electrocardiographic correlation, *J Ultrasound Med* (1992) **11**:263–8.

Bolondi L, Bassi SL, Gaiani S et al, Liver cirrhosis: changes of Doppler waveform of hepatic veins, *Radiology* (1991) **178**:513–16.

Buonamico P, Sabba C, Echo Doppler duplex scanner and color in the study of portal hypertension, *J Clin Gastroenterol* (1991) **13**:342–7.

Foshager MC, Ferral H, Finlay DE et al, Color Doppler sonography of transjugular intrahepatic portosystemic shunts (TIPS), *AJR* (1994) **163**:105–11.

Fraser-Hill MA, Atri M, Bret PM et al, Intrahepatic portal venous system: variations demonstrated with duplex and color Doppler US, *Radiology* (1990) **177**:523–6.

Golli M, Mathieu D, Anglade M et al, Focal nodular hyperplasia of the liver: value of color Doppler US in association with MR imaging, *Radiology* (1993) **187**:113–17.

Golli M, Van Nhieu J, Mathieu D et al, Hepatocellular adenoma: color Doppler US and pathologic correlations, *Radiology* (1994) **190**:741–744.

Goyal AK, Pokharna DS, Sharma SK, Effects of a meal on normal and hypertensive portal venous systems: a quantitative ultrasonographic assessment, *Gastrointest Radiol* (1989) **14**:164–6.

Grant EG, Tessler F, Perrella R, Color Doppler invaluable in imaging liver vessels, *Diagnostic Imaging* (1989) **11**:90–4.

Grant E, Perrella R, Tessler F. Budd-Chiari syndrome: the results of duplex and color Doppler imaging, *AJR* (1989) **152**:377–81.

Grant EG, Tessler FN, Gomes AS et al, Color Doppler imaging of portosystemic shunts, *AJR* (1990) **154**:393–7.

Kawasaki T, Moriyasu F, Kimura T et al, Hepatic function and portal hemodynamics in patients with liver cirrhosis, *Am J Gastroenterol* (1990) **85**:1160–4.

Koslin DB, Mulligan SA, Berland LL, Duplex assessment of the portal venous system, *Semin Ultrasound, CT, MR* (1992) **13**:22–33.

Lafortune M, Patriquin J, Pomier G, Hemodynamic changes in portal circulation after portosystemic shunts: use of duplex sonography in 43 patients, *AJR* (1987) **149**:701–6.

Lee D, Ko Y, Yoon Y, Lim J, Sonography and color Doppler imaging of Budd-Chiari syndrome of membranous obstruction of the inferior vena cava, *J Ultrasound Med* (1994) **13**:159–63.

Leen E, Goldberg JA, Robertson J et al, Detection of hepatic metastases using duplex/color Doppler sonography, *Ann Surg* (1991) **214**:599–604.

Lencioni R, Caramella D, Bartolozzi C. Hepatocellular carcinoma: use of color Doppler US to evaluate response to treatment with percutaneous ethanol injection, *Radiology* (1995) **194**:113–18.

Li D, Dong B, Wu Y, Yan K, Image-directed and color Doppler studies of gallbladder tumors, *J Clin Ultrasound* (1994) **22**:551–5.

McGrath F, Lee S, Gibney R, Color Doppler imaging of the cystic artery, *J Clin Ultrasound* (1992) **20**:433–8.

Numata K, Tanaka K, Mitsui K et al, Flow characteristics of hepatic tumors at color Doppler sonography: correlation with arteriographic findings, *AJR* (1993) **160**:515–21.

Ralls PW. Color Doppler sonography of the hepatic artery and portal venous system, *AJR* (1990) **155**:517–25.

Ralls PW, Mayekawa DS, Lee KP et al, The use of color Doppler sonography to distinguish dilated intrahepatic ducts from vascular structures, *AJR* (1989) **152**:291–2.

Ralls PW, Johnson MB, Lee KP et al, Color Doppler sonography in hepatocellular carcinoma, *Am J Physiol Imaging* (1991) **6**:57–61.

Ralls PW, Johnson MB, Radin DR et al, Budd-Chiari syndrome: detection with color Doppler sonography, *AJR* (1992) **159**:113–16.

Tanaka S, Kitamura T, Fujita M et al, Color Doppler flow imaging of liver tumors, *AJR* (1990) **154**:509–14.

Tanaka K, Inoue S, Numata K et al, Color Doppler sonography of hepatocellular carcinoma before and after treatment by transcatheter arterial embolization, *AJR* (1992) **158**:541–6.

Tanaka K, Numata K, Okazaki H et al, Diagnosis of portal vein thrombosis in patients with hepatocellular carcinoma: efficacy of color Doppler sonography compared with angiography, *AJR* (1993) **160**:1279–83.

Tessler FN, Gehring BJ, Gomes AS et al, Diagnosis of portal vein thrombosis: value of color Doppler imaging, *AJR* (1991) **157**:293–6.

RENAL APPLICATIONS

Alexander AA, Merton DA, Mitchell DG et al, Rapid diagnosis of renal vein thrombosis using color Doppler imaging, *J Clin Ultrasound* (1993) **21**:468–71.

Baker SM, Middleton WD, Color Doppler sonography of ureteral jets in normal volunteers: importance of the relative specific gravity of urine in the ureter and bladder, *AJR* (1992) **159**:773–5.

Beduk Y, Erden I, Gogus O et al, Evaluation of renal morphology and vascular function by color flow Doppler sonography immediately after extracorporeal shock wave lithotripsy, *J Endourol* (1993) **7**:457–60.

Berland L, Koslin D, Routh W, Keller F, Renal artery stenosis: prospective evaluation of diagnosis with duplex US compared with angiography, *Radiology* (1990) **174**:421–3.

Bude R, Rubin J, Adler R, Power versus conventional color Doppler sonography: comparison in the depiction of normal intrarenal vasculature, *Radiology* (1994) **192**:777–80.

Burge HJ, Middleton WD, McClennan BL, Hildebolt CF, Ureteral jets in healthy subjects and in patients with unilateral ureteral calculi: comparison with color Doppler US, *Radiology* (1991) **180**:437–42.

Cox IH, Erickson. SJ, Foley WD, Dewire DM, Ureteric jets: evaluation of normal flow dynamics with color Doppler sonography, *AJR* (1992) **158**:1051–5.

Deane C, Cowan N, Giles J et al, Arteriovenous fistulas in renal transplants: color Doppler ultrasound observations, *Urol Radiol* (1992) **13**:211–17.

Denys A, Hélénon O, Souissi M et al, Color and pulsed Doppler of renal masses. Angiographic and anatomo-pathological correlation, *J Radiologie* (1991) **72**:599–608.

Desberg A, Paushter D, Lammert G et al, Renal artery stenosis: evaluation with color Doppler flow imaging, *Radiology* (1990) **177**:749–53.

Dubbins PA, Renal artery stenosis: duplex Doppler evaluation, *Br J Radiol* (1986) **59**:225–9.

Eggli KD, Eggli D, Color Doppler sonography in pyelonephritis, *Pediatr Radiol* (1992) **22**:422–5.

Grenier N, Douws C, Morel D et al, Detection of vascular complications in renal allografts with color Doppler flow imaging, *Radiology* (1991) **178**:217–23.

Healy D, Neumyer M, Renal artery stenosis: diagnosis with color duplex US, *Radiology* (1990) **176**:877–8.

Hélénon D, El Helou N, Thervet E et al, Significance of hypoperfused territories demonstrated by color Doppler ultrasonography following renal transplantation, *Transplant Proc* (1994) **26**:299.

Hélénon O, Attlan E, Legendre C et al, Gd-DOTA-enhanced MR imaging and color Doppler US of renal allograft necrosis. *RadioGraphic* (1992) **12**:21–33.

Hélénon O, Thervet E, Correas J et al, Renal allograft necrosis: value of color Doppler ultrasound and Gd-DOTA-enhanced magnetic resonance imaging, *Transplant Proc* (1994) **26**:300.

Hübsch PJS, Mostbeck G, Barton PP et al, Evaluation of arteriovenous fistulas and pseudoaneurysms in renal allografts following percutaneous needle biopsy, *J Ultrasound Med* (1990) **9**:95–100.

Ikegami M, Tahara H, Hara V et al, Tissue characterization of renal transplant rejection by color Doppler, *Transplant Proc* (1994) **26**:941–2.

Jafri SZ, Madrazo BL, Miller JH, Color Doppler ultrasound of the genitourinary tract. *Curr Opin Radiol* (1992) **4**:16–23.

Jain S, Pinheiro L, Nanda NC et al, Noninvasive assessment of renal artery stenosis by combined conventional and color Doppler ultrasound, *Echocardiography* (1990) **7**:679–88.

Johnson CP, Foley WD, Gallagher LS et al, Evaluation of renal transplant dysfunction using color Doppler sonography, *Surg Gynecol Obstet* (1991) **173**:279–84.

Kier R, Taylor K, Feyock A, Ramos I, Renal masses: characterization with Doppler US, *Radiology* (1990) **176**:703–7.

Martensson O, Duchek M, Translabial ultrasonography with pulsed colour-Doppler in the diagnosis of female urethral diverticula, *Scand J Urol Nephrol* (1994) **28**:101–4.

Mulligan SA, Koslin DB, Berland LL, Duplex evaluation of native renal vessels and renal allografts, *Semin Ultrasound, CT, MR* (1992) **13**:40–52.

Needleman L, Ultrasonography of renal transplants. In: Resnick, Rifkin ML, eds *Ultrasonography of the Urinary Tract*, 3rd edn (Williams & Wilkins: Baltimore, 1991) 436–56.

Patriquin H, Doppler examination of the kidney in infants and children, *Urol Radiol* (1991) **12**:220–7.

Platt JF, Duplex Doppler evaluation of native kidney dysfunction: obstructive and nonobstructive disease, *AJR* (1992) **158**:1035–42.

Platt JF, Rubin JM, Ellis JH, DiPietro MA, Duplex Doppler US of the kidney: differentiation of obstructive from nonobstructive dilatation, *Radiology* (1989) **171**:515–17.

Renowden SA, Duplex and colour flow sonography in the diagnosis of post-biopsy arteriovenous fistulae in the transplant kidney, *Clin Radiol* (1992) **45**:233–7.

Schwerk W, Restrepo I, Stellwaag M et al, Renal artery stenosis: grading with image-directed Doppler US evaluation of renal resistive index, *Radiology* (1994) **190**:785–90.

Stavros AT, Parker SH, Yakes WF et al, Segmental stenosis of the renal artery: pattern recognition of tardus and parvus abnormalities with duplex sonography, *Radiology* (1992) **184**:487–92.

Sullivan RR, Johnson MB, Lee KP, Ralls PW, Color Doppler sonographic findings in renal vascular lesions, *J Ultrasound Med* (1991) **10**:161–5.

Visser MO, Leighton JO, Bor MVD, Walther FJ, Renal bloodflow in neonates: quantification with color flow and pulsed Doppler US, *Radiology* (1992) **183**:441–4.

Willi UV, Pediatric genitourinary imaging, *Curr Opin Radiol* (1991) **3**:936–45.

Yura T, Yuasa S, Sumikura T et al, Doppler sonographic measurement of phasic renal artery bloodflow velocity in patients with chronic glomerulonephritis, *J Ultrasound Med* (1993) **12**:215–19.

Goerg C, Schwerk W, Color Doppler imaging of focal splenic masses, *Eur J Radiol* (1994) **18**:214–19.

Golzarian J, Braude P, Bank W, Case report: colour Doppler demonstration of pseudoaneurysms complicating pancreatic pseudocysts, *Br J Radiol* (1994) **67**:91–3.

Itoh K, Suzuki O, Yasuda Y, Aihara T, Evaluation of bloodflow in tumor masses by using 2D-Doppler color flow mapping—case reports, *Angiology* (1987) **38**:705–11.

Iwase H, Kyogane K, Suga S, Morise K, Endoscopic ultrasonography with color Doppler function in the diagnosis of rectal variceal bleeding, *J Clin Gastroenterol* (1994) **19**:227–30.

Kahn L, Kamen C, McNamara M Jr, Variable color Doppler appearance of pseudoaneurysm in pancreatitis. *AJR* (1994) **162**:187-188.

Koslin DB, Muligan SA, Berland LL, Duplex assessment of the splanchnic vasculature, *Semin Ultrasound, CT, MR* (1992) **13**:34–9.

Lam A, Firman K, Value of sonography including color Doppler in the diagnosis and management of long standing intususception, *Pediatr Radiol* (1992) **22**:112–14.

Merton DA, Needleman L, Alexander AA et al, Lipoblastoma: diagnosis with computed tomography, ultrasound and color Doppler imaging, *J Ultrasound Med* (1992) **11**:549–52.

Nghiem D, Ludrosky L, Young J, Evaluation of pancreatic circulation by duplex color Doppler flow sonography, *Transplant Proc* (1994) **26**:466.

Quillin S, Siegel M, Color Doppler US of children with acute lower abdominal pain, *Radiographics* (1993) **13**:1281–93.

Quillin S, Siegel M, Appendicitis: efficacy of color Doppler sonography, *Radiology* (1994) **191**:557–60.

Quillin S, Siegel M, Gastrointestinal inflammation in children: color Doppler ultrasonography, *J Ultrasound Med* (1994) **13**:751–6.

Taylor GA, Perlman EJ, Scherer LR et al, Vascularity of tumors in children: evaluation with color Doppler imaging, *AJR* (1991) **157**:1267–71.

Wilson SR, Thurston WA, Gastrointestinal sonography, *Curr Opin Radiol* (1992) **4**:69–77.

MISCELLANEOUS APPLICATIONS (PANCREAS, SPLEEN, GASTROINTESTINAL, AND TUMORS)

Altorjay I, Erdelyi L, Newest method for the detection of chronic intestinal ischemia: color Doppler sonography, *Orvosi Hetilap* (1992) **133**:2025–8.

PROSTATE AND OTHER ENDORECTAL APPLICATIONS

Alexander AA, To color Doppler image the prostate or not: that is the question, *Radiology* (1995) **195**:11–13.

Alexander AA, Liu JB, Palazzo JP et al, Endorectal color and duplex imaging of the normal rectal wall and rectal masses. *J Ultrasound Med* (1994) **13:**509–15.

Kelly IMG, Lees WR, Rickards D, Prostate cancer and the role of color Doppler US, *Radiology* (1993) **189:**153–56.

Newman JS, Bree RL, Rubin JM, Prostate cancer: diagnosis with color Doppler sonography with histologic correlation of each biopsy site, *Radiology* (1995) **195:**86–90.

Rifkin MD, Sudakoff GS, Alexander AA, Prostate: techniques, results, and potential applications of color Doppler US scanning, *Radiology* (1993) **186:**509–13.

INTRAOPERATIVE APPLICATIONS

Avila NA, Shawker TH, Choyke PL, Oldfield EH, Cerebellar and spinal hemangioblastomas: evaluation with intraopertive gray-scale color Doppler flow US, *Radiology* (1993) **188:**143–7.

Babcock DS, Barr LL, Crone KR, Intraoperative uses of ultrasound in the pediatric neurosurgical patient, *Pediatric Neurosurgery* (1992) **18:**84–91.

Barr LL, Babcock DS, Crone KR, Berger TS, Ball WS, Prenger EC, Color Doppler US imaging during pediatric neurosurgical and neuroradiological procedures, *Radiology* (1991) **181:**567–71.

Duncan WJ, Tyrell MJ, Bharadwaj B, Iyengar SKS, Intraoperative Doppler flow studies: emphasis on colour mapping, *Can J Surg* (1988) **31:**313–18.

Harris DD, Ruckle HC, Gaskill DM Wang Y, Hadley HR, Intraoperative ultrasound: determination of the presence and extent of vena caval tumor thrombus, *Urology* (1994) **44:**189–93.

Kasai H, Makuuchi M, Kawasaki S, Ishizone S, Kitahara S et al, Intraoperative color Doppler ultrasonography for partial-liver transplantation from living donors in pediatric patients, *Transplantation* (1992) **54:**173–5.

Lantz EJ, Charboneau JW, Hallett JW, Dougherty MJ, James EM, Intraoperative color Doppler sonography during renal artery revascularization, *AJR* (1994) **162:**859–63.

Machi J, Sigel B, Intraopertive ultrasonography (Review), *Radiol Clin North Am* (1992) **30:**1085–103.

Machi J, Sigel B, Kurohiji T et al, Operative color Doppler imaging for general surgery, *J Ultrasound Med* (1993) **12:**455–61.

Machi J, Sigel B, Kurohiji T et al, Operative color Doppler imaging for vascular surgery, *J Ultrasound Med* (1992) **11:**65–71.

Rubin JM, Hatfield MK, Chandler WF, Black KL, DiPietro MA, Intracerebral arteriovenous malformations: intraoperative color Doppler flow imaging, *Radiology* (1989) **170:**219–22.

Yamashita Y, Kurohiji T, Hayashi J, Kimitsuki H et al, Intraoperative ultrasonography during laparoscopic cholecystectomy, *Surg Laparosc Endosc* (1993) **3:**167–71.

Chapter 5   Color flow imaging in obstetrics and gynecology

John S Pellerito and Beth R Gross

INTRODUCTION

Color flow imaging (CFI) is quickly becoming a routine part of the ultrasound examination of the female pelvis. Multiple obstetric and gynecologic applications are currently performed utilizing this technique. Obstetric applications include identification of placental and umbilical cord abnormalities as well as diagnosis of congenital anomalies. The combination of color and pulsed Doppler with endovaginal scanning has proven particularly useful for gynecologic evaluations. Endovaginal color flow imaging (EVCF) is used to identify the dominant ovarian follicle or corpus luteal cyst, detect ectopic pregnancy and spontaneous abortion, localize small retained products of conception, characterize adnexal masses, and diagnose ovarian torsion. EVCF also aids in the diagnosis of different types of uterine abnormalities, including endometritis, fibroids, pelvic venous congestion syndrome, and endometrial carcinoma.

EVCF also provides several advantages over gray scale endovaginal sonography (EVS) alone. EVCF allows quick localization of tissue vascularity for pulsed Doppler examination and assessment of local hemodynamics. This improves the identification of placental flow associated with normal intrauterine pregnancy, ectopic pregnancy, spontaneous abortion and retained products of conception compared to transabdominal scanning or EVS alone. EVCF also permits enhanced detection of abnormal tissue perfusion characteristics associated with ovarian and endometrial carcinoma. Through Doppler spectral analysis and waveform characterization of flow patterns, specific diagnoses are made, eliminating the need for computed tomography (CT) or magnetic resonance imaging (MRI) in many cases.

TECHNIQUE

CFI should be considered a dynamic technique which requires adjustment of the color flow parameters according to the indication for examination. Most manufacturers provide color flow preset levels which are used as a general guide or starting point for each examination. These parameters, including color velocity range (pulse repetition frequency, PRF), color gain and color wall filter, are adjusted to enhance color flow information and decrease surrounding noise. To further optimize the color flow examination, the focal zone should be placed at the level of interest.

Color amplitude imaging (CAI) or 'power Doppler' ultrasound is a new CFI modality which produces color flow images based on the integrated Doppler power spectrum. This color mode provides an extended dynamic range which improves the visualization of tissue vascularity. Color amplitude images do not provide velocity or directional information. They are less angle dependent and do not demonstrate aliasing. CAI enhances diagnosis of placental and congenital abnormalities, ovarian torsion, retained products of conception, and uterine and ovarian malignancy.

VASCULAR ANATOMY AND HEMODYNAMICS

Color flow examination requires knowledge of the vascular anatomy and hemodynamic changes of the female pelvis. The vessels most frequently examined in the pelvis include the iliac, uterine and ovarian

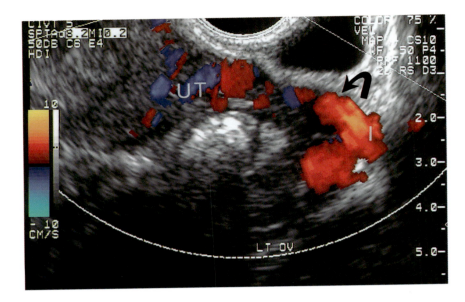

a

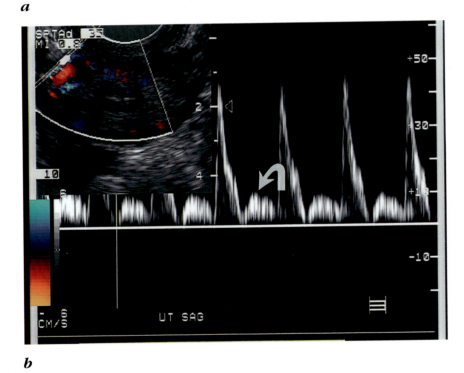

b

Figure 5.1 *Uterine artery. (a) The uterine artery (arrow) originates from the internal iliac artery (I) and courses toward the lower uterine segment (UT). (b) Pulsed Doppler sampling reveals a high-impedance signal with a characteristic diastolic notch (arrow).*

arteries and veins. The uterine artery is a branch of the internal iliac artery. The uterine artery penetrates into the myometrium at the lower uterine segment (Fig. 5.1). Uterine artery branches course toward the fundus and cervix. Color and pulsed Doppler sampling of the uterine artery reveals high-impedance, low-diastolic flow. Branches also cross

the broad ligament to supply the ovary (Fig. 5.2). There is a gradual decrease in resistance to flow during pregnancy due to invasion of the uterine spiral arteries by the growing placenta.

Each ovary receives a dual blood supply. The ovarian artery originates from the abdominal aorta and descends to the pelvis. The ovary also receives

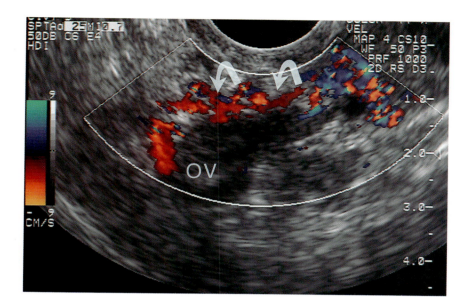

Figure 5.2 *Uterine branches. Uterine artery branches (arrows) cross the broad ligament and penetrate into the right ovary (OV).*

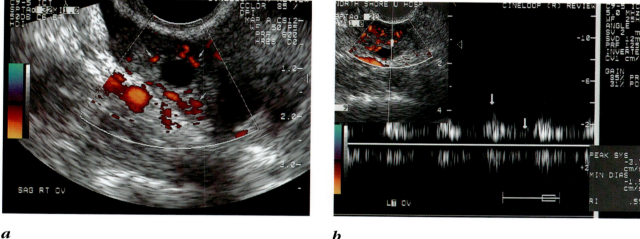

a   *b*

Figure 5.3 *Normal ovary—follicular phase. (a) CAI demonstrates multiple intraovarian vessels (arrows). (b) Pulsed Doppler reveals low-velocity signals with little flow in diastole.*

branches from the uterine artery. Flow patterns observed during color and pulsed Doppler sampling of the ovary depend on the phase of the ovulatory cycle. During the follicular phase, low-velocity, high-impedance waveforms are usually obtained (Fig. 5.3).

The luteal phase coincides with the extrusion of the mature oocyte and formation of the corpus luteal cyst. Thickening of the cyst walls is seen during gray scale imaging. CFI demonstrates a ring of vascularity

('ring of fire' pattern) around the luteal cyst (Fig. 5.4). Pulsed Doppler shows a marked increase in peak systolic and end-diastolic velocities. The increased velocities are related to neovascularization of the corpus luteum required for oocyte maturation and hormonal activity.

Color and pulsed Doppler signals obtained from a postmenopausal ovary typically have low peak systolic velocities, similar to ovaries in the follicular

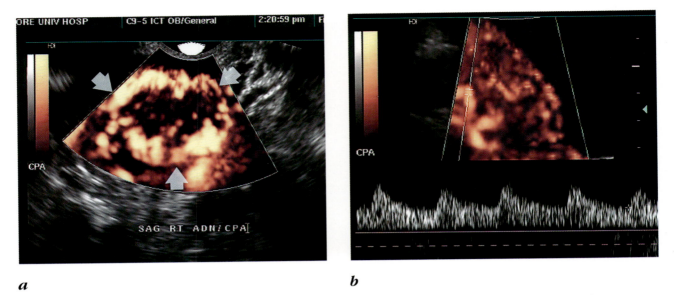

a   *b*

Figure 5.4 *Corpus luteal cyst. (a) A typical 'ring of fire' flow pattern (arrows) is noted around the corpus luteum during CAI. (b) Pulsed Doppler reveals low-impedance flow.*

phase. These vessels may be very difficult to visualize with conventional color flow settings. Low color velocity scale (PRF) and color wall filter adjustments may be necessary to detect postmenopausal ovarian blood flow. CAI improves the visualization of ovarian flow, particularly in postmenopausal women. Since postmenopausal ovaries no longer ovulate, they remain relatively quiescent and are associated with little or no diastolic flow.

OBSTETRIC APPLICATIONS

UMBILICAL CORD ABNORMALITIES

During obstetric ultrasonography, CFI and, more recently, CAI have refined our ability to examine the umbilical cord and placental circulation. Identification of the normal placental cord insertion (Fig. 5.5) is necessary during periumbilical fetal blood sampling and fetal transfusion procedures. CFI assists in the assessment of abnormal cord insertions such as marginal (Fig. 5.6), velamentous cords and vasa previa. Vasa previa is a type of velamentous insertion wherein the umbilical vessels, unsupported by placental tissue or umbilical cord, traverse the fetal

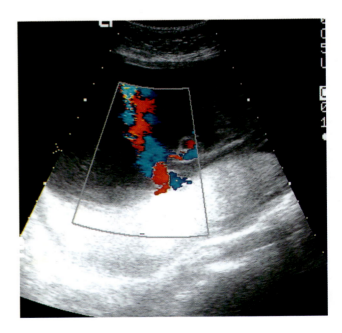

Figure 5.5 *Normal placental cord insertion. Color flow image of a normal cord insertion onto the central placental surface.*

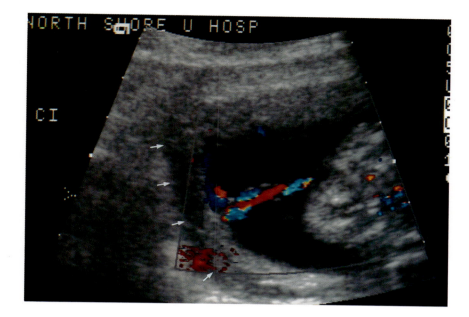

Figure 5.6 *Marginal cord insertion. The umbilical cord inserts at the edge of the placenta (arrows).*

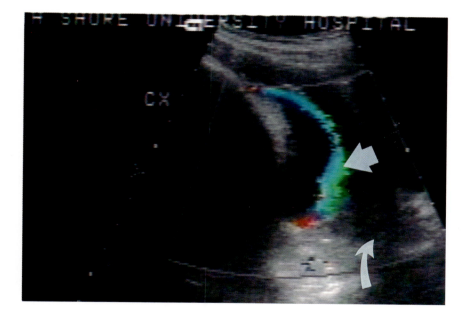

Figure 5.7 *Vasa previa. Transabdominal sagittal color flow image demonstrates umbilical vessels (arrow) covering the cervix (curved arrow).*

membranes of the lower uterine segment in front of the presenting fetal part. Correct diagnosis of this entity prenatally can prevent exsanguination of the fetus from rupture of the umbilical vessels during delivery. Several authors have suggested using EVCF in the evaluation of patients at risk for vasa previa, including low-lying to marginal placenta previa, velamentous cord insertion, succenturiate lobe of the placenta and multiple gestations. CFI and pulsed Doppler can readily delineate umbilical vessels crossing the internal cervical os (Fig. 5.7).

Single nuchal cords are common, being encountered during 20% of births. The presence of cord around the fetal neck and shoulder may be associ-

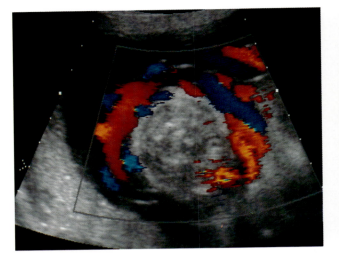

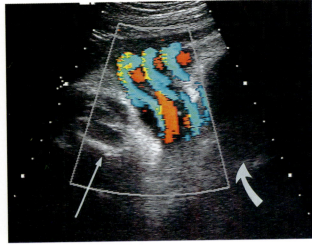

Figure 5.8 *Single nuchal cord. Transverse image through the fetal nuchal region demonstrates a single loop of umbilical cord wrapped around the fetal neck.*

Figure 5.9 *Triple nuchal cord. Sagittal color flow image reveals three loops of umbilical cord around the fetal neck, confirmed at the time of delivery (arrow, fetal shoulder; curved arrow, fetal head).*

ated with fetal heart rate decelerations, especially when oligohydramnios is present. Rarely, a tight nuchal cord may cause fetal strangulation. CFI aids in the diagnosis of single and multiple nuchal cords (Figs. 5.8 and 5.9). Antepartum or intrapartum identification of single or multiple nuchal cords impacts on obstetric management when this finding is consid-

ered in conjunction with other evidence of fetal compromise.

A transverse scan through the fetal pelvis will normally demonstrate both umbilical arteries coursing around the bladder (Fig. 5.10). The recognition of a two-vessel cord is important because of its association with an increased risk of congenital anomalies.

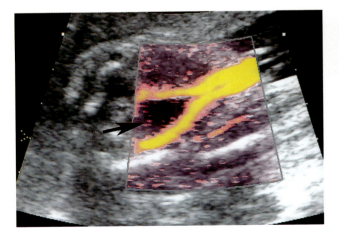

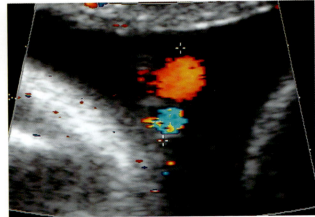

Figure 5.10 *Normal fetal cord insertion. CAI demonstrates two umbilical arteries entering the abdomen and coursing lateral to the fetal bladder (arrow).*

Figure 5.11 *Two-vessel umbilical cord. Transverse image through the umbilical cord reveals a single umbilical artery and vein.*

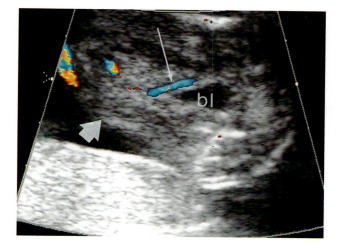

Figure 5.12 *Single umbilical artery. CFI demonstrates a single umbilical artery (long arrow) entering the fetal pelvis at the level of the bladder (bl), in this fetus with an omphalocele (short arrow).*

CFI of the umbilical cord allows for earlier diagnosis of a single umbilical artery (Figs 5.11 and 5.12). Intrinsic cystic masses of the umbilical cord are usually detected during the second and third trimesters. These cysts are associated with abdominal wall defects and chromosomal abnormalities. Color

flow evaluation of umbilical masses distinguishes cysts from vascular structures (Fig. 5.13).

CFI also allows for visualization of communicating placental vessels during the evaluation of monochorionic pregnancies with twin–twin transfusion syndrome and acardiac twins. Identification of these anastomotic vessels is necessary prior to laser coagulation during fetoscopy. This is illustrated in a case of a twin–twin transfusion syndrome associated with adjacent insertions of both umbilical cords, with a thin intervening membrane (Fig. 5.14). Similarly, we diagnosed an amorphous acardiac twin by demonstrating the insertion of a thin cord from the acardiac twin onto the site of the cord insertion of the normal twin (Fig. 5.15).

PLACENTAL ABNORMALITIES

CFI is also useful for identification of abnormal placental development such as placenta accreta. Placenta accreta is a term used to describe abnormal placental invasion of the myometrium. Invasion of the trophoblastic tissue may be superficial (accreta), deep (increta), or through the myometrium to the serosal surface (percreta). The diagnosis of placenta accreta permits for both intensive pregnancy surveillance and preparation of the obstetric and anesthesia teams for a high-risk cesarean section. Gray scale findings suggestive of placenta accreta include

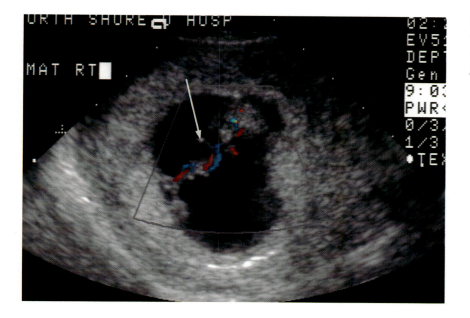

Figure 5.13 *Umbilical cord cyst. Transverse image of an umbilical cord cyst (arrow) in a 13-week pregnancy.*

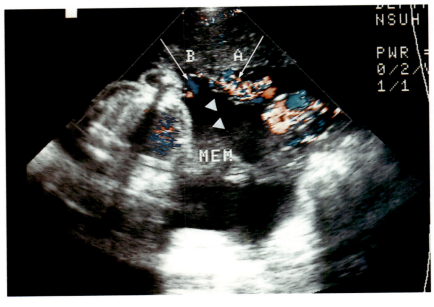

a

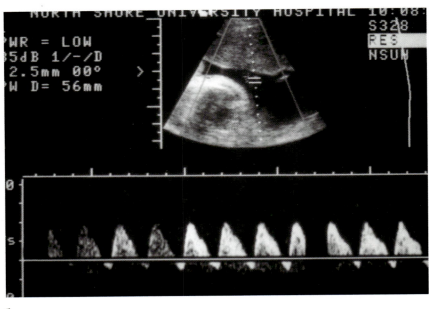

b

Figure 5.14 *Twin–twin transfusion syndrome. (a) CFI demonstrates both umbilical cords inserting into the placenta (arrows), with a thin intervening membrane (arrowheads). The recipient cord (right) is larger than the donor cord. (b) Pulsed Doppler evaluation of the donor umbilical cord demonstrates abnormal arterial waveforms with reversal of flow in diastole.*

absence of the normal retroplacental lucent zone, thinning or disruption of the hyperechoic uterine–bladder interface, or a focal exophytic mass. CFI demonstrated the retroplacental vascularity that represents a continuum of lacunar flow from the placenta through the myometrial layer without an intervening clear space. These findings are striking when a placenta percreta is present (Fig. 5.16).

Color flow evaluation of a placental mass is extremely helpful for the diagnosis of chorioangioma. Chorioangiomata are the most common placental tumors, occurring in 1% of all pregnancies. These

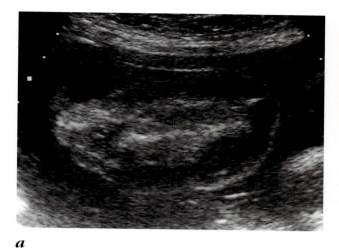

a

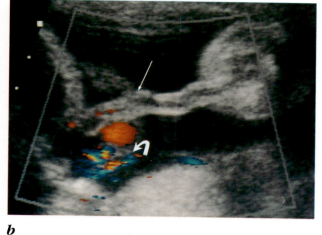

b

c

Figure 5.15 *Acardia. (a) An amorphous acardiac twin is identified. The co-twin was normal. (b) CFI shows the placental insertion of the thin cord of the acardiac twin (arrow) adjacent to the normal cord of the co-twin (curved arrow). (c) Gross specimen of the placental surface demonstrates the thin acardiac (arrows) and normal twin cords. (Reprinted with permission from* The Fetus, **4**:3, 1994.)

tumors are associated with non-immune hydrops. Large lesions are associated with adverse perinatal and maternal outcomes. CFI demonstrates hypervascularity in portions of the mass fed by anomalous branches of chorionic vessels arising from the umbilical cord insertion (Fig. 5.17).

UTEROPLACENTAL CIRCULATION

CFI and CAI improve visualization of small vessels in the placenta. Prior studies of the umbilical–placental circulation have focused primarily on the umbilical cord (Fig. 5.18). Abnormal systolic to diastolic (*S/D*)

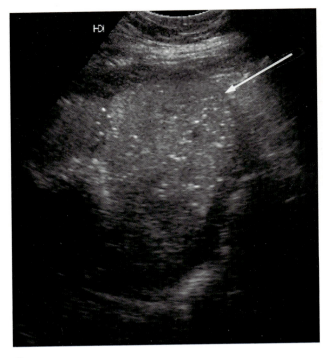

a

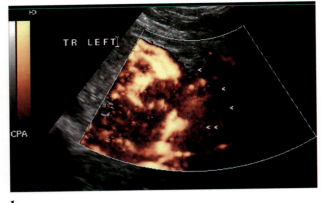

b

Figure 5.16 *Placenta percreta. (a) Transverse image through the uterus in a patient with prior myomectomy and cesarian sections demonstrates focal loss of the normal retroplacental lucent zone from invasion of placental tissue (arrow). (b) CAI demonstrates increased vascularity related to trophoblastic invasion through the myometrium (arrows), which was confirmed at delivery.*

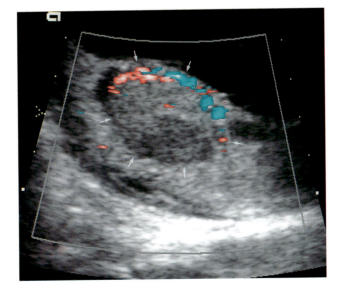

Figure 5.17 *Chorioangioma. This patient presented with polyhydramnios and preterm labor. CFI demonstrates a solid placental mass with peripheral vascularity (arrows).*

flow velocity ratios are reflective of elevated placental flow resistance in pathologic states, commonly associated with fetal growth restriction or hypertension (Fig. 5.14). Giles et al reported that the elevation of vascular resistance of the umbilical artery is a reflection of the obliteration of the tertiary villous arterioles. Improved visualization of intraplacental vessels with CFI has been described in normal and growth retarded pregnancies. With the advent of CAI, we have a powerful tool for investigating the placental villous architecture in normal and compromised fetuses (Fig. 5.19).

CFI allows for easy localization of vessels in the uterine circulation. Early diastolic notching is a normal feature of the uterine arterial waveform prior to 26 weeks of gestation (Fig. 5.20). During the third trimester, the vascular impedance decreases and results in loss of the diastolic notch. The presence of a diastolic or, less commonly, a systolic notch in the hypertensive third trimester patient has been reported to be a predictor of poor pregnancy outcome. Since uteroplacental insufficiency is suspect in pregnancies complicated by hypertension and growth restriction, many investigators have studied uterine arterial velocimetry, with variable results.

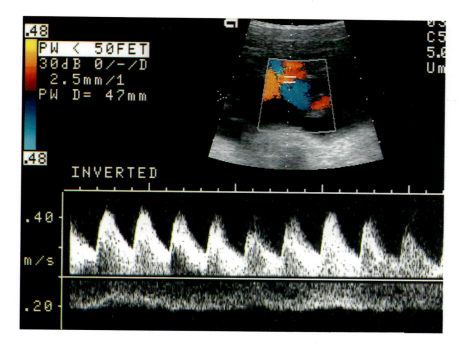

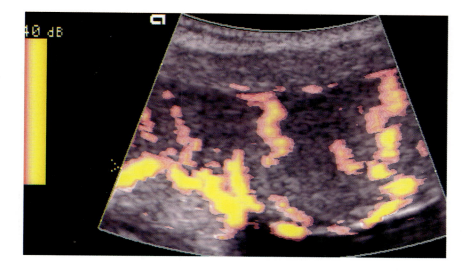

Figure 5.18 *Umbilical artery Doppler. Pulsed Doppler evaluation reveals normal spectral waveforms from the umbilical artery in this 28-week gestation; umbilical venous waveform is seen below the baseline.*

Figure 5.19 *Normal placenta. CAI demonstrates normal placental vasculature in this third trimester pregnancy.*

FETAL CIRCULATION

The investigation of intrafetal vessels has also been pursued in growth-restricted fetuses. It is postulated that the 'brain-sparing' effect which occurs in the setting of fetal hypoxia is associated with decreased vascular resistance in the fetal cerebral circulation, as manifest by Doppler studies of the internal carotid artery and middle cerebral artery. CFI allows for identification of the circle of Willis and aids in the pulsed Doppler interrogation of intracerebral vessels (Fig. 5.21). Conversely, Doppler analysis of the fetal abdominal aorta and renal arteries reveals increased vascular resistance in growth-restricted fetuses.

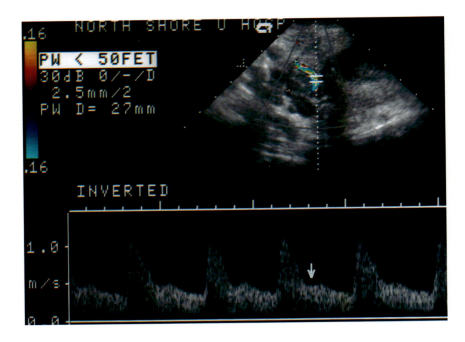

Figure 5.20 *Uterine artery. Normal color Doppler examination of the uterine artery in a 13 week gestation reveals a diastolic notch.*

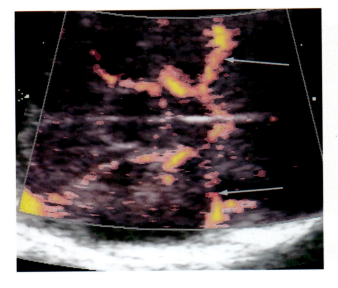

Figure 5.21 *Middle cerebral artery. Color amplitude image demonstrates the middle cerebral arteries (arrows) in the circle of Willis.*

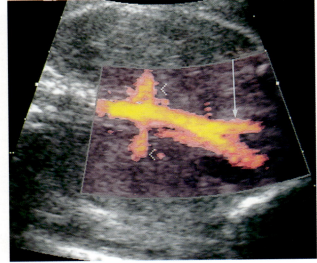

Figure 5.22 *Aorta and renal arteries. CAI of the fetal abdomen depicts the aorta through the iliac bifurcation (long arrow) and the renal arteries (arrowheads).*

Identification of small fetal vessels such as the renal arteries is difficult without the use of CFI (Fig. 5.22). The fetal venous circulation may also provide clues to abnormal fetal development. For example, the ductus venosus is a trumpet-shaped vessel, less than 2 mm in width, which delivers a high-velocity jet of oxygenated blood from the umbilical vein into the inferior vena cava across the foramen ovale. This physiological shunt has diagnostic potential in compromised fetuses, including those with hydrops,

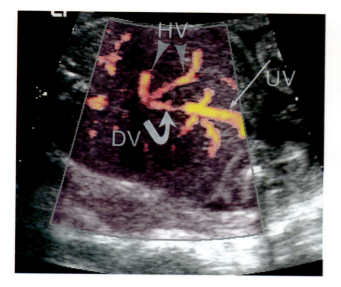

Figure 5.23 *Ductus venosus. Transverse color amplitude image through the fetal liver demonstrates the ductus venosus (DV) between the umbilical vein (UV) and inferior vena cava (IVC). Note the hepatic veins (HV).*

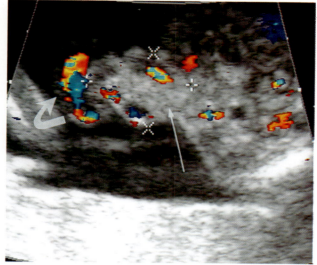

Figure 5.24 *Omphalocele. Color flow examination shows umbilical cord insertion (curved arrow) into the herniated abdominal sac (straight arrow).*

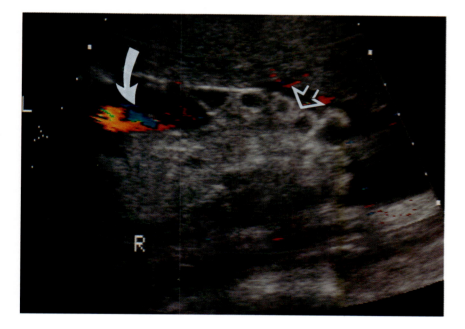

Figure 5.25 *Gastroschisis. CFI shows insertion of the umbilical cord (curved arrow) to the left of the free-floating bowel loops (open arrow).*

congenital heart disease and growth restriction. Identification of the ductus venosus is greatly enhanced with CFI, allowing for differentiation between the ductus venosus and neighboring hepatic veins (Fig. 5.23).

FETAL ANOMALIES

CFI is valuable in the diagnosis of fetal anomalies, especially during the evaluation of abdominal wall abnormalities.

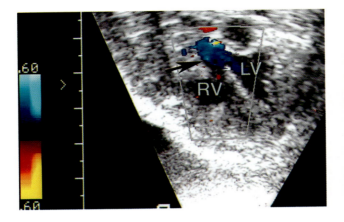

Figure 5.26 *Overriding aorta. Transverse color flow image through the fetal heart shows the outflow jet (arrow) from the left (LV) and right (RV) ventricles into the overriding aorta.*

Evaluation of fetal abdominal wall defects can be difficult when fluid-filled bowel is intermingled with umbilical vessels. CFI allows for delineation of herniated viscera into the base of the umbilical cord associated with an omphalocele (Fig. 5.24), as opposed to herniation adjacent to the cord insertion associated with gastroschisis (Fig. 5.25). CFI is an important component of the fetal heart evaluation (Fig. 5.26). Copel et al found that CFI is helpful in the determination of cardiac anomalies by providing additional directional flow information, especially when the great vessels were abnormal.

GYNECOLOGIC APPLICATIONS

ECTOPIC PREGNANCY

Ectopic pregnancy is an uncommon complication of first trimester pregnancy. The incidence of ectopic pregnancy is increasing due to pelvic inflammatory disease, in vitro fertilization programs and use of Clomid and Pergonal. Any process which produces scarring or obstruction of the fallopian tube predisposes to ectopic pregnancy. This includes infection, prior tubal surgery or instrumentation, endometriosis and prior ectopic pregnancy.

Ectopic pregnancy presents as a sac-like mass or extrauterine embryo in 54% of cases. CFI increases the sensitivity for the diagnosis of ectopic pregnancy

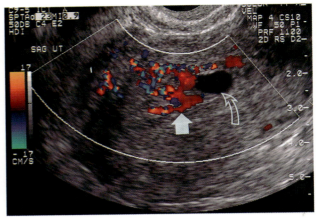

a

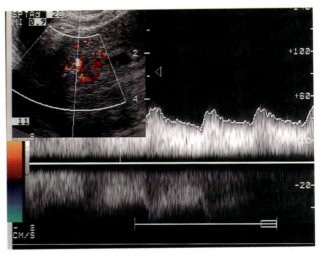

b

Figure 5.27 *Placental flow. (a) EVCF shows a gestational sac within the endometrial canal (arrow). Placental flow is seen within the trophoblast adjacent to the sac (arrowhead). (b) Pulsed Doppler demonstrates low-impedance signals consistent with placental flow.*

through the identification of placental flow in a solid or complex adnexal mass. In a recent study, EVCF demonstrated placental flow in 85% of ectopic pregnancies. Placental flow is recognized as low-impedance (persistent forward diastolic flow) signal localized to the site of placentation in the uterus or adnexa (Fig. 5.27). The low resistance to bloodflow into the intervillous space accounts for the observed low-impedance waveform. The identification of

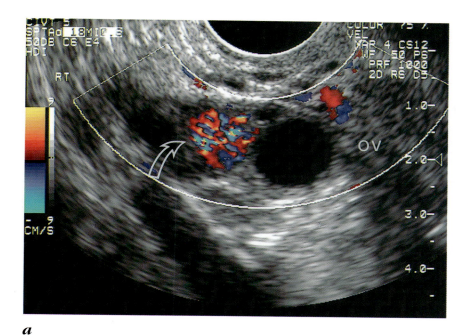

a

Figure 5.28 *Ectopic pregnancy. This patient presented with slowly rising hCG titers, right adnexal pain and no evidence of an intrauterine pregnancy. (a) CFI reveals an area of intense vascularity (arrow) adjacent to the right ovary (OV) representing placental flow from an ectopic pregnancy. (b) Pulsed Doppler sampling shows low-resistance placental flow.*

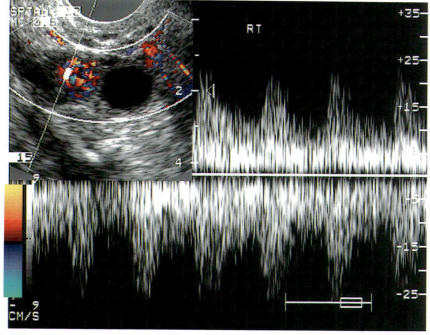

b

placental flow in a mass separate from the ovary confirms the diagnosis of ectopic pregnancy. Ectopic pregnancies may be identified on the basis of placental flow alone even in the absence of a well-defined mass (Fig. 5.28). EVCF is utilized to evaluate the efficacy of treatment of ectopic pregnancy. This is particularly valuable after administration of methotrexate. In a pregnant patient, the detection of placental flow in the adnexa, with or without mass, should suggest ectopic pregnancy.

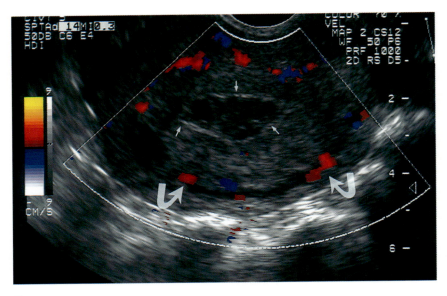

a

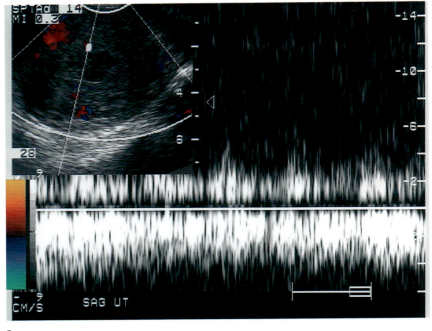

b

Figure 5.29 *Pseudogestational sac. (a) Color flow examination of the endometrial canal reveals an irregular, avascular sac (straight arrows). Color flow is seen in the myometrial arcuate vessels (curved arrows). (b) Pulsed Doppler interrogation confirms absence of placental flow in sac.*

CFI is also useful in characterizing pseudogestational sacs associated with ectopic pregnancies. A pseudosac is recognized as an irregular sac or endometrial thickening representing a decidual reaction from elevated hCG titers. Pseudogestational sacs do not demonstrate a double decidual sac sign, yolk sac, fetal pole or placental flow (Fig. 5.29). The absence of placental flow within an intrauterine sac increases the likelihood of ectopic pregnancy and should prompt a thorough examination of the adnexae.

Identification of placental flow also aids in the diagnosis of spontaneous abortion and gestational trophoblastic neoplasia. Intrauterine placental flow is

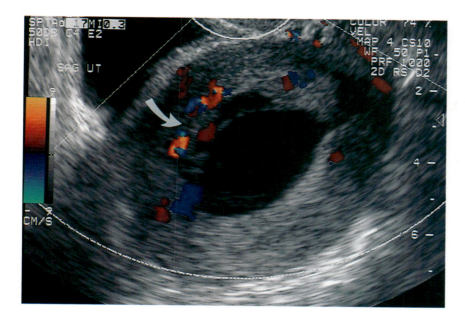

Figure 5.30 *Spontaneous abortion. This patient presented with vaginal bleeding and positive hCG titers. An irregular endometrial sac is seen with peripheral vascularity (arrow) but no fetal pole.*

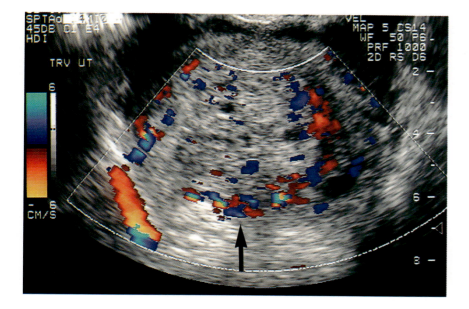

Figure 5.31 *Gestational trophoblastic neoplasia. An echogenic, heterogeneous mass is identified in the uterus in this patient with markedly elevated hCG titers. CFI reveals hypervascularity (arrow) within the endometrium and myometrium due to an invasive mole.*

recognized as a low-impedance signal with a peak systolic velocity of 21 cm/s or greater with an angle of insonation of 0°. In the absence of a normal intrauterine pregnancy, differentiation between an intra- or extrauterine gestation can be extremely difficult. By the detection of intrauterine placental flow, a confident diagnosis of spontaneous or incomplete abortion is made, regardless of the appearance of the adnexa (Fig. 5.30).

Gestational trophoblastic neoplasia may present as a complex or solid uterine mass. Patients will present with elevated serum hCG titers. CFI and pulsed Doppler demonstrate hypervascular flow within the uterus with markedly increased peak systolic velocities (Fig. 5.31).

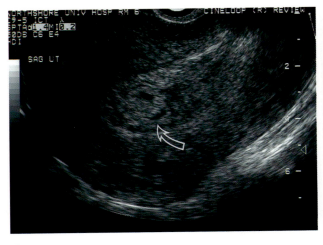

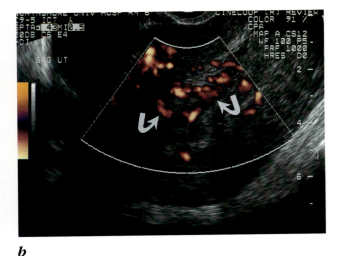

a   *b*

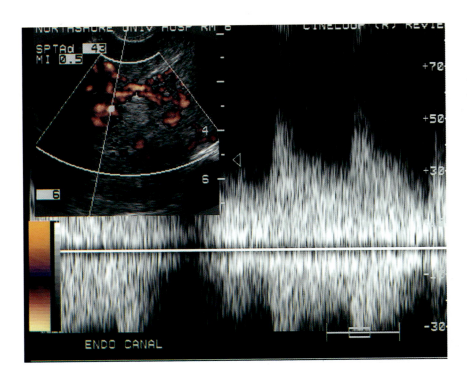

c

Figure 5.32 *Retained products of conception. This patient presented with vaginal bleeding and persistently elevated bCG titers following delivery. (a) Longitudinal image of the uterus demonstrates minimal mass and fluid in the endometrial canal (arrow). (b) CAI shows foci of increased vascularity (arrows) within the endometrial canal. (c) Spectral tracings reveal a high-velocity, low impedance flow pattern consistent with retained placental tissue.*

RETAINED PRODUCTS OF CONCEPTION

Retained products of conception may also demonstrate placental flow. Sonographic findings associated with retained products of conception include an irregular gestational sac, endometrial thickening, and fluid or debris in the endometrial canal. CFI is useful in the diagnosis of retained products by identifying residual trophoblastic tissue and placental flow. Placental flow may be found in the endometrial canal even in the absence of appreciable tissue or mass. Utilizing a peak systolic velocity cutoff of 21 cm/s,

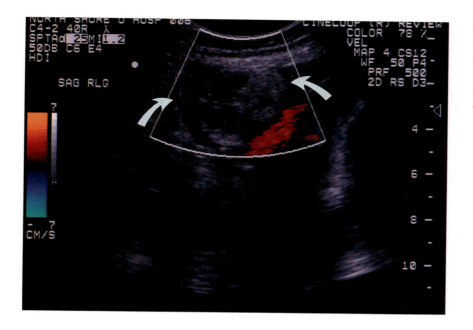

Figure 5.33 *Ovarian torsion. A heterogeneous mass is seen in the right adnexal region. No color flow is seen within the mass (arrows). A torsed dermoid was found at laparoscopy.*

EVCF can distinguish retained products of conception from residual blood clot or complete abortion. Due to its increased sensitivity to flow, CAI may improve the recognition of small retained products of conception (Fig. 5.32).

OVARIAN TORSION

The diagnosis of ovarian torsion relies on the failure to detect arterial flow from within ovarian parenchyma. Most patients with torsion present with

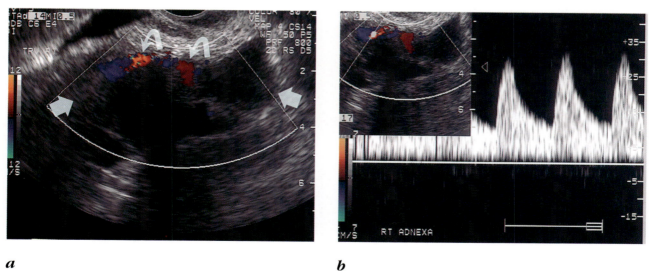

a   *b*

Figure 5.34 *Ovarian cancer. (a) A predominantly solid right adnexal mass (arrows) is seen with areas of abnormal vascularity (curved arrows). (b) Spectral analysis reveals high-velocity, low-impedance waveforms without an early diastolic notch, consistent with malignant neovascularity.*

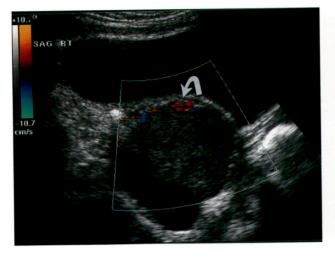

a

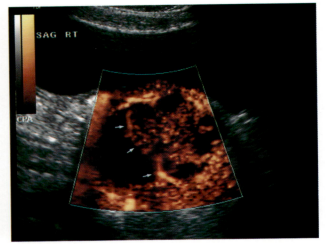

b

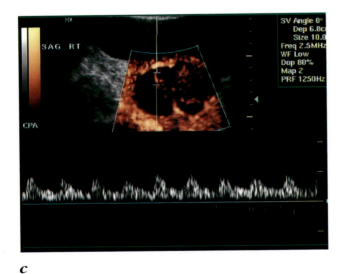

c

Figure 5.35 *Ovarian cancer. (a) CFI reveals a predominantly solid, complex mass with scant peripheral vascularity (arrow). The findings suggest a hemorrhagic cyst. (b) CAI shows marked internal vascularity (arrows) consistent with a solid neoplasm. (c) There is low-impedance flow within the solid component, consistent with tumor vascularity.*

a solid or cystic ovarian mass which serves as the focal point for torsion. The absence of flow within the torsed ovary during CFI, CAI and pulsed Doppler is diagnostic (Fig. 5.33). All color flow parameters must be optimized to ensure that the absence of flow is not related to technical factors, including high PRF, high wall filter or low color gain settings. Arterial flow may be seen only around the periphery of the ovary with chronic torsion due to reactive inflammation. Decreased vascularity may be seen within the ovary with partial torsion.

CHARACTERIZATION OF ADNEXAL MASSES

CFI and pulsed Doppler can demonstrate malignant neovascularity associated with adnexal cancers. Color flow signals representing abnormal vascularity are identified within the complex and solid components of ovarian tumors. CFI permits identification of abnormal vessels and assists in placement of the sample volume for pulsed Doppler examination. Spectral tracings from ovarian cancer demonstrate high-veloc-

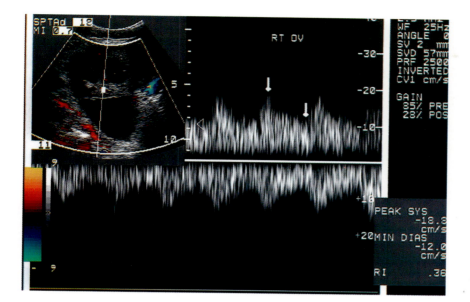

Figure 5.36 *Metastatic ovarian cancer. Color flow is identified within the solid portion of a complex right adnexal mass. Pulsed Doppler demonstrates low-impedance flow consistent with malignant neovascularity.*

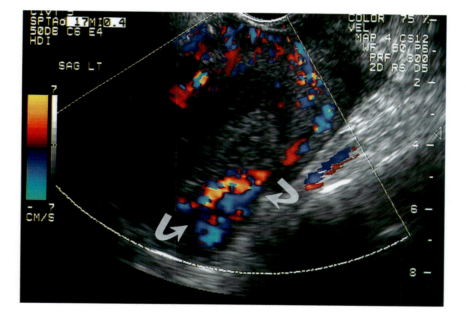

Figure 5.37 *Uterine fibroid. EVCF demonstrates a focal area of increased vascularity (arrows) marking the site of a fundal fibroid.*

ity and/or low-impedance monophasic (continuous) waveforms with no diastolic notch (Fig. 5.34). CAI appears to improve visualization of malignant vascularity compared to conventional CFI (Fig. 5.35).

An endovaginal color flow scoring system was developed to differentiate benign from malignant adnexal masses. EVCF criteria include an elevated ovarian volume, complex morphologic features, elevated peak systolic velocity (PSV >25 cm/s) or low resistive index (RI ≤0.4) and presence of color flow within solid components (Fig. 5.36). In a recent study of 807 EVCF examinations, the EVCF scoring system demonstrated a sensitivity of 94% and specificity of 92% for the detection of pelvic malignancy.

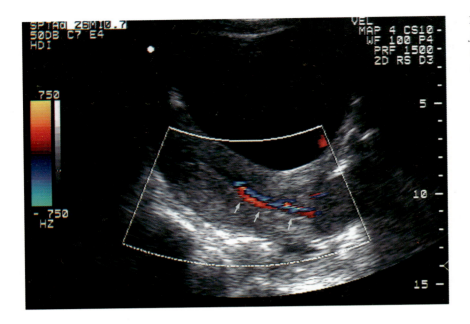

Figure 5.38 *Uterine polyp. Color flow image demonstrates the location of a polyp (arrows) in the endometrial canal.*

The role of EVCF in ovarian cancer screening is not yet defined. Criteria for the identification of early ovarian cancer in the absence of an adnexal mass have not been determined. In addition, data are not available that prove screening alters mortality. Screening large numbers of patients is costly and the appropriate screening intervals are unknown. While EVCF promises earlier detection of ovarian cancer, multicenter trials are needed to justify this application.

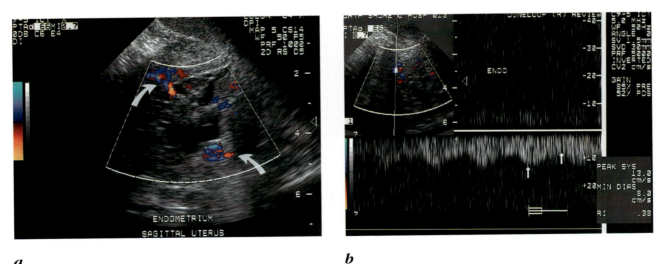

a   *b*

Figure 5.39 *Endometrial cancer. (a) Tumor vessels (arrows) are seen within a thickened, heterogeneous endometrium in this postmenopausal patient. (b) Pulsed Doppler reveals low-impedance flow (RI = 0.38) compatible with malignant neovascularity.*

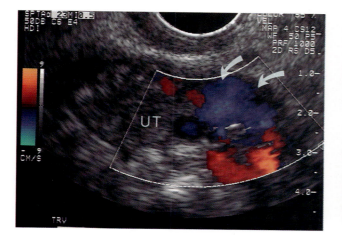

Figure 5.40 *Pelvic congestion syndrome. Enlarged, tortuous pelvic veins (arrow) are noted adjacent to the uterus (UT).*

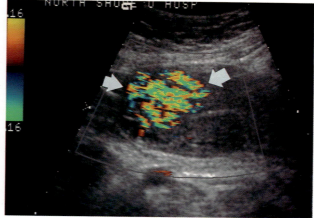

Figure 5.41 *Uterine arteriovenous malformation. A vascular mass (arrows) is identified in the fundal region which proved to be a uterine arteriovenous malformation at surgery.*

UTERINE ABNORMALITIES

CFI is assuming a larger role in the evaluation of uterine abnormalities. CFI may enhance the definition of fibroids (Fig. 5.37) or endometrial polyps (Fig. 5.38) by demonstrating increased vascularity within the mass. EVCF is also utilized to display abnormal vascularity associated with endometrial carcinoma (Fig. 5.39). This is particularly useful in the evaluation of postmenopausal bleeding in patients with a thickened endometrium. The detection of low-impedance bloodflow within a thickened endometrium during pulsed Doppler examination is suspicious for endometrial carcinoma. Enlarged, tortuous parauterine vessels are seen in association with the pelvic congestion syndrome (Fig. 5.40). Patients with this syndrome may present with complaints of non-specific pelvic pain. Unusual vascular lesions, including uterine vascular malformations, are also identified with CFI (Fig. 5.41).

In conclusion, multiple applications of CFI are already defined. Attention to technique and understanding of color flow parameters is key to maximum sensitivity. Integration of clinical and sonographic information as well as recognition of pitfalls improves diagnostic accuracy and reduces misinterpretation.

FURTHER READING

Abuhamad AZ, Copel JA, Color applications and limitations in obstetrics. In: Copel JA, Reed KL, eds, *Doppler Ultrasound in Obstetrics and Gynecology* (Raven Press: New York, 1995) 87–93.

Aoki S, Hata T, Hata K et al, Doppler color flow mapping of an invasive mole, *Gynecol Obstet Invest* (1989) **27**:52–4.

Arts H, van Eyck J, Antenatal diagnosis of vasa previa by transvaginal color Doppler sonography, *Ultrasound Obstet Gynecol* (1993) **3**:276–8.

Bourne TH, Transvaginal color Doppler in gynecology, *Ultrasound Obstet Gynecol* (1991) **1**:359–73.

Bourne TH, Campbell S, Steer C et al, Transvaginal color flow imaging: a possible new screening technique for ovarian cancer, *BMJ* (1989) **299**:1367–70.

Bourne TH, Campbell S, Whitehead MI et al, Detection of endometrial cancer in postmenopausal women by ultrasonography and color flow imaging, *BMJ* (1990) **301**:369.

Chou MM, Ho ESC, Hwang SF et al, Prenatal diagnosis of placental chorioangioma: contribution of color Doppler ultrasound, *Ultrasound Obstet Gynecol* (1994) **4**:332–4.

Copel JA, Morotti R, Hobbins JC et al, The antenatal diagnosis of congenital heart disease using fetal echocardiography: is color flow mapping necessary?, *Obstet Gynecol* (1991) **78**:1–8.

Dillon EH, Feyock AL, Taylor KJW, Pseudogestational sacs: Doppler US differentiation from normal or abnormal intrauterine pregnancies, *Radiology* (1990) **176**:359–64.

Dillon EH, Quedens-Case C, Ramos IM et al, Endovaginal pulsed and color flow Doppler in first trimester pregnancy, *Ultrasound Med Biol* (1993) **19**:517–25.

Feinstein SJ, Lodeiro JG, Vintzileos AM et al, Intrapartum ultrasound diagnosis of nuchal cords as a decisive factor in management, *Am J Obstet Gynecol* (1985)**153**:308–9.

Finberg H, Williams JW, Placenta accreta: prospective sonographic diagnosis in patients with placenta previa and prior Cesarean section, *J Ultrasound Med* (1992) **11**:333–43.

Fleischer AC, Rodgers WH, Rao BK et al, Assessment of ovarian tumor vascularity with transvaginal color Doppler sonography, *J Ultrasound Med* (1991) **10**:295–7.

Fleischer AC, Rodgers WH, Kepple DM et al, Color doppler sonography of ovarian masses: a multiparameter analysis, *J. Ultrasound Med* (1993) **12**:41–8.

Frede TE, Ultrasonic visualization of varicosities in the female genital tract, *J Ultrasound Med* (1984) **3**:365–9.

Giles WB, Trudinger BJ, Baird PJ, Fetal umbilical artery flow velocity waveforms and placental resistance: pathological correlation, *Br J Obstet Gynaecol* (1985) **92**:31–8.

Halvie MA, Silver TM, Ovarian torsion: sonographic evaluation, *J Clin Ultrasound* (1989) **17**:327–32.

Hamper UM, Sheth S, Abbas, FM et al, Transvaginal color doppler sonography of adnexal masses: differences in blood flow impedance in benign and malignant lesions, *AJR* (1993) **160**:1225–8.

Harding JA, Lewis DF, Major CA et al, Color flow Doppler — a useful instrument in the diagnosis of vasa previa, *Am J Obstet Gynecol* (1990) **163**:1566–8.

Hata K, Hata T, Senoh D et al, Change in ovarian arterial compliance during the human menstrual cycle assessed by Doppler ultrasound, *Br J Obstet Gynaecol* (1990) **97**:163.

Hata K, Toshiyuki H, Ritsuto F et al, An accurate antenatal diagnosis of vasa previa with transvaginal color Doppler sonography, *Am J Obstet Gynecol* (1994) **171**:265–7.

Hecher K, Ville Y, Nicolaides KH, Color Doppler ultrasonography in the identification of communicating vessels in twin–twin transfusion syndrome and acardiac twins, *J Ultrasound Med* (1995) **14**:37–40.

Hirata GI, Masaki DI, O'Toole M et al, Color flow mapping and Doppler velocimetry in the management of a placental chorioangioma associated with nonimmune fetal hydrops, *Obstet Gynecol* (1993) **81**:850–2.

Hsieh FJ, Kuo PL, Ko TM et al, Doppler velocimetry of intraplacental fetal arteries, *Obstet Gynecol* (1991) **77**:478–82.

Kirkinen P, Kurmanavichius J, Nuch A et al, Blood flow velocities in human intraplacental arteries, *Acta Obstet Gynecol Scand* (1994) **73**:220–4.

Kiserud T, Eik-Nes SH, Blaas HK et al, Ultrasonographic velocimetry of the fetal ductus venosus, *Lancet* (1991) **338**:1412–14.

Kiserud T, Eik-Nes SH, Hellevik LR et al, Ductus venosus — a longitudinal Doppler velocimetric study of the human fetus, *J Matern Fetal Invest* (1992) **2**:5–11.

Mari G, Deter R, Middle cerebral artery flow velocity waveforms in normal and small-for-gestational-age fetuses, *Am J Obstet Gynecol* (1992) **166**:1262–70.

Matta WHM, Stabile I, Shaw RW et al, Doppler assessment of uterine blood flow changes in patients with fibroids receiving the gonadotropin-releasing hormone agonist Buserelin, *Fertil Steril* (1988) 1083–5.

Megier P, Desroches A, prenatal color Doppler diagnosis of placenta previa accreta, *Ultrasound Obstet Gynecol* (1994) **4**:437.

Nyberg DA, Mahony BS, Luthy D et al, Single umbilical artery: prenatal detection of concurrent anomalies, *J Ultrasound Med* (1991) **10**:247–52.

Pattison RC, Norman K, Odendaal HJ, The role of Doppler velocimetry in the management of high risk pregnancies: a randomized controlled trial, *J Matern Fetal Invest* (1993) **3**:182.

Pellerito JS, Taylor KJW, Ectopic pregnancy. In: Copel JA, Reed KL, eds, *Doppler Ultrasound in Obstetrics and Gynecology* (Raven Press: New York; 1995) 41–53.

Pellerito JS, Taylor KJW, Quedens-Case C et al, Ectopic pregnancy: evaluation with endovaginal color flow imaging, *Radiology* (1992) **183**:407–11.

Pellerito JS, Taylor KJW, Case CQ, Current applications of endovaginal color flow imaging, *Radiology* (1994) **193**(P):395.

Pellerito JS, Taylor KJW, Quedens-Case C et al, Endovaginal color flow scoring system: a sensitive indicator of pelvic malignancy, *Radiology* (1994) **193(P)**:276.

Pellerito JS, Troiano RN, Quedens-Case C et al, Common pitfalls of endovaginal color flow imaging, *Radiographics* (1995) **15**:37–47.

Rosado WM Jr, Trambert MA, Gosink BB et al, Adnexal torsion: diagnosis by using Doppler sonography, *AJR* (1992) **159**:1251–3.

Rosemund RL, Kepple DM, Transvaginal color Doppler sonography in the prenatal diagnosis of placenta accreta, *Obstet Gynecol* (1992) **80**:508–10.

Rotmensch S, Liberati M, Luo JS et al, Villous artery flow velocity waveforms and color Doppler flow patterns in placentas of growth-retarded fetuses, *Am J Obstet Gynecol* (1993) **168**:292.

Rotmensch S, Liberati M, Santolaya-Forgas, J et al, Uteroplacental and intraplacental circulation. In: Copel JA, Reed KL, eds, *Doppler Ultrasound in Obstetrics and Gynecology* (Raven Press: New York; 1995) 115–24.

Rubin JM, Bude RO, Carson PL et al, Power Doppler US: a potentially useful alternative to mean frequency-based color Doppler US, *Radiology* (1994) **190**:853–6.

Schulman H, Fleischer A, Stern W et al, Umbilical velocity wave ratios in human pregnancy, *Am J Obstet Gynecol* (1984) **148**:985–9.

Sepulveda W, Pryde PG, Greb AE et al, Prenatal diagnosis of umbilical cord pseudocysts, *Ultrasound Obstet Gynecol* (1994) **4**:147–50.

Skibo LK, Lyons EA, Levi CS, First trimester umbilical cord cysts, *Radiology* (1992) **182**:719–22.

Strong TH, Sarno AP, Paul RH, Significance of intrapartum amniotic fluid volume in the presence of nuchal cord, *J Reproductive Med* (1992) **37**:718–20.

Taylor KJW, Schwartz PE, Screening for early ovarian cancer, *Radiology* (1994) **192**:1–10.

Taylor KJW, Burns PN, Wells PNT. Ultrasound Doppler flow studies of the ovarian and uterine arteries, *Br J Obstet Gynaecol* (1985) **92**:240–6.

Taylor KJW, Schwartz PE, Kohorn EI, Gestational trophoblastic neoplasia: diagnosis with Doppler US, *Radiology* (1987) **165**:445–8.

Taylor KJW, Ramos I, Carter D et al, Correlation of Doppler US tumor signals with neovascular morphologic features, *Radiology* (1988) **166**:57–62.

Thaler I, Weiner Z, Itskovits J, Systolic or diastolic notch in uterine artery blood flow velocity waveforms in hypertensive pregnant patients: relationship to outcome, *Obstet Gynecol* (1992) **80**:277–82.

Tonge HM, Wladimiroff JW, Noordam MJ et al, Blood flow velocity waveforms in the descending fetal aorta: comparison between normal and growth-retarded pregnancies, *Obstet Gynecol* (1986) **67**:851–4.

Trudinger BJ, Giles WB, Cook CM et al, Fetal umbilical artery flow velocity waveforms and placental resistance: clinical significance, *Br J Obstet Gynaecol* (1985) **92**:23–30.

Verdel MJC, Exalto N, Tight nuchal coiling of the umbilical cord causing fetal death, *J Clinical Ultrasound* (1994) **22**:64–6.

Vyas S, Nicolaides KH, Campbell S, Renal artery flow-velocity waveforms in normal and hypoxic fetuses, *Am J Obstet Gynecol* (1989) **161**:168–72.

Wladimiroff JW, Tonge HM, Stewart PA, Doppler ultrasound assessment of cerebral blood flow in the human fetus, *Br J Obstet Gynaecol* (1986) **93**:471–5.

Chapter 6 **Superficial parts**

William D Middleton and Daniel A Merton

INTRODUCTION

Color flow imaging (CFI) is particularly effective in imaging bloodflow in vessels of superficial structures because high-frequency transducers can be employed. The Doppler frequency shift is proportional to the transmitted frequency, with higher-frequency probes resulting in larger Doppler frequency shifts which are easier to separate from background noise. More importantly, the strength of the reflection from small, moving scatterers (e.g. red blood cells) is proportional to the fourth power of the transmitted frequency. Hence, a doubling of the transducer frequency (e.g. from 3.5 to 7.0 MHz) will result in a 16-fold increase in signal strength. This effect also facilitates detection of low-velocity flow in the small vessels of superficial organs.

To date, the superficial organ in which CFI has made the greatest impact is the testis. However, CFI can, at times, be a useful addition to conventional gray scale imaging in the evaluation of the thyroid, breast, eye and orbit, and neonatal brain. Additionally, evaluation of superficial masses occurring throughout the body can often be accomplished more efficiently and thoroughly (and diagnostic confidence levels improved) with CFI than by gray scale or duplex imaging alone. Other superficial-parts applications are still being discovered, as advances in technology such as color amplitude imaging (CAI) (also known as 'power Doppler') improve our abilities to assess bloodflow and, more importantly, pathologies that alter flow in both large and small vessels. These applications include evaluation of tendons, muscles, joints and very superficial structures such as the skin and subcutaneous tissues.

SCROTUM AND TESTIS

CFI is excellent at displaying the anatomic relationships of normal testicular vessels. Unlike most other organs, the largest arteries of the testis are capsular vessels that travel on the surface of the testis (Fig. 6.1a). The capsular arteries then supply branches called centripetal arteries that enter the testicular parenchyma and course toward the mediastinum (Fig. 6.1a,b). The centripetal arteries then arborize into recurrent rami that course away from the mediastinum (Fig. 6.1b). Traditional anatomic wisdom suggested that it was unusual for major branches of the testicular artery to enter the testis through the mediastinum. However, CFI studies have shown that transmediastinal arteries are actually present in 50% of testes (Fig. 6.1c). Intratesticular veins are not visualized as frequently as intratesticular arteries. However, with improvements in conventional color flow sensitivity and the development of CAI, it is now possible to detect intratesticular veins in many patients (Fig. 6.2).

In the past, ultrasound has had little role in evaluating patients with acute scrotal pain because there was a great deal of overlap in the gray scale findings of testicular torsion and scrotal inflammatory processes such as epididymitis and orchitis. CFI has made it relatively easy to distinguish these conditions in most post-pubertal men. As one would expect, torsion or other causes of ischemia produce asymmetrically diminished (Fig. 6.3) or absent (Fig. 6.4) bloodflow to the affected testis. If the ischemia is not reversed quickly, infarction of the testis occurs which, in turn, can produce an inflammatory reaction in the peritesticular tissues (Fig. 6.5). In addition to

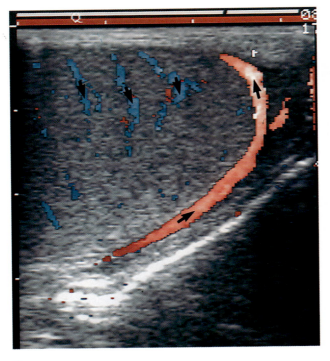

a

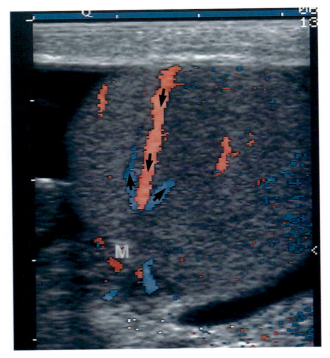

b

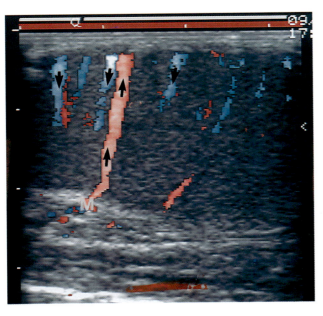

c

Figure 6.1 *Normal testicular vascular anatomy. Longitudinal color flow image of the lower pole of a normal testis (a) demonstrates a capsular artery in red at the periphery of the testis and several centripetal arteries in blue within the testis. Flow direction is as indicated by the arrows. Transverse color flow image of the testis (b) demonstrates a centripetal artery in red with bloodflow directed towards the mediastinum (M). Two small recurrent rami branches of the centripetal artery are demonstrated in blue. Flow direction is indicated by the arrows. Longitudinal view of the testis (c) demonstrates a transmediastinal artery in red passing through the mediastinum of the testis (M) and extending to the opposite side of the testicular parenchyma. Although previously thought to be an unusual normal variant, transmediastinal arteries can be seen with CFI in approximately 50% of testes. Also shown are multiple centripetal arteries in blue. Flow direction is indicated by the arrows.*

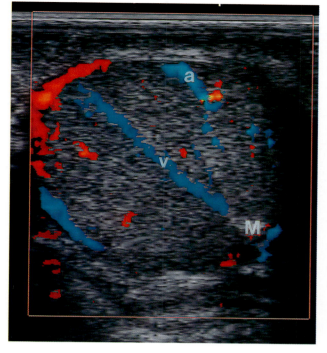

a

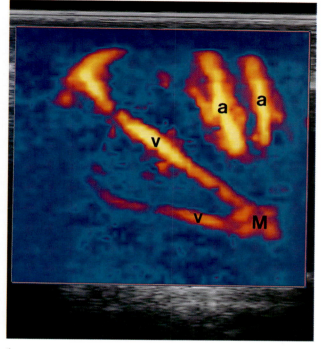

b

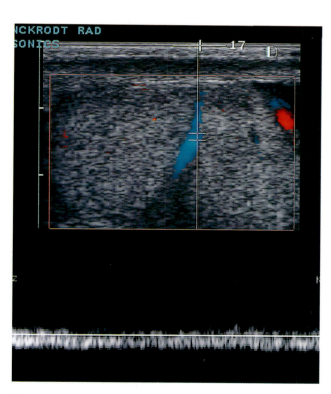

c

Figure 6.2 *Testicular veins. Transverse color flow image of the testis (a) demonstrates two intratesticular vessels, both displayed as blue, indicating flow away from the transducer and, in this case, flow towards the mediastinum (M). The smaller, more anterior vessel is a centripetal artery (a) and the larger vessel that is deeper in the testis is a testicular vein (v). Improved low-flow sensitivity with CFI has made it possible to identify intratesticular veins more often. Color amplitude image of the same testis (b) demonstrates similar vascular anatomy but shows an additional centripetal artery (a) as well as an additional testicular vein (v). Longitudinal color flow image of the testis and accompanying pulsed Doppler waveform (c) shows an intratesticular vessel color-encoded blue. This flow was directed away from the transducer and towards the mediastinum. Based on the CFI appearance, this could represent either a centripetal artery or an intratesticular vein. Waveform analysis is needed in cases such as this in order to determine the type of vessel being imaged. In this case, the pulsed Doppler waveform confirmed that this represented an intratesticular vein.*

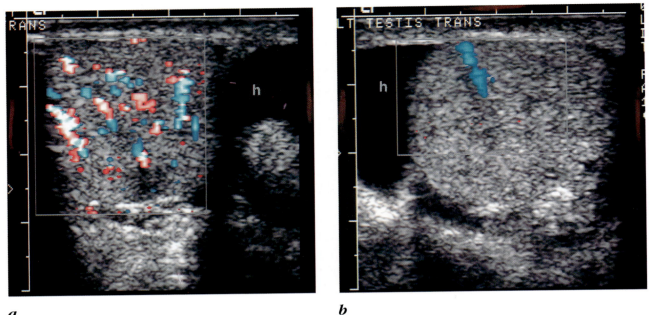

a   *b*

Figure 6.3 *Acute testicular torsion. Transverse color flow image of the asymptomatic right testis (a) demonstrates multiple intratesticular vessels and normal echogenicity. Also seen is a hydrocele (h) on the left side (right side of image). Transverse color flow image of the left testis (b) demonstrates a reactive hydrocele (h). The testis appeared normal on gray scale and had echogenicity similar to the right side. However, only a single intratesticular vessel could be visualized. These findings are consistent with testicular torsion. Subsequent scrotal exploration confirmed left testicular torsion with a viable left testis.*

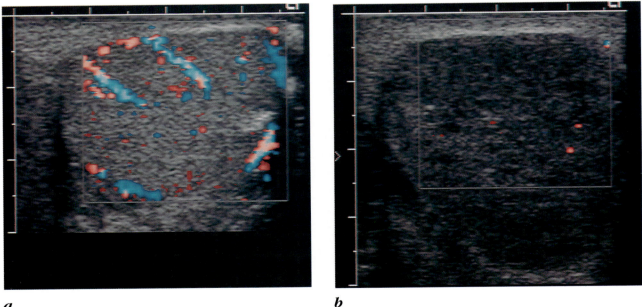

a   *b*

Figure 6.4 *Delayed testicular torsion. Transverse color flow image of the asymptomatic testis (a) demonstrates normal echogenicity and detectable flow in multiple intratesticular vessels. Transverse color flow image of the symptomatic testis (b) demonstrates minimal color noise but no detectable intratesticular vessels. In addition, the testis is enlarged, hypoechoic and somewhat inhomogeneous. These findings are consistent with an infarcted testis. At scrotal exploration, the testis was found to be torsed and infarcted with hemorrhagic necrosis.*

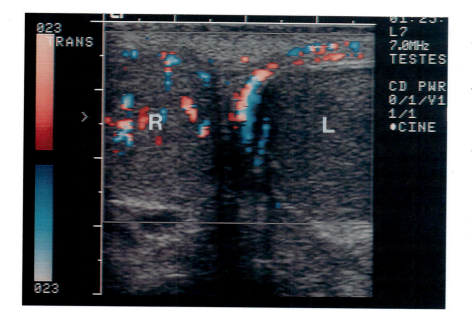

Figure 6.5 *Testicular infarction following inguinal hernia repair. Transverse color flow image of the right (R) and left (L) testes. Normal flow is seen in the right testis but no bloodflow is detected in the left testis. Increased flow is seen around the left testis secondary to peritesticular hyperemia associated with the inflammatory response due to testicular infarction. Also note the decreased echogenicity of the left testis which is indicative of infarction.*

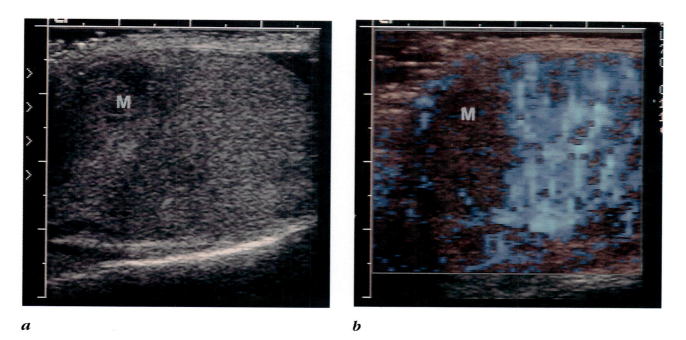

a   *b*

Figure 6.6 *Epididymo-orchitis with focal testicular infarction. Longitudinal color flow image of the testis (a) demonstrates a poorly marginated region of decreased echogenicity in the upper pole of the testis that simulates an intratesticular mass (M). Longitudinal color amplitude image (b) shows that there is increased vascularity in the normal portion of the testis and no flow in the abnormal portion of the testis. These findings, in conjunction with the patient's clinical history, are consistent with epididymo-orchitis with focal testicular infarction due to venous outflow obstruction. This would be an unusual appearance for a tumor, since the vast majority of tumors of this size would have detectable internal vessels. Nevertheless, lesions such as this should be followed to resolution with serial follow-up sonograms.*

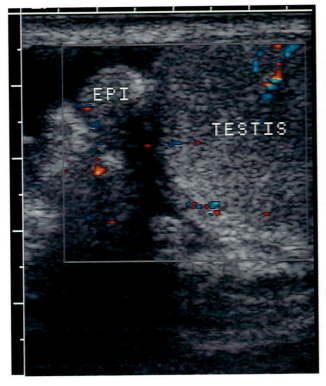

a

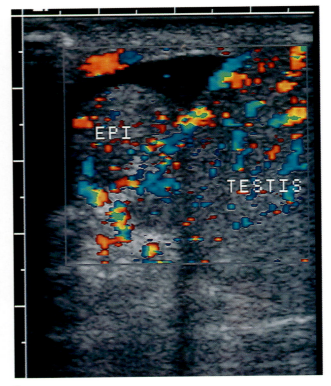

b

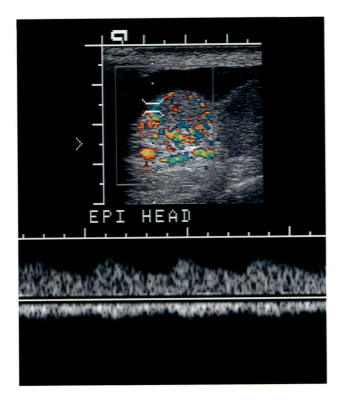

c

Figure 6.7 *Epididymo-orchitis. Longitudinal color flow image of the asymptomatic left testis (a) demonstrates a normal-sized epididymal head (EPI) adjacent to the upper pole of the testis. No vascularity is seen in the epididymal head, which is a normal finding. Longitudinal color flow image of the symptomatic right side (b) demonstrates enlargement of the epididymal head and multiple detectable vessels within the epididymal head (EPI). This is consistent with hypervascularity due to epididymitis. The testis is also hypervascular compared to the contralateral side, consistent with associated orchitis. Color flow image of the symptomatic epididymal head with associated pulsed Doppler waveform (c) again demonstrates epididymal hypervascularity. The waveform confirms a low-resistance-type arterial pattern above the baseline and a venous pattern below the baseline. These findings also support the diagnosis of epididymitis.*

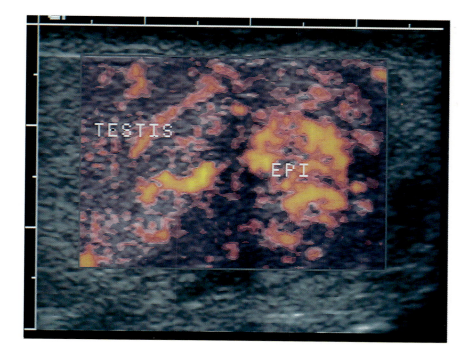

Figure 6.8 *Epididymitis. Longitudinal color amplitude image of the lower pole of the testis and the tail of the epididymis (EPI) shows hypervascularity of the epididymal tail. This developed after an episode of trauma and is consistent with post-traumatic epididymitis.*

torsion, testicular ischemia can be caused by trauma or as a postoperative complication (Fig. 6.5). Epididymitis can also produce testicular ischemia by compressing the peritesticular veins and decreasing the venous outflow. This effect may be focal or diffuse (Fig. 6.6).

Epididymitis and orchitis, on the other hand, produce inflammation and hyperemia of the epididymis and testis (Figs 6.7 and 6.8). Epididymitis may involve the epididymis diffusely or focally, whereas orchitis is generally diffuse. In the unusual cases where orchitis is focal, it can simulate a testicular tumor sonographically (Fig. 6.9). Associated findings that favor a diagnosis of focal orchitis include involvement of the epididymis, laboratory signs of infection, testicular tenderness, and lack of a palpable mass.

CFI plays only a minor role in evaluation of palpable testicular masses. For the most part, any palpable scrotal mass that is shown on sonography to be solid or complex and intratesticular in location is likely to be a tumor and needs to be removed. Initially, there was hope that CFI could help to distinguish benign and malignant testicular lesions and to differentiate the various types of malignant testicular tumors. Unfortunately, the color flow findings depend more on the size of the tumor than on the histology. Tumors larger than 1.5 cm are usually hypervascular (Figs 6.10–6.13) and tumors equal to or less than 1.5 cm are hypovascular or avascular. One situation where CFI is somewhat helpful is when a large intratesticular lesion is shown to be hypovascular. This suggests that the lesion is something other than a tumor and, if the clinical circumstances are appropriate, lesions such as these can be treated conservatively and followed with serial sonograms (Fig. 6.6). Another potential area where CFI can be helpful is in patients with lymphoma or leukemia who have diffuse bilaterally symmetric tumor infiltration of the testes. This abnormality can be difficult to detect with gray scale sonography but is usually easily detected with CFI due to the associated testicular hypervascularity.

CFI is also useful for the evaluation of suspected varicoceles. The underlying abnormality is incompetent valves in the testicular vein that allow retrograde bloodflow into the pampiniform plexus. This generally causes enlargement of the veins in the plexus and may cause infertility. On CFI, the dilated peritesticular veins are visualized as tortuous tubular structures, usually located lateral, superior and posterior to the testis. At rest, the flow in the veins is usually

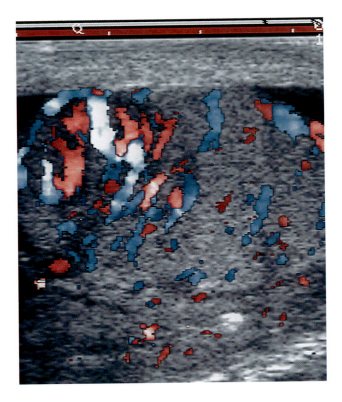

Figure 6.9 *Focal orchitis. Longitudinal color flow image of the symptomatic testis demonstrates a vague zone of decreased echogenicity in the upper pole. There is marked focal hypervascularity in this region of abnormality. Although this appearance is non-specific and could be seen with neoplastic disorders, this patient also had an enlarged hypervascular epididymis, which makes an inflammatory etiology more likely. In addition, the patient's clinical history was consistent with an inflammatory/infectious process. The abnormality seen on sonography corresponded with an area of tenderness on physical examination but no palpable mass. In a case such as this, follow-up examination should be performed following appropriate antibiotic treatment to ensure that the focal testicular abnormality resolves.*

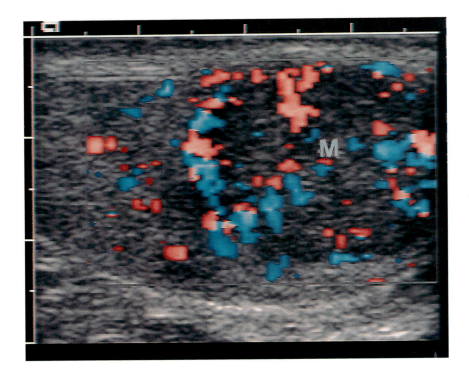

Figure 6.10 *Seminoma. Longitudinal color flow image of the testis demonstrates a homogeneous hypoechoic mass (M) in the lower pole which is hypervascular compared to the adjacent testicular parenchyma. Unlike the previous case of focal orchitis, this mass was readily palpable as a firm lower pole lesion and was non-tender. The combined findings on sonography and physical examination support the diagnosis of a testicular tumor, and orchiectomy was performed confirming the presence of a seminoma.*

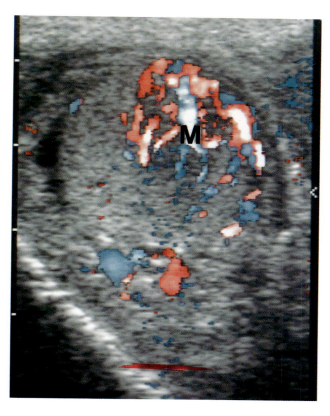

Figure 6.11 *Testicular lymphoma. Transverse color flow image of the lower pole of the testis demonstrates marked focal hypervascularity in a poorly marginated hypoechoic mass (M). The imaging appearance of this abnormality is quite similar to the example of focal orchitis shown in Fig. 6.8. However, this patient did not demonstrate clinical signs of infection and this lesion was firm and readily palpable. Orchiectomy was performed and pathology revealed focal testicular lymphoma.*

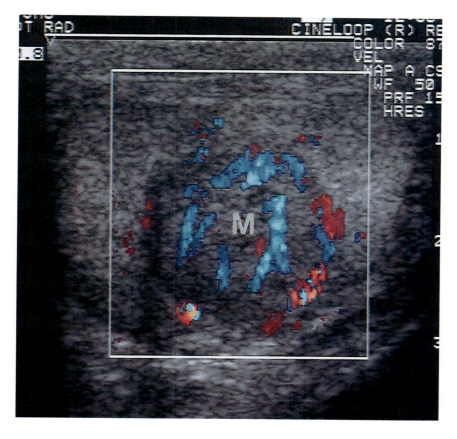

Figure 6.12 *Benign Leydig cell tumor. Transverse color flow image of the testis demonstrates a slightly hypoechoic mass (M) in the testis. This mass is hypervascular when compared to the adjacent testicular parenchyma. Its appearance is similar to the case of seminoma, lymphoma and focal orchitis seen in the previous figures. An orchiectomy was performed and this lesion was shown to be a benign Leydig cell tumor.*

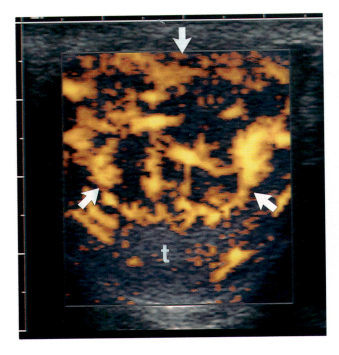

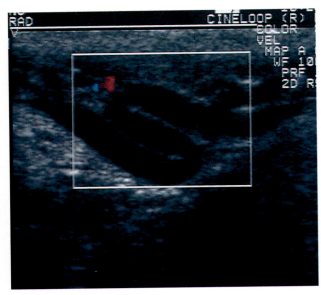

a

Figure 6.13 *Metastatic disease to the testis. Transverse color amplitude image of the testis demonstrates a hypoechoic mass (arrows) with intense hypervascularity when compared to the normal adjacent testicular parenchyma (t). This patient had a history of rhabdomyosarcoma of the maxillary sinus. The gray scale and color flow appearance of the testicular lesion is consistent with either metastatic disease to the testis or a primary testicular neoplasm. Orchiectomy was performed and metastatic rhabdomyosarcoma to the testis was confirmed.*

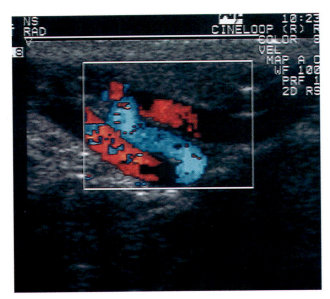

b

too slow to be detected with CFI (Fig. 6.14a). However, during a Valsalva maneuver, the rapid retrograde flow increases the flow velocity to the point where it becomes detectable (Fig. 6.14b). A transient rush of retrograde flow is commonly seen in the peritesticular veins of normal individuals. One study has suggested that the augmented flow during Valsalva should last for 1 second or more before considering the diagnosis of a varicocele. In the setting of infertility, if a varicocele is not detected with the patient supine, the examination should be performed with the patient upright. This increases hydrostatic pressure in the veins and can accentuate the abnormal findings of a varicocele. In general,

Figure 6.14 *Varicocele. Longitudinal color flow image of the left peritesticular tissues (a) demonstrates a dilated tortuous tubular structure. At rest, no flow was detected within this vessel despite 'low-flow' parameter settings. A similar view obtained when the patient performed a Valsalva maneuver (b) demonstrates augmented flow within this vessel which makes it readily detectable with CFI. These findings are consistent with a left testicular varicocele.*

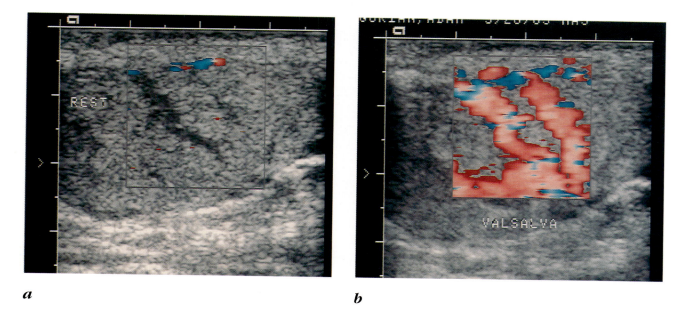

a   *b*

Figure 6.15 *Intratesticular varicocele. Longitudinal color flow image of the testis obtained at rest (a) demonstrates several linear hypoechoic structures within the testicular parenchyma that contain no detectable bloodflow. A similar view obtained during a Valsalva maneuver (b) shows readily apparent flow within these structures secondary to Valsalva-induced flow augmentation. These findings are consistent with an intratesticular varicocele.*

varicoceles are confined to the peritesticular veins. However, in unusual situations, varicoceles can also involve intratesticular veins (Fig. 6.15).

THYROID AND PARATHYROID

CFI evaluation of thyroid disease has yet to find a well-defined role. As in the testis, there is hope that it can add information to help differentiate benign and malignant processes. However, to date there is little convincing evidence that this is possible. Both benign and malignant thyroid nodules tend to be hypervascular, and the overlap in appearances is significant (Figs 6.16 and 6.17). Occasionally, CFI can help identify or demarcate isoechoic thyroid nodules (Fig. 6.18). Although CFI can determine the vascularity of diffuse diseases of the thyroid (Figs 6.19 and 6.20), it is yet to be shown that this information is clinically useful.

Ultrasound is frequently used to identify enlarged parathyroid glands in patients with hyperparathyroidism. Since parathyroid adenomas are typically hypervascular, CFI can occasionally add diagnostic confidence that a nodule visualized on gray scale sonography is in fact a parathyroid adenoma (Fig. 6.21).

BREAST

Similar to other superficial-parts applications, color flow evaluation of female breast masses has been investigated as one method of distinguishing benign from malignant disease. Unfortunately, CFI of breast lesions has proven to be more of a challenge to researchers attempting to establish criteria that would reliably enable this important differentiation. As in other applications, significant overlap exists in both the qualitative CFI appearance and quantitative hemodynamics of benign and malignant breast tumors (Fig. 6.22). In fact, in a recent study with large numbers of proven breast pathologies, gray scale ultrasound findings were determined to be most beneficial for the sonographic differentiation of benign from malignant lesions, and CFI contributed

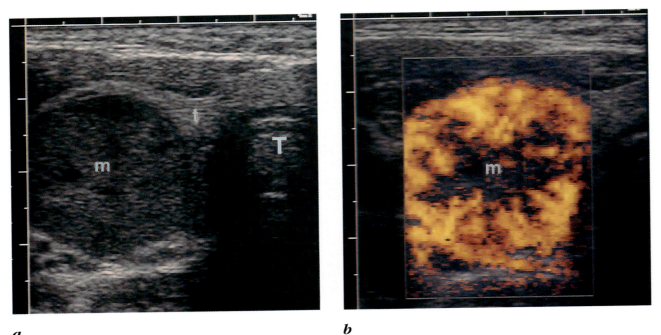

a   *b*

Figure 6.16 *Follicular thyroid carcinoma. (a) Transverse gray scale image of the right lobe of the thyroid demonstrates a slightly inhomogeneous hypoechoic mass (m) replacing much of the right lobe of the thyroid. Some adjacent normal thyroid parenchyma (t) is seen in the right lobe and the thyroid isthmus. The trachea (T) is seen medially. (b) Transverse color amplitude image of the same mass demonstrates intense hypervascularity primarily in the peripheral aspect of the mass.*

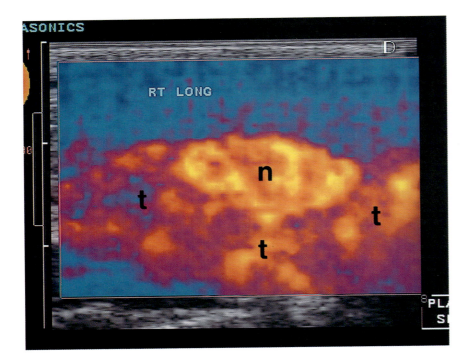

Figure 6.17 *Benign nodular hyperplasia of the thyroid. Longitudinal color amplitude image of the right lobe of the thyroid demonstrates mild increased vascularity of the normal thyroid parenchyma (t) when compared to the tissues adjacent to the thyroid. A focal oval-shaped nodule (n) with increased vascularity is seen in the superficial aspect of the thyroid. Because this patient had undergone previous radiation therapy for acne, this lesion was resected and was proven to represent benign nodular hyperplasia.*

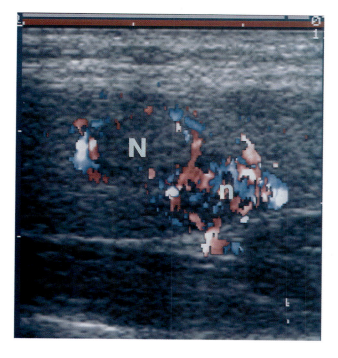

Figure 6.18 *Benign thyroid nodules. Longitudinal color flow image of the left lobe of the thyroid demonstrates a hypoechoic hypervascular nodule located in the posterior inferior aspect of the gland (n). In addition, an isoechoic nodule (N) is seen slightly superiorly. This nodule was very difficult to detect on gray scale imaging and the peripheral hypervascularity seen with CFI provided increased diagnostic confidence that there was in fact a nodule present. Fine-needle aspiration of both lesions demonstrated benign cells and colloid material but no evidence of malignancy.*

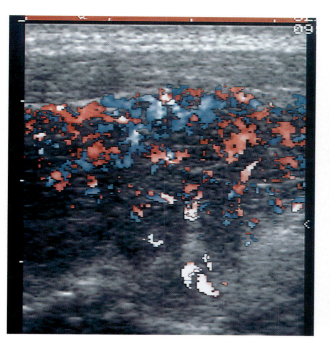

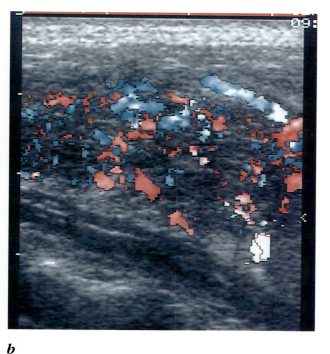

a   *b*

Figure 6.19 *Grave's disease. Longitudinal color flow image of the right lobe of the thyroid (a) demonstrates decreased echogenicity of the thyroid parenchyma as well as marked diffuse hypervascularity. A similar view of the left lobe of the thyroid (b) shows similar findings. Diffuse hypervascularity in a thyroid gland that is enlarged and homogeneously hypoechoic is very characteristic of Grave's disease.*

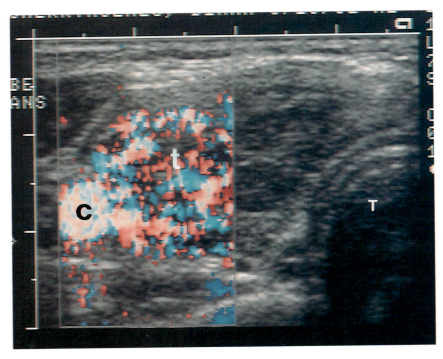

a

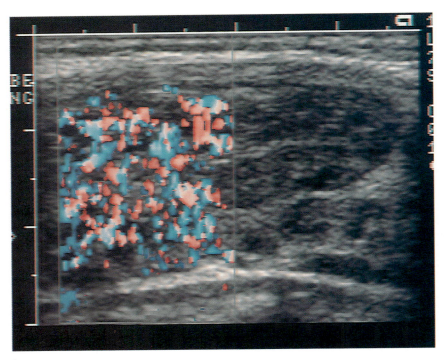

b

Figure 6.20 *Hashimoto's thyroiditis. Transverse color flow image of the right lobe of the thyroid (a) demonstrates marked hypervascularity of the thyroid gland (t) as well as decreased echogenicity and inhomogeneous echo pattern. Also seen in this view are the trachea (T) and common carotid artery (C). Longitudinal color flow image of the right lobe of the thyroid (b) again demonstrates marked hypervascularity as well as inhomogeneity and decreased echogenicity of the right lobe. These findings are typical of Hashimoto's thyroiditis.*

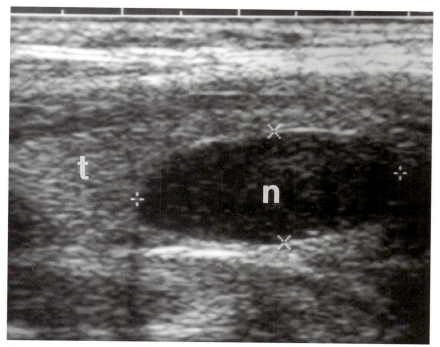

a

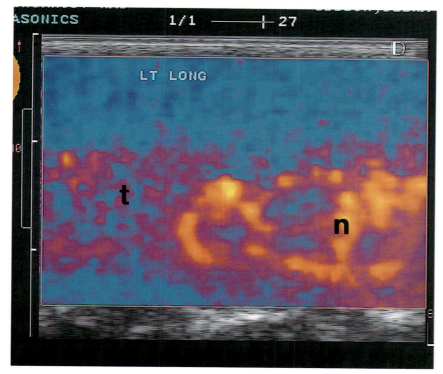

b

Figure 6.21 *Parathyroid adenoma. Longitudinal gray scale image of the left neck (a) demonstrates an oval-shaped hypoechoic nodule (n) posterior to the thyroid (t). A color amplitude image of the same area (b) demonstrates mild increased vascularity of the thyroid (t) when compared to the adjacent tissues. The hypoechoic nodule seen on gray scale evaluation is even more hypervascular than the adjacent thyroid. These findings are consistent with a parathyroid adenoma and this was confirmed at surgical exploration.*

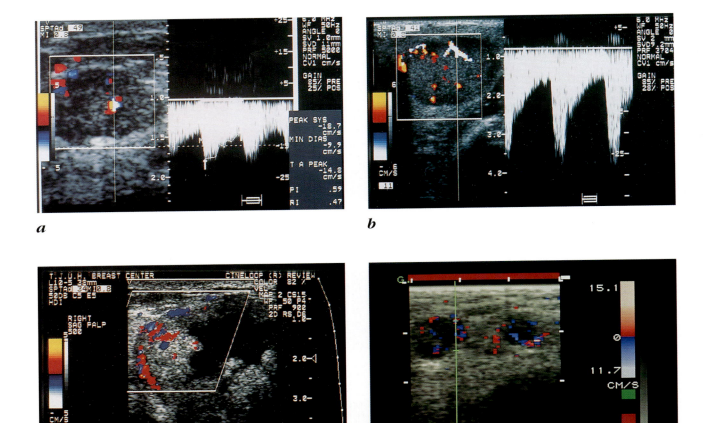

a

b

c

d

Figure 6.22 *Color flow images of breast lesions. This well-circumscribed mass (a) represents a fibroadenoma with an unusually high level of vascularity. In a different patient (b) another well-circumscribed mass was thought to be benign, based on the gray scale appearance. However, findings of increased flow signals and high systolic shifts on spectral analysis raised the suspicion of malignancy. Histopathologic examination revealed invasive ductal carcinoma. In another patient an unusual-appearing breast mass (c) consisting of solid and cystic components was confirmed as a benign hydradenoma. In a fourth patient (d) multiple small hypoechoic breast masses were identified with gray scale imaging. CFI detected bloodflow primarily around the periphery of the lesions. These masses were proven to represent multiple foci of lymphoma. Courtesy of C. Piccoli.*

little to the identification of breast cancers. One potential sign of malignancy that is detectable by CFI with pulsed spectral Doppler comprises high-frequency shifts and reduced pulsatility of bloodflow, which are presumably related to arteriovenous (AV) shunts known to occur in malignancies. Compared to duplex Doppler alone, CFI provides a more reliable global assessment of flow within any mass, including those of the breast. However, the identification of AV shunts is both operator and equipment dependent. Furthermore, even with meticulous scanning and proper equipment selection and optimization, the lack of AV shunting within a lesion is not a reliable indication of a benign entity.

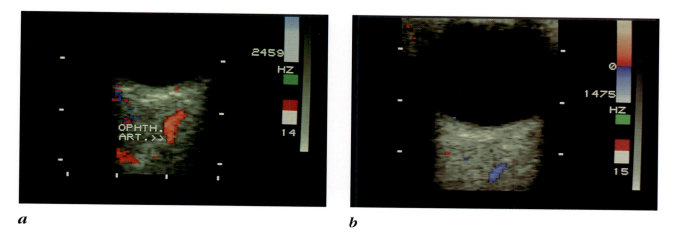

a   *b*

Figure 6.23 *CFI permits rapid assessment of flow in the OA, which is most commonly identified in the nasal aspect of the orbit. (a) Transverse color flow image of normal flow direction (i.e. out of the orbit) in the right OA. (b) In a different patient with known right internal carotid artery occlusion, retrograde flow (color-coded blue) is detected in the right OA.*

EYE AND ORBIT

CFI is useful for a variety of ophthalmologic indications. Often, establishing the presence or absence of flow within an abnormal-appearing area can be the important first step in deriving a correct diagnosis, and CFI can provide this information in the most cost-effective and least traumatic manner. Because of the high level of flow sensitivity obtainable with currently available color flow systems and other factors of superficial scanning already discussed, flow within the major vessels of the eye and orbit can routinely be visualized using CFI.

The CFI examination is performed through the closed eyelid using a small amount of sterile acoustic coupling. Various gazes are used to position the eye and facilitate CFI examination of the vessels of the globe and orbit. In cases of suspected venous aneurysms, a Valsalva maneuver may be necessary to cause dilatation of the aneurysmal vessel segment.

The ophthalmic artery (OA) can be identified in variable locations within the orbit, but it is most consistently visualized slightly medial to and crossing the optic nerve (Fig. 6.23). The central retinal artery (CRA), along with its accompanying vein, can be

seen within the optic nerve and, at times, the CRA can be traced from its terminal retinal branches posteriorly to its origin from the OA (Fig. 6.24). The retinal arteriolar vessels, because of their small size and close proximity to one another, are usually depicted with CFI as a 'retinal blush' along the posterior aspect of the globe. The short and long posterior ciliary arteries can be visualized adjacent to the optic nerve. With CFI, separation of the choroidal and retinal arterioles cannot usually be accomplished unless there is retinal detachment. Bloodflow in the superior and inferior ophthalmic veins and venae vorticosae may, at times, also be detected (Fig. 6.25).

Specific indications for ophthalmologic CFI include suspected cavernous sinus fistula, or arterial occlusions, venous thromboses, or varices in the vessels of the eye or orbit (Figs 6.26 and 6.27). Additionally, CFI can be used in cases when the clinician is unable to directly visualize the posterior portions of the eye and orbit due to intraocular hemorrhage or other causes. In these cases CFI can provide information on orbital pathologies such as tumors or retinal detachment and may help to differentiate these entities (Figs 6.28 and 6.29). Finally, many non-invasive vascular laboratories commonly use CFI to determine the direction of flow in the ophthalmic arteries as part of

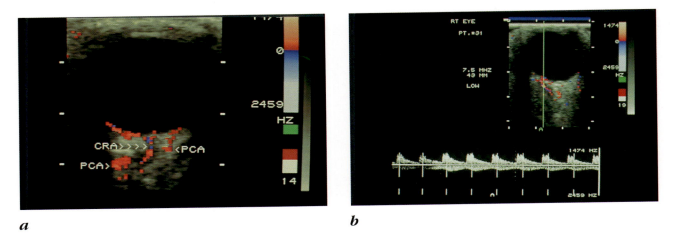

a *b*

Figure 6.24 *(a) Color flow image of the central retinal artery (CRA) located within the optic nerve. The CRA provides flow to the retina and the short and long posterior ciliary arteries (PCA) supply the choroid. Bloodflow in the retinal and choroidal arteriolar vessels results in a 'retinal blush' depiction of flow at the back of the globe. (b) Pulsed spectral Doppler analysis of a normal CRA (above the baseline) and central retinal vein (below the baseline).*

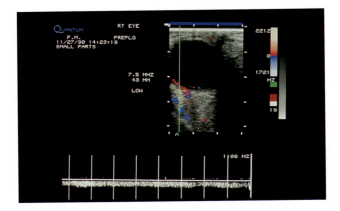

Figure 6.25 *Sagittal color flow image of the superior ophthalmic vein demonstrating a typical venous waveform on spectral Doppler.*

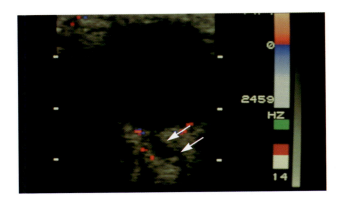

Figure 6.26 *CRA occlusion. In a patient with a recent episode of acute blindness, CFI identifies no flow in the CRA consistent with an occlusion of this vessel. Note the reduced echogenicity of the optic nerve (arrows) in this patient, and patency of the posterior ciliary arteries.*

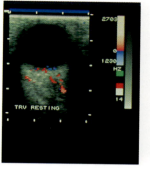

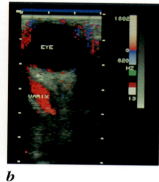

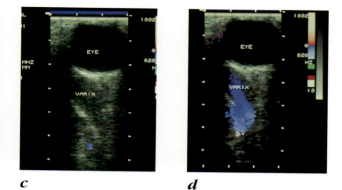

a   *b*   *c*   *d*

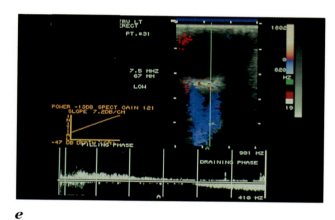

e

Figure 6.27 *Orbital varix. This patient presented to the ophthalmologist complaining of exophthalamos during physical exertion. Color flow image (a) of the eye appears normal with the patient in a resting state. During a Valsalva maneuver (b) afferent blood (color-coded red) slowly distends an orbital varix. At the point of maximum distention (c) venous stasis is present within the varix and no flow is detected. Upon release of Valsalva (d) efferent bloodflow is detected (color-coded blue). Spectral Doppler analysis (e) demonstrates the varix's filling phase (flow above the baseline) and draining phase (flow below the baseline). CFI is a useful means of evaluating in real time the hemodynamics of orbital varices, which can confirm the initial clinical diagnosis.*

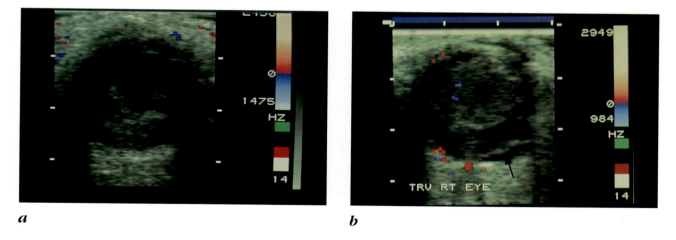

a   *b*

Figure 6.28 *CFI can be used to identify neovascularity in orbital tumors when present. This additional information may help to determine the etiology. (a) This patient recently had trauma to the eye. Internal echoes are identified with gray scale imaging within the normally anechoic vitreous body, suggesting intraocular hemorrhage. No flow could be detected with CFI, thereby increasing the confidence level of the diagnosis. (b) In a different patient thought to have intraocular hemorrhage, CFI identifies flow signals within the abnormal echogenic area within the globe. This patient was subsequently found to have a ciliary body tumor and retinal detachment (arrow).*

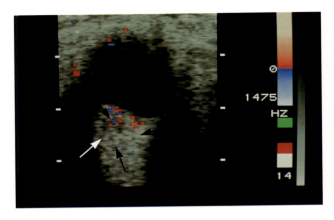

a

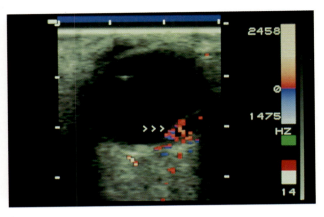

b

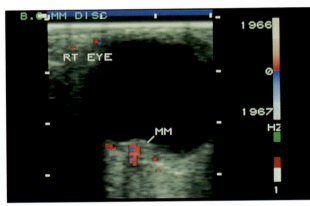

c

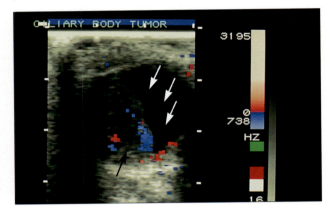

d

Figure 6.29 *Examples of orbital tumors. Color flow images of: (a) an orbital hemangioma (arrows) which appears echogenic on gray scale imaging; and (b) a hypervascular malignant melanoma (arrowheads) located along the medial aspect of the eye. (c) A small malignant melanoma (MM) located on the optic disk (note the flow in the distal CRA). (d) A large ciliary body tumor (arrows). (e) A color flow image and spectral Doppler waveform from a leiomyoma located in the anterior portion of the globe.*

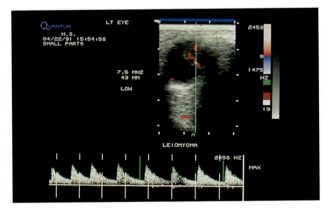

e

the complete cerebrovascular duplex Doppler examination. While CFI can reliably perform this task in a time-efficient manner, consideration should be given to the acoustic output level of the scanner being employed. The United States Food and Drug Administration recommends a much lower power output level for ophthalmic applications (17 mW/cm² spatial peak temporal average (SPTA) than for carotid applications (720 mW/cm² SPTA). The operator is obliged to utilize as low as is reasonably achievable

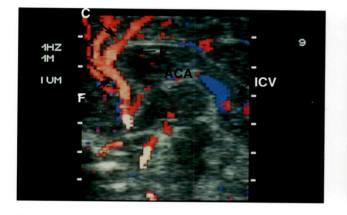

a

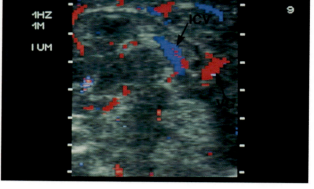

b

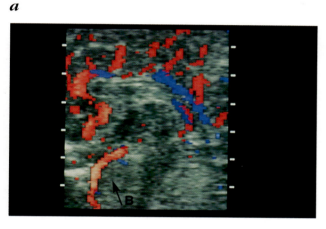

c

Figure 6.30 *Midline longitudinal color flow images of the neonatal brain obtained from the anterior fontanelle. (a) This image demonstrates portions of the internal carotid artery within the carotid siphon and the anterior cerebral artery (ACA) within the interhemispheric fissure. The frontopolar (F), callosomarginal (C) and pericallosal (P) branches can be identified. Flow in the proximal pericallosal artery is well visualized; however, flow in the segment that runs parallel to the corpus callosum is not seen, because of its flow direction in relation to the beam. Posteriorly, flow in the internal cerebral vein (ICV) is detected (color-coded blue). (b) This image better demonstrates the distal component of an ICV and the great cerebral vein of Galen (VG). Color coding changes from blue in the ICV, to black, and then to red in the vein of Galen as it courses superiorly towards the straight sinus (not seen). (c) This image demonstrates flow in the basilar artery (B) anterior to the pons, and other vasculature structures already described.*

(ALARA) acoustic power levels during all diagnostic ultrasound examinations. This responsibility is especially important when evaluating the delicate tissues of the eye.

NEONATAL BRAIN

As with conventional gray scale ultrasound, one limitation of performing CFI of the newborn brain is the restricted access provided by the fontanelles that are used as acoustic windows to view brain structure. Typically, the anterior fontanelle is utilized for these examinations. With the ultrasound probe placed in this location, the bloodflow direction in major intracranial vessels such as the internal carotid, basilar and distal (A-2 segments) anterior cerebral arteries is almost parallel with the ultrasound beam (i.e. a 0° angle), which provides ample visualization of flow in these vessels (Figs 6.30–6.35). The antero-lateral fontanelle, however, because of its lateral position on the skull, should when necessary be used to provide the most complete visualization of the circle of Willis, including the middle, posterior and proximal (A-1 segments) portions of the anterior cerebral arteries (Fig. 6.36).

Sector or tightly curved linear array transducers with frequencies of 5.0–7.5 MHz are preferred

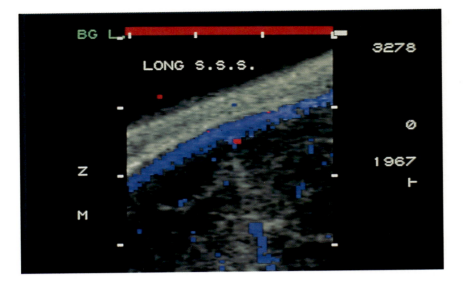

Figure 6.31 *Midline longitudinal color flow image demonstrating the superior sagittal sinus (SSS). Because of its superficial location and perpendicular flow direction, a wedge-shaped acoustic standoff is needed to provide an adequate Doppler angle to acquire flow information. When clinically indicated, CFI can be used to non-invasively evaluate for intracranial venous thrombosis in neonates.*

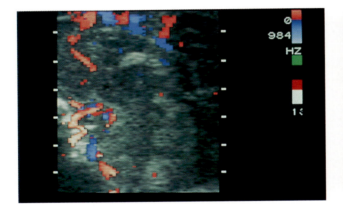

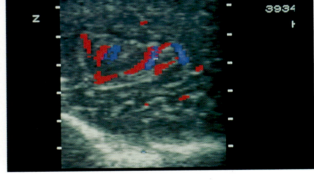

Figure 6.32 *Longitudinal color flow image obtained slightly to the left of midline demonstrating the internal carotid artery coursing through the carotid siphon. The short posterior communicating artery is identified with normal flow direction from the internal carotid artery to the posterior cerebral artery. Bloodflow in the cavernous sinus (color coded blue) is seen posterior to the internal carotid artery.*

Figure 6.33 *Parasagittal color flow image of the Sylvian fissure demonstrating branches of the middle cerebral artery (precentral, central and parietal arteries) on the lateral surface of the brain.*

because they provide high resolution, a small transducer footprint (needed to access the fontanelles), and a wide field of view which will provide more complete visualization of brain anatomy. Power output levels of the ultrasound system must be considered when scanning the pediatric patient, especially during neurosonographic examinations.

Focal cystic-appearing masses sometimes detected during routine gray scale imaging of the neonatal brain may represent a benign cyst or a life-threatening vascular malformation (Fig. 6.37). CFI can provide the necessary information to make the distinction between these two entities at the newborn's bedside, thereby providing a means of obtaining definitive diagnosis without requiring the infant to be taken out of the critical care setting. The so-called vein of Galen

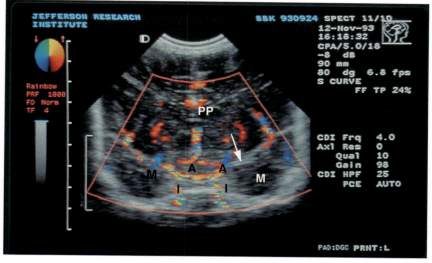

a

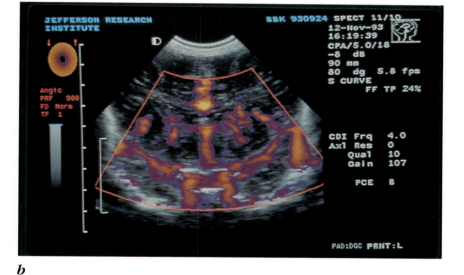

b

c

Figure 6.34 *Coronal conventional color (a) and color amplitude (b) images of a newborn's brain obtained from the anterior fontanelle. The supraclinoid portions of the internal carotid arteries (I) course laterally to terminate in the anterior (A) and middle (M) cerebral arteries. Lenticulostriate arteries are seen arising from the horizontal portion of the middle cerebral arteries, while the paired pericallosal arteries (P) are seen in cross-section within the interhemispheric fissure. In the conventional CFI mode, internal carotid artery flow through the siphon is aliased and there is a flow void (arrow) in the mid-portion of the left middle cerebral artery due to the poor Doppler angle for flow in this vessel segment. In the color amplitude image there is no aliasing, better flow continuity, and an overall improvement in visualization of intracranial vasculature. A coronal color flow image (c) obtained in a plane slightly posterior to those above in a different patient demonstrates flow in the cavernous sinuses (CS). Portions of the supraclinoid internal carotid arteries are also seen.*

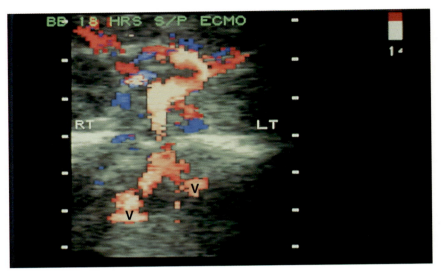

a

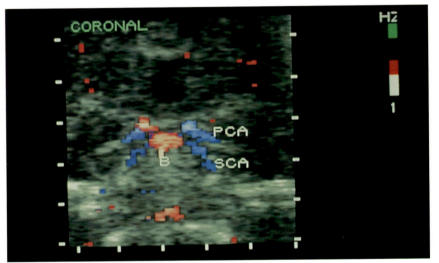

b

Figure 6.35 *Coronal color flow images of the posterior cranial circulation. (a) The vertebral arteries (v) can be seen inferior to the foramen magnum joining at midline to form the single basilar artery. (Note: in this oblique view portions of the anterior circle of Willis can also be seen.) (b) In a slightly different section the distal basilar artery terminates in the superior cerebellar arteries (SCA) and posterior cerebral arteries (PCA), separated by the tentorium (c). In a different patient a tortuous basilar artery is identified.*

c

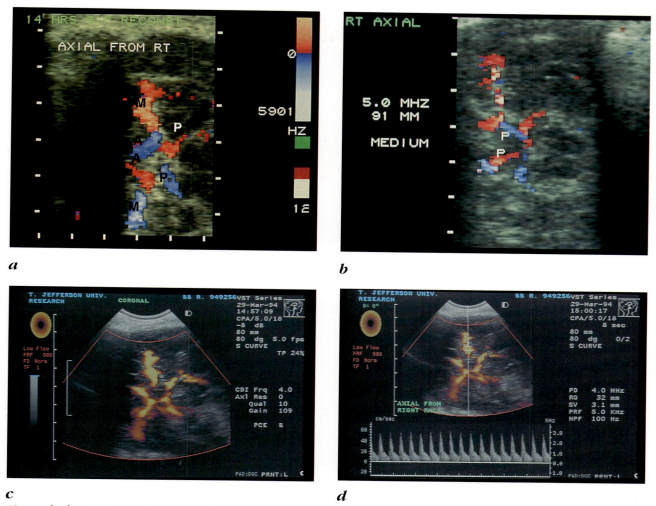

Figure 6.36 *Axial color flow images of the circle of Willis in term neonates obtained through the anterolateral fontanelle. (a) The normal flow direction in the middle cerebral arteries (M) and posterior cerebral arteries (P) is opposite to that of the ipsilateral anterior cerebral arteries (A). In a scan plane (b) slightly inferior to image (a), the posterior communicating arteries (P) can be identified with flow directed from the internal carotid arteries posteriorly towards the posterior cerebral arteries. In a different patient (c), CAI is used to visualize flow through the circle of Willis, and guides for pulsed spectral Doppler (d), which demonstrates a normal middle cerebral artery waveform.*

aneurysm (VGA), which is actually an arterio-venous (AV) communication, typically presents on gray scale imaging as an anechoic mass inferior and slightly posterior to the splenium of the corpus callosum (Fig. 6.38). The mass may compress adjacent, otherwise normal structures such as the cerebral ventricles, or aqueducts. CFI of a VGA will demonstrate a focal dilatation of the affected vessel segment with a swirling flow pattern in color. CFI may be used to

determine the location of the major feeding (arterial) vessels of the VGA. New therapeutic techniques use angiographic-guided embolization of the afferent vessels to reduce the flow of blood through the abnormal AV communication and thereby reduce the degree of the patient's right heart volume overload (Fig. 6.39). Pulsed Doppler spectral analysis of afferent VGA vessels will typically demonstrate low pulsatility (i.e. high diastolic flow component) as a

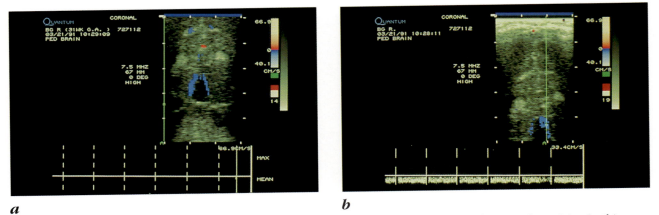

a *b*

Figure 6.37 *CFI is ideally suited to differentiate intracranial cysts from abnormalities of a vascular origin. In this case a midline cystic structure was detected during a routine gray scale examination. Coronal color flow image (a) demonstrates flow within the internal cerebral veins but no flow within a cystic area (c). A pulsed Doppler evaluation (b) confirms normal internal cerebral vein flow. This probably represents a benign cyst near the quadrigeminal cystern.*

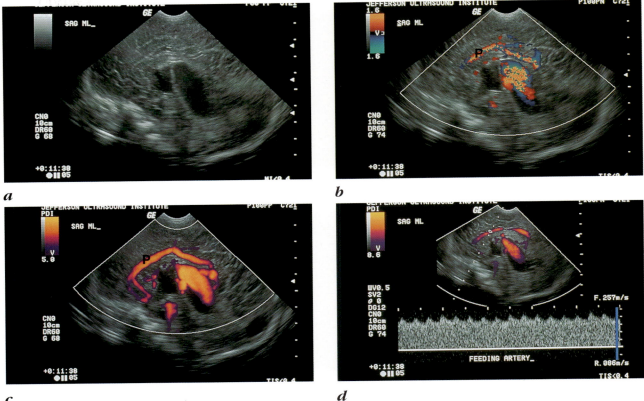

a *b*

c *d*

Figure 6.38 *Vein of Galen aneurysm (VGA). Sagittal (a) gray scale image of a term neonate with clinical signs of right heart volume overload and a cranial bruit. There is a large midline hypoechoic mass (M) posterior to the third ventricle. Conventional color (b) and color amplitude (c) imaging demonstrate a prominent pericallosal artery (P) and flow within the mass consistent with a diagnosis of a VGA. Pulsed Doppler spectral analysis (d) identifies an abnormal waveform, particularly the elevated diastolic component, obtained from the pericallosal artery, one of the primary afferent VGA vessels. Note the lack of aliasing artifacts and improved flow mapping characteristics of the color amplitude image.*

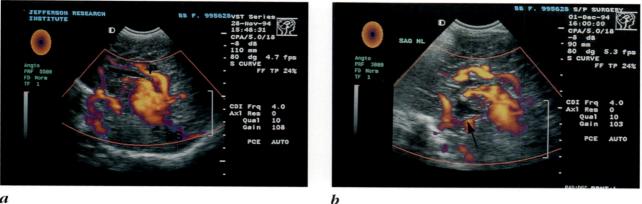

Figure 6.39 *Pre- and post-embolization of a vein of Galen aneurysm (VGA). Sagittal color amplitude image (a) obtained prior to embolization demonstrates some of the afferent and efferent vessels, the pericallosal artery (P) and straight sinus (SS) respectively, and the VGA with compression of the third ventricle (not seen). There was also compression of the lateral ventricles. The embolization procedure was performed under angiographic guidance and was promptly concluded when the infant's cardiac status sufficiently improved. Post-embolization sagittal color amplitude image (b) demonstrates a slight reduction in the size of the VGA and decompression of the third ventricle (arrow). Although the VGA is still present the flow signal intensity and conspicuity of the afferent and efferent vessels has been reduced. While at 1 year of age this infant is clinically stable, additional therapeutic procedures may be necessary.*

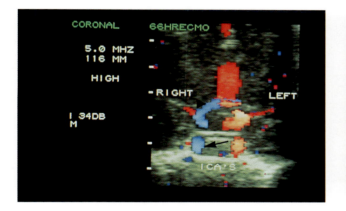

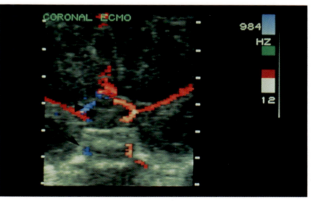

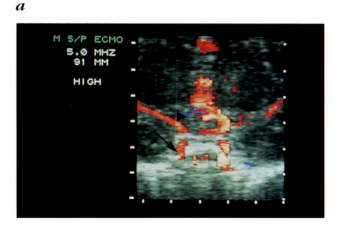

Figure 6.40 *Compensatory bloodflow patterns in infants with RCCA ligation for ECMO. These collateral flow patterns are identified best with coronal CFI of the anterior portion of the circle of Willis. The anterior communicating artery dominant pattern (a) is identified as retrograde right internal carotid artery flow (arrow). The posterior communicating artery (PcoA) dominant pattern (b) is identified as antegrade distal right internal carotid artery flow (distal to the PcoA) but reversed proximal right internal carotid artery flow (arrow). The external carotid artery dominant pattern (c) is identified when flow in the entire right internal carotid artery is antegrade (arrow). In all of these examples, bloodflow in the right A-1 portion of the anterior cerebral artery (arrow heads) is retrograde (color-coded blue).*

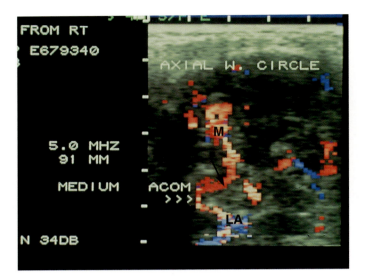

Figure 6.41 *Axial color flow image of the circle of Willis obtained from the right side of an infant on ECMO. Color flow image of collateralization via the anterior communicating artery (ACOM) resulting in retrograde flow in the A-1 portion of the right anterior cerebral artery (arrow). Compare this image to those of the normal circle of Willis in Fig. 7.36. LA, left anterior cerebral artery; M, right middle cerebral artery.*

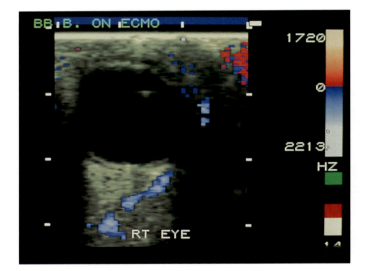

Figure 6.42 *Many infants treated with ECMO ultimately establish sufficient vascular collateralization to result in an external carotid artery (ECA) dominant flow pattern (see Fig. 6.40). These collaterals may occur spontaneously, or require days or even weeks to develop. This transverse color flow image of the right orbit identifies retrograde flow in the right ophthalmic artery from collateralizing ECA branches (flow away from the probe is color-coded blue). In this patient there was antegrade intracranial internal carotid artery flow (not shown).*

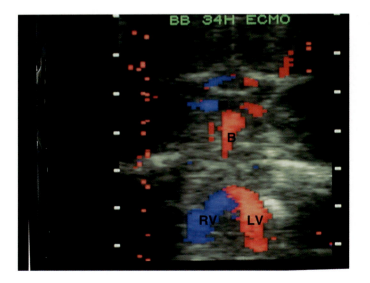

Figure 6.43 *During ECMO this infant had reduced pulses in his right upper extremity, which was cyanotic. CFI of the intracranial circulation detected reversed flow in the right vertebral artery (RV) (a 'subclavian steal' phenomenon), but antegrade left vertebral artery (LV) and basilar artery (B) flow. This flow pattern reverted back to normal when the arterial cannula that was in the RCCA was removed after completion of ECMO. Using the smallest possible arterial cannula size may help to avoid subclavian steals in ECMO infants whose cranial blood supply is already compromised by RCCA ligation.*

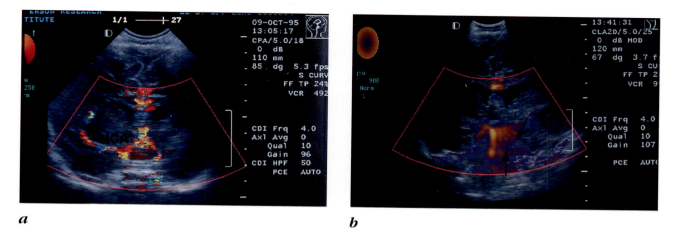

Figure 6.44 *Middle cerebral artery (MCA) infarction. These color flow images were obtained from a 3-month-old infant who had been on ECMO. (a) Flow is seen in the right MCA but is not detected in the left MCA. A magnetic resonance angiogram confirmed infarction of the left MCA territory, which was thought to be a result of an embolic event that occurred during ECMO. On a color amplitude image of the posterior intracranial circulation (b) increased flow is detected in the region of the left posterior cerebral artery (arrows), presumably related to collateral flow in vessels supplying viable brain tissue adjacent to the left MCA territory. Liquefaction of a large portion of the left hemisphere was identified with gray scale imaging.*

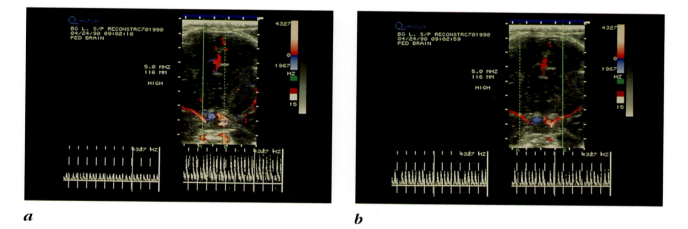

Figure 6.45 *Dual spectral Doppler waveforms from the (a) internal carotid arteries (ICA) and (b) middle cerebral arteries (MCA) in an infant after ECMO and reconstruction of the RCCA. Compared to the left ICA, the right ICA flow is diminished. However, MCA flow remains symmetric because of persistent collateral flow from left to right through the anterior communicating artery (note the retrograde flow direction in the A-1 segment of the right anterior cerebral artery). A Doppler ultrasound examination identified greater than 50% stenosis at the RCCA reconstruction site.*

result of reduced peripheral resistance. CFI-guided pulsed Doppler spectral analysis should be used to differentiate afferent VGA vessels from those feeding normal brain tissue, which demonstrate a higher degree of pulsatility. Pulsed Doppler spectral analysis

with the sample volume placed within a VGA will demonstrate a turbulent flow signal as a result of flow separations within the dilated vein. From a clinical management perspective, the differentiation of these lesions from simple cysts is an important one, and the

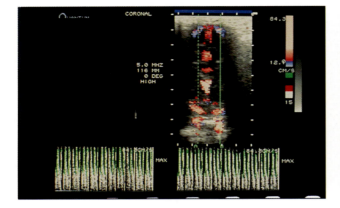

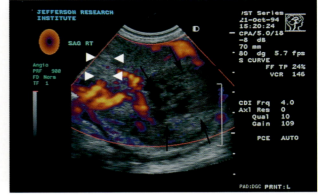

Figure 6.46 *Dual spectral Doppler waveforms obtained from the internal carotid arteries (ICA) in an infant 3 months after ECMO and reconstruction of the RCCA. In this case there is symmetric flow in the ICAs. A Doppler ultrasound evaluation of this infant's RCCA demonstrated no evidence of stenosis. All of the intracranial arteries had antegrade flow.*

Figure 6.47 *Parasagittal color amplitude image of a premature infant brain demonstrating a large area of cystic periventricular leukomalcia (PVL) without flow (arrows). Additionally, no flow was demonstrable in the more normal-appearing anterior cortex (arrow heads) which later also developed PVL. CAI may provide a means of predicting the viability of brain tissue prior to the development of degenerative changes detectable with gray scale imaging.*

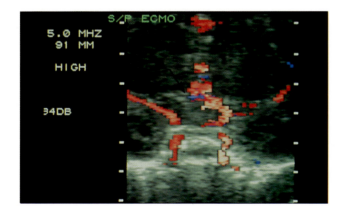

Figure 6.48 *Hypoplasia of an intracranial vessel identified using CFI. The right proximal (A-1) segment of the anterior cerebral artery (ACA) (arrow) was not seen in either the coronal (shown here) or axial views, and was presumed to be hypoplastic or atretic. In this situation both distal segments of the ACAs (A-2) are perfused via a single A-1 segment with collateral flow through the anterior communicating artery to the right A-2 segment. The A-1 segment of the ACA is particularly prone to this abnormality.*

addition of CFI to a gray scale ultrasound examination can greatly reduce the chance of a false-negative examination.

Extracorporeal membrane oxygenation (ECMO) therapy is a temporary heart–lung bypass used for term newborns suffering from reversible lung damage due to meconium aspiration, diaphragmatic hernia and other causes. During venoarterial ECMO, deoxygenated blood is routed from the right atrium of the heart (via a cannula in the right jugular vein) to the ECMO circuit. Within the ECMO circuit, carbon dioxide is removed and the blood is oxygenated, medicated, warmed and then returned to the infant's systemic circulation at the aortic arch via a cannula in the right common carotid artery (RCCA). During ECMO the RCCA is ligated, thereby creating a variety of compensatory collateral flow patterns of both the intra- and extracranial arterial circulations. Although primarily investigational, CFI has been used to determine the collateral flow patterns which maintain perfusion to the brain territories normally supplied by the RCCA (Figs 6.40–6.42). Another potential consequence of ECMO is partial stenosis or occlusion of the right subclavian artery by the arterial cannula crossing this vessel's origin. In this case, bloodflow to the right upper extremity is provided by the right

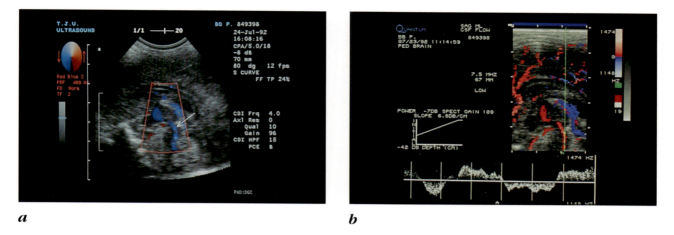

a

b

Figure 6.49 *CFI detection of CSF flow dynamics. A sagittal midline color flow image (a) detects CSF flow directed inferiorly through the aqueduct of Sylvius (arrow). In a different patient (b) CSF flow is better characterized with pulsed Doppler spectral analysis. Note the directional changes in response to increased intra-abdominal pressure resulting from gentle manual compression of the neonate's abdomen.*

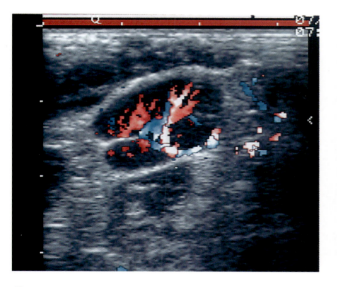

a

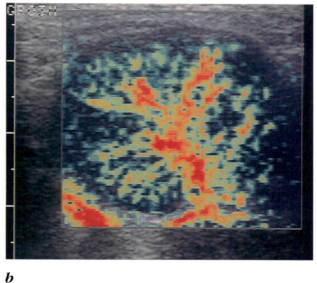

b

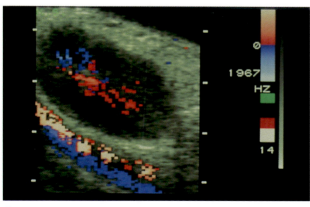

c

Figure 6.50 *Lymphadenopathy. (a) Transverse color flow image of the neck demonstrates a slightly enlarged cervical lymph node. The vascularity to this node is increased but the architectural pattern is normal, with vessels radiating out from a central hilum. This appearance may be seen in lymphoma (as in this case) and in benign inflammatory processes. (b) An oblique color amplitude image of the groin in another patient with lymphoma shows an enlarged hypervascular node with preservation of the normal branching pattern. (c) In a third case, CFI identifies the normal vascular architecture within one of multiple palpable masses of the groin of a 7-year-old girl. Bloodflow in the femoral artery and vein is also demonstrated. In this case lymphadenitis was the result of 'cat-scratch fever'.*

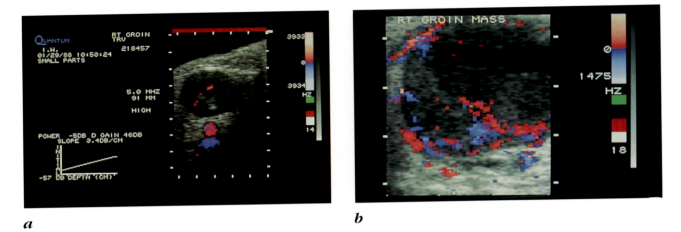

Figure 6.51 *Metastatic lymphadenopathy. (a) This patient presented to ultrasound with a palpable pulsating mass of the groin which suggested a pseudoaneurysm resulting from recent cardiac catheterization. Gray scale evaluation detected several hypoechoic masses overlying the femoral artery. CFI detected multiple vessels randomly distributed throughout the lesions. No central hilum or vascular branching could be demonstrated. Further inquiry revealed a history of urinary bladder (transitional cell) cancer. These masses were surgically confirmed as metastatic lymphadenopathy from bladder cancer. The importance of a thorough physical history is exemplified by this case. (b) In a different patient a large groin mass was detected during ultrasound evaluation of the lower extremities to rule out venous thrombosis. This patient's history of uterine cervical cancer contributed to a diagnosis of metastatic lymphadenopathy. CFI demonstrated abundant flow around the periphery of the lesion, with an area of suspected central necrosis. There was compression of the femoral vein by this mass which presumably resulted in venous stasis and deep vein thrombosis (not shown).*

vertebral artery; the so-called 'subclavian steal' phenomenon (Fig. 6.43). The significance of this finding has not been completely determined; however, using the smallest arterial cannula possible appears to reduce its incidence. CFI may also be useful in the detection of vascular insults related to ECMO, such as emboli that result in intracranial vascular occlusions (Fig. 6.44). In some cases, following the completion of ECMO and cannula removal, the RCCA is surgically reconstructed (Figs 6.45 and 6.46). Well established as a means of assessing the adult extracranial circulation, CFI is, too, ideally suited to determine the functional status of the child's RCCA reconstruction site and can be used serially to monitor the cerebrovascular status of these individuals.

CFI is currently being included in a variety of other pediatric neurosonographic investigations. In the future CFI may improve our understanding of the etiology of intracranial hemorrhage and hypoxic brain injuries in premature infants (Fig. 6.47). Additionally, the effects of trauma, hydrocephalus or other congenital anomalies (Fig. 6.48) on brain perfu-sion may be better understood with the use of CFI, possibly when combined with other diagnostic studies such as electroencephalography. Finally, cerebrospinal fluid (CSF) flow can be detected using currently available CFI systems (Fig. 6.49). At this time the particular benefits and applications of this utilization of CFI remain to be determined.

OTHER SUPERFICIAL PARTS

Peripheral lymph nodes are generally well imaged with ultrasound. A variety of gray scale criteria have been developed to help distinguish benign and malignant lymphadenopathy. Specific color flow vascular patterns have also been investigated but a consensus regarding its utility has not yet been established. In general, metastatic disease tends to result in a distorted vascular architecture within the node, while inflammatory disease and lymphoma preserve the normal architecture of lymph node vessels

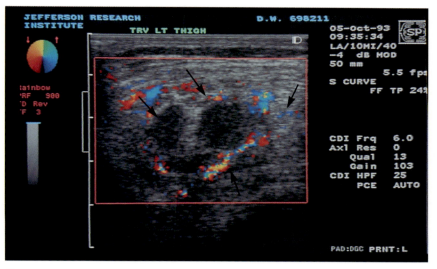

a

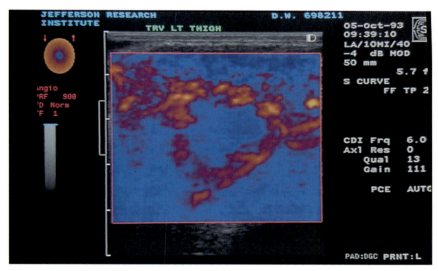

b

c

Figure 6.52 *Conventional (a) and color amplitude (b) images of a thigh abscess (arrows). There is increased flow around the mass periphery, consistent with reactive hyperemia, and no flow detected centrally. Pulsed Doppler spectral analysis (c) demonstrates an abnormal arterial waveform with increased diastolic flow and reduced pulsatility. In this case the CFI information suggested an inflammatory process, as opposed to a simple fluid collection, which resulted in more aggressive clinical management. Needle aspiration confirmed the ultrasound diagnosis.*

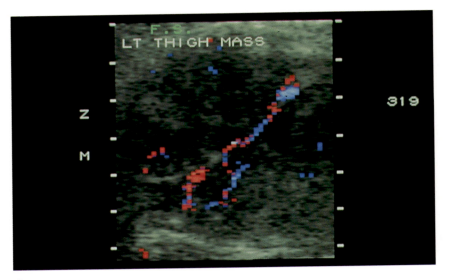

a

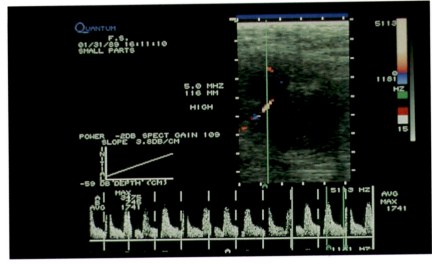

b

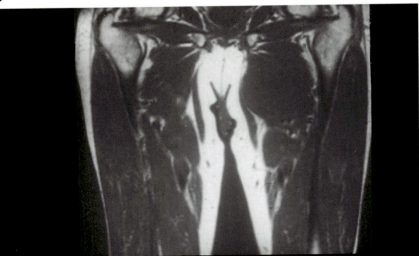

c

Figure 6.53 *Liposarcoma. This elderly patient presented for ultrasound evaluation of a palpable firm mass in the medial aspect of the thigh thought to be the result of previous trauma from a fall. Gray scale imaging demonstrated a focal mass of mixed echogenicity. CFI (a) identified multiple vessels coursing through this area but no increase in flow at the periphery. CFI-guided pulsed Doppler (b) better characterized the flow. There is an abnormal spectral signal with increased diastolic flow and reduced pulsatility. While these are non-specific findings, they suggest the presence of a neoplasm. A magnetic resonance imaging study (c), while consistent with the ultrasound diagnosis, was no more specific. At surgery a large, well-circumscribed liposarcoma was excised.*

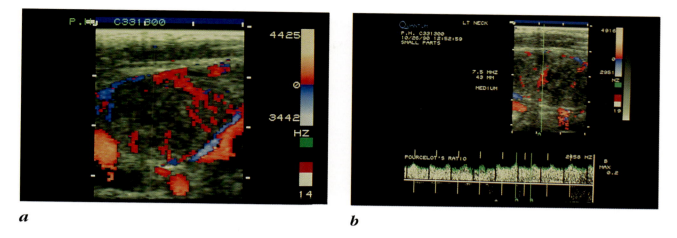

a   b

Figure 6.54 *Metastatic papillary carcinoma. This patient was referred for ultrasound evaluation of a large palpable mass located at the base of the neck thought to be related to the thyroid. CFI (a) identified a hypervascular solid mass lateral to and separate from the thyroid. The thyroid gland itself appeared sonographically normal. Spectral Doppler analysis (b) demonstrated a markedly abnormal arterial waveform consisting of an elevated diastolic component yielding a very low Pourcelot's ratio of 0.2. This was histopathologically confirmed as metastatic papillary carcinoma in the supraclavicular nodes.*

branching from a central echogenic hilum. These changes can be detected with CFI (Figs 6.50 and 6.51). Furthermore, by using CFI one may avoid mistaking enlarged lymph nodes for other entities such as iatrogenic pseudoaneurysms.

Tumors and other masses such as hematomas, seromas and abscesses occurring in a superficial location can be evaluated with CFI to obtain information on the presence of vessels, the relative vascularity of the mass, the origin of its vascular supply, and its effect on surrounding structures (Figs 6.52–6.55). The color flow data can also be used to guide sample volume placement for pulsed Doppler spectral analysis, which can better characterize bloodflow. The results of the color and spectral Doppler evaluation, while often non-specific, may provide additional information on which to base a diagnosis.

High-resolution ultrasound is becoming increasingly accepted as a valuable non-invasive means of evaluating musculoskeletal disorders. CFI adds information to the gray scale examination by determining the presence of associated hyperemia. This may indicate an inflammatory process (Figs 6.56–6.58) or, alternatively, can be used to help distinguish complex fluid collections such as intratendinous hematomas from solid tissue such as granulation tissue (Fig. 6.59).

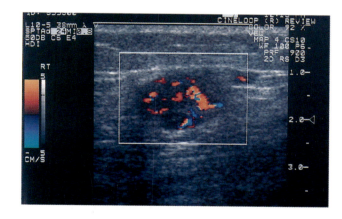

Figure 6.55 *Malignant melanoma metastasis. This patient, with a history of malignant melanoma, was referred to ultrasound to evaluate the site of previous resection of a subcutaneous metastasis. There was no palpable abnormality. A hypoechoic mass was detected with gray scale imaging. Further evaluation with CFI demonstrated abnormal vascularity in the mass. These findings were suspicious for recurrent disease. Surgical resection confirmed melanoma metastasis to the subcutaneous fat. In the future, ultrasound with CFI may serve as a screening device to detect locally recurrent disease in patients with melanoma. Courtesy of L. Nazarian.*

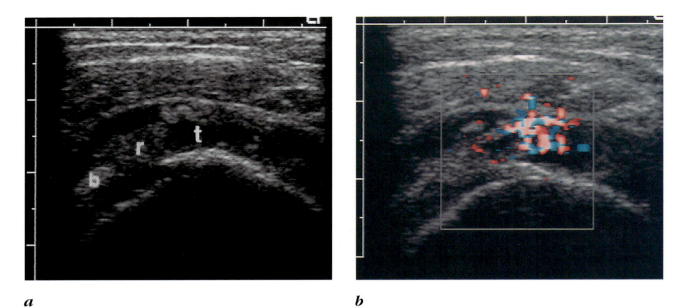

a   *b*

Figure 6.56 *Rotator cuff tear with inflammation. (a) Transverse gray scale image of the rotator cuff demonstrates an anechoic rotator cuff tear (t) in the region of the supraspinatous tendon. A normal portion of the rotator cuff (r) and the intra-articular portion of the biceps tendon (b) is also identified. (b) Transverse color flow image in a similar area demonstrates focal intense hypervascularity in the region of the rotator cuff tear indicative of an inflammatory component to the tear.*

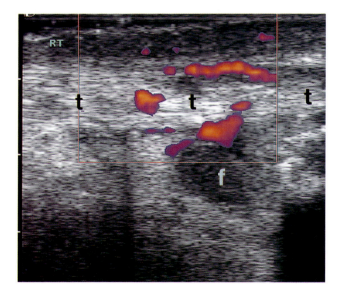

Figure 6.57 *Achilles tendonitis. Longitudinal color amplitude image of the right Achilles tendon (t) demonstrates peritendinous fluid (f) and hyperemia around the tendon.*

During invasive procedures such as needle biopsies, CFI may be used to select a needle path which will avoid puncture of native or tumor vessels and, therefore, reduce the likelihood of extensive bleeding or other complications (Fig. 6.60). Additionally, CFI used during biopsy procedures may direct the investigator to locations which will most likely provide a diagnostically adequate pathology specimen and help to avoid sampling areas of necrosis or cystic components of tumors which may yield inadequate specimens.

CONCLUSION

CFI is complementary to gray scale ultrasound for the evaluation of a variety of superficial structures. The use of high-frequency transducers improves spatial resolution and color flow sensitivity, resulting in exceptional anatomic detail and bloodflow assessment of structures such as the testis, eye and thyroid. Additionally, data obtained with CFI can enhance the evaluation of palpable masses and strengthen the

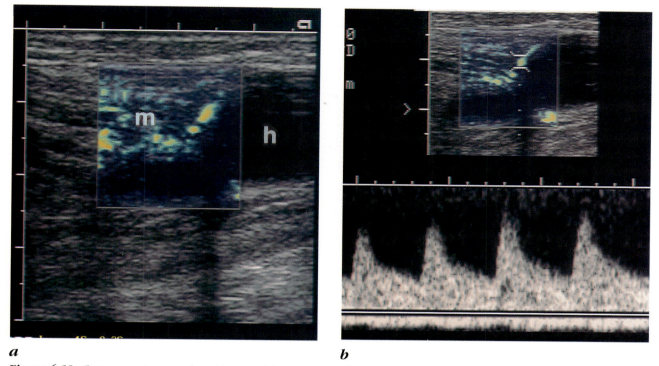

a *b*

Figure 6.58 *Gastrocnemius muscle rupture and hematoma with associated hyperemia. (a) Longitudinal color amplitude image of the gastrocnemius muscle (m) demonstrates a fluid collection representing a hematoma (h) adjacent to the retracted edge of the torn muscle tissue. Hyperemic flow is seen in the edge of the torn muscle. (b) A similar color flow image with pulsed Doppler waveform shows low-resistance arterial flow in the edge of the torn muscle. This low-resistance-type flow is unusual for an extremity artery and provides collaborative information regarding the inflammatory reaction at the edge of the torn muscle.*

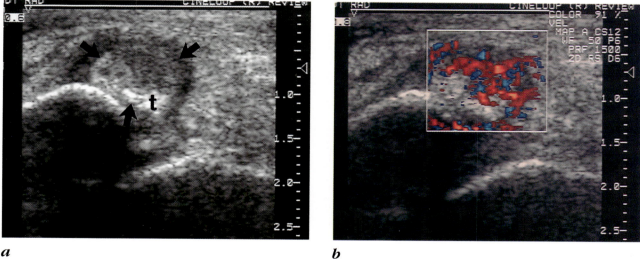

a *b*

Figure 6.59 *Partial tear of the posterior tibial tendon with granulation tissue. (a) Transverse gray scale image of the posterior tibial tendon (arrows) demonstrates hyperechoic region in the tendon representing normal tendonous fibers (t). In addition, there is a prominent hypoechoic portion in the tendon that could represent either hematoma or granulation tissue. (b) Transverse color flow image at the same level demonstrates that the hypoechoic component to the tendon is intensely hypervascular. This is indicative of granulation tissue rather than intratendinous hematoma.*

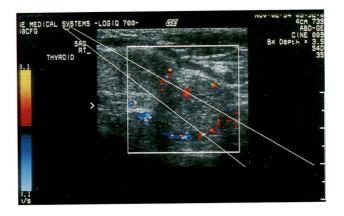

Figure 6.60 *CFI guidance during needle biopsy. During fine-needle aspiration of a thyroid mass, CFI facilitates selection of a path which will avoid major tumor vessels and thereby reduce the likelihood of excessive bleeding or other complications.*

confidence level of the sonographic diagnosis. New CFI applications such as the evaluation of the musculoskeletal system are now becoming more widely practiced. Future advances in technology will continue to improve the sensitivity of CFI systems and reduce some of the operator dependence which exists today. These improvements, possibly combined with other factors and new imaging techniques, may further expand the range of applications for CFI of superficial parts.

FURTHER READING

SCROTUM AND TESTIS

Atkinson GO Jr, Patrick LE, Ball TI Jr, Stephenson CA, Broecker BH, Woodard JR, The normal and abnormal scrotum in children: evaluation with color Doppler sonography, *AJR* (1992) **158**:613–17.

Burks DD, Markey BJ, Burkhard TK, Balsara ZN, Haluszka MM, Canning DA, Suspected testicular torsion and ischemia: evaluation with color Doppler sonography, *Radiology* (1990) **175**:815–21.

Casal, M et al, Varicocele evaluation with Doppler color sonography before and after percutaneous treatment, *Semin Intervent Radiol* (1990) **7**:222–5.

Horstman WG, Middleton WD, Melson GL, Scrotal inflammatory disease: color Doppler US findings, *Radiology* (1991) **179**:55–9.

Horstman WG, Middleton WD, Melson GL, Siegel BA, Color Doppler US of the scrotum, *RadioGraphics* (1991) **11**:941–57.

Horstman WG, Melson GL, Middleton WD, Andriole GL, Testicular tumors: findings with color Doppler US, *Radiology* (1992) **185**: 733–7.

Lerner RM, Mevorach RA, Hulbert WC, Rabinowitz R. Color Doppler US in the evaluation of acute scrotal disease, *Radiology* (1990) **176**:355–8.

Meza MP, Amundson GM, Aquilina JW, Reitelman C, Color flow imaging in children with clinically suspected testicular torsion, *Pediatr Radiol* (1992) **22**:370–3.

Middleton WD, Bell MW, Analysis of intratesticular arterial anatomy with emphasis on transmediastinal arteries, *Radiology* (1993) **189**:157–60.

Middleton WD, Siegel BA, Melson GL, Yates CK, Andriole GL, Acute scrotal disorders: prospective comparison of color Doppler US and testicular scintigraphy, *Radiology* (1990) **177**:177–81.

Petros JA, Andriole GL, Middleton WD, Picus DA, Correlation of testicular color Doppler ultrasonography, physical examination and venography in the detection of left varicoceles in men with infertility, *J Urol* (1991) **145**:785–8.

Ralls PW, Larsen D, Johnson MB, Lee KP, Color Doppler sonography of the scrotum, *Semin Ultrasound, CT, MR* (1991) **12**:109–14.

THYROID AND PARATHYROID

Fobbe F, Finke R, Reichenstein E, Schleusener H, Wolf KJ, Appearance of thyroid diseases using color-coded duplex sonography, *Eur J Radiol* (1989) **9**:29–31.

Gooding GAW, Clark OH, Use of color Doppler imaging in the distinction between thyroid and parathyroid lesions, *Am J Surg* (1992) **164**:51–6.

Ralls PW, Mayekawa DS, Lee KP et al, Color-flow Doppler sonography in Graves disease: 'thyroid inferno', *AJR* (1988) **150**:781–4.

BREAST

Carson P, Adler DD, Fowlkes J, Harnist K, Rubin J, Enhanced color flow imaging of breast cancer vasculature: continuous wave Doppler and three-dimensional display, *J Ultrasound Med* (1992) **11**:377–85.

Cosgrove DO, Bamber JC, Davey JB, McKinna JA, Sinnett HD, Color Doppler signals From breast tumors — work in progress, *Radiology* (1990) **176**:175–80.

Piccoli C, Current utilization and future techniques of breast ultrasound, *Curr Opin Radiol* (1992) **4**:139–45.

EYE AND ORBIT

Erickson SJ, Hendrix LE, Massaro BM et al, Color Doppler flow imaging of the normal and abnormal orbit, *Radiology* (1989) **173**:511–16.

Lieb WE, Shields JA, Cohen SM et al, Color Doppler imaging in the management of intraocular tumors, *Ophthalmology* (1990) **97**:1660–4.

Lieb WE, Cohen SM, Merton DA, Shields JA, Mitchell DG, Goldberg BB, Color Doppler imaging of the eye and orbit, *Arch Ophthalmol* (1991) **98**:548–52.

Wong AD, Cooperberg PL, Ross WH, Araki DN, Differentiation of detached retina and vitreous membrane with color flow Doppler, *Radiology* (1991) **178**:429–31.

NEONATAL BRAIN

Alexander AA, Mitchell DG, Merton DA et al, Cannula-induced vertebral steal in neonates during extracorporeal membrane oxygenation: detection with color Doppler US, *Radiology* (1992) **182**:527–30.

Circillo SF, Schmidt KG, Silverman NH et al, Serial ultrasonic evaluation of neonatal vein of Galen malformations to assess the efficacy of interventional neuroradiology procedures, *Neurosurgery* (1990) **27**:544–8.

DeAngelis GA, Mitchell DG, Merton DA et al, Right common carotid artery reconstruction in neonates after extracorporeal membrane oxygenation: color Doppler imaging, *Radiology* (1992) **182**:521–5.

Govaert P, Voet D, Achten E et al, Noninvasive diagnosis of superior sagittal sinus thrombosis in a neonate, *Am J Perinatol* (1992) **9**:201–4.

Mitchell DG, Needleman L, Merton DA et al, Neonatal brain color Doppler imaging Part I: technique and vascular anatomy, *Radiology* (1988) **1667**:303–6.

Mitchell DG, Merton DA, Desai H et al, Neonatal brain color Doppler imaging Part II: Altered flow patterns from extracorporeal membrane oxygenation, *Radiology* (1988) **1667**:307–10.

Mitchell DG, Merton DA, Mirsky PJ, Needleman L, Circle of Willis in newborns: color Doppler imaging of 53 healthy full-term infants, *Radiology* (1989) **172**:201–5.

Tatsuno M, Uchida K, Okuyama K, Kawauchi A, Color Doppler flow imaging of CSF flow in an infant with intraventricular hemorrhage, *Brain Dev* (1992) **14**:110–13.

Taylor GA, Intracranial venous system in the newborn: evaluation of normal anatomy and flow characteristics with color Doppler US, *Radiology* (1992) **183**:449–52.

Taylor GA, Walker LK, Intracranial venous system in newborns treated with extracorporeal membrane oxygenation: Doppler US evaluation after ligation of the right jugular vein, *Radiology* (1992) **183**:453–6.

Van Bel F, Van Zwieten PHT, Den Ouden LL, Contribution of color Doppler flow imaging to the evaluation of the effect of indomethacin on cerebral hemodynamics, *J Ultrasound Med* (1990) **9**:107–9.

OTHER SUPERFICIAL PARTS

Merton DA., Ultrasound examination of invasive procedure puncture site complications: a review of scan techniques and benefits of color Doppler imaging, *J Diagn Med Sonogr* (1993) **9**:297–305.

Mitchell DG, Merton DA, Liu JB, Goldberg BB, Superficial masses with color flow Doppler imaging, *J Clin Ultrasound* (1991) **19**:550–60.

Newman JS, Adler RS, Bude RO, Rubin JM, Detection of soft-tissue hyperemia: value of power doppler sonography, *AJR* (1994) **163**:385–9.

Swischuck LE, Desai PB, John SD, Exuberant blood flow in enlarged lymph nodes:findings on color flow Doppler, *Pediatr Radiol* (1992) **22**:419–21.

Chapter 7 Peripheral vascular color flow imaging

Tina L Nack and Colin R Deane

INTRODUCTION

Color flow imaging (CFI) has become a powerful tool in peripheral vascular sonography. By creating a spatial map of the presence, absence, direction and magnitude of scatterer motion, CFI can provide an eloquent summary of bloodflow throughout the scan field. This information can be used to differentiate vascular and non-vascular structures (such as a hematoma from a pseudoaneurysm), demonstrate intravascular flow voids (thrombus, hyperplasia and atherosclerosis), and detect small vessels (tumor flow, parenchymal flow). As a result of its ability to depict flow events throughout a vessel lumen, CFI is also useful in guiding sample volume placement, for example in stenotic vessels where it clearly depicts the stenotic jet and post-stenotic turbulence guiding sample volume placement to document the spectral effects of arterial stenosis (Table 7.1). Despite the strengths of color displays of bloodflow, final vascular diagnoses are rarely made without the use of spectral Doppler and the detailed, quantitative information which it provides.

Table 7.1 Spectral manifestations of arterial stenosis.

Primary effects	Increased peak systolic velocity (PSV) (jet) at the stenotic site
Secondary effects	Downstream separation/turbulence, eddies
	Diminished downstream flow velocity and pulsatility
	Increased upstream flow pulsatility
Tertiary effects	Changes in flow direction and increased flow in collateral vessels

This chapter covers those areas which are conventionally described as peripheral vascular scanning applications, including cerebrovascular (carotid, vertebral and intracranial arteries), peripheral arterial (lower extremity graft surveillance, scanning the lower extremity arterial tree and scanning arterial injuries and malformations), upper and lower extremity venous scanning (ruling out deep venous thrombosis, evaluating chronic venous disease and placing and maintaining temporary central venous access), and dialysis graft and fistula evaluation.

TRANSDUCERS

As most peripheral vascular scanning allows large areas of skin contact and minimal depth, linear transducers are the transducers of choice in most applications. These transducers not only afford a large field of view in the near and far field, but also allow for a greater uniformity of color flow and spectral Doppler angle throughout the region of interest. The availability of beam steering also provides a greater flexibility of angles of insonation. These factors not only make the color image more comprehensible by reducing the number of variables introduced by the interaction of vector velocity (direction and magnitude of bloodflow) and angle of the scan lines (parallel in a linear transducer, variable in a sector image format), but also make it easier for the operator to maintain a constant angle when using spectral Doppler. The latter is important as it may be desirable to obtain all measurements at, for example, 60° when applying diagnostic criteria using absolute numbers which were generated using a 60° Doppler angle (such as with the most popularly applied internal carotid artery stenosis diagnostic criteria), or to maintain the same angle of insonation for each measurement when using stenosis criteria which rely on ratios (such as those for grading peripheral stenoses). Even when angle correcting and using angles less than 70°, intrinsic spectral broadening can cause overestimation of velocities (approximately 15–20% overestimation at 60° as compared to 0°). This error has been incorporated into the absolute velocity criteria which have been generated at 60° angles.

Sector transducers are the transducers of choice, however, when scanning around bony impediments such as the mandible, clavicle or sternum, when skin surface is limited (bandages or sutures), or when a large field of view is required deeper in the field, such as when evaluating a large mass which is not superficial.

CEREBROVASCULAR

CAROTID ARTERIES

Although there is some variation between populations, atherosclerotic carotid artery disease is seen at greatest frequency in the proximal internal carotid artery and carotid bulb. Disease in this region has been demonstrated to be correlated with subsequent neurologic events.

The good ultrasound access to the common carotid and proximal internal carotid arteries permits imaging of the lumen and allows for accurate placement of the pulsed Doppler sample volume. In this way, a clear image of the plaque can usually be obtained and velocity increases caused by disease can be accurately measured. Duplex ultrasound of the carotid arteries is clearly indicated in patients with transient ischemic attacks (TIAs) and/or cerebral vascular accidents (CVAs), in asymptomatic patients with a bruit on physical examination, and as follow-up in patients with known disease or prior endarterectomy or angioplasty to rule out progression or recurrence. If internal carotid artery (ICA) stenosis is discovered on initial evaluation, entry into medical or surgical therapy can be based on the results of the duplex examination, although it is common practice in some centers to obtain arteriography prior to endarterectomy.

The left CCA is the second great vessel originating from the arch, while the right CCA arises from the brachiocephalic artery, which is the first great vessel. Occasionally, the left CCA will arise from the brachiocephalic artery as well. The CCA runs cephalad up the neck lying posterio-lateral to the thyroid and medial to the internal jugular vein (Figs 7.1–7.3). At the mid cervical level or above (there is great variation) the carotid

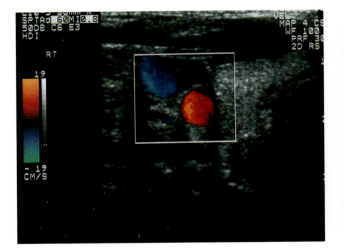

Figure 7.1 *Common carotid artery (CCA), transverse view. The jugular vein is anterior and lateral to the carotid artery and is readily identified by its irregular shape. The CCA is circular in cross-section.*

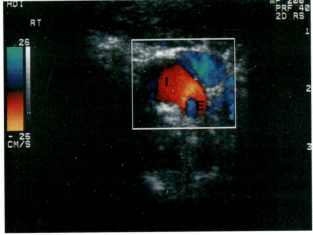

Figure 7.2 *Carotid bulb, transverse view. The arterial cross sectional area is enlarged when compared with the CCA. The entrance to the ICA (I) is upper left of the bulb and the external carotid artery (E) is deeper and to the right in the image. In both entrance regions, secondary flows produce regions of blue coded flow.*

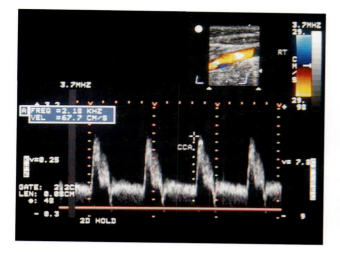

Figure 7.3 *CCA flow waveform. The CCA waveform contains elements of both the external carotid artery (ECA) and internal carotid artery (ICA) waveforms, with rapid acceleration, a post-systolic notch and forward flow throughout diastole.*

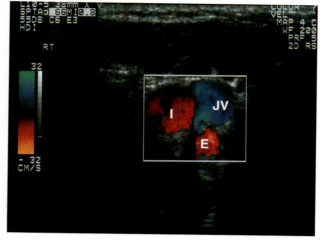

Figure 7.4 *ICA (I), ECA (E) and jugular vein (JV), transverse view. Distal to the bifurcation, flow is not yet uniform in the ICA. In this example, the ICA lies lateral and anterior to the ECA. The ICA is usually larger than the ECA.*

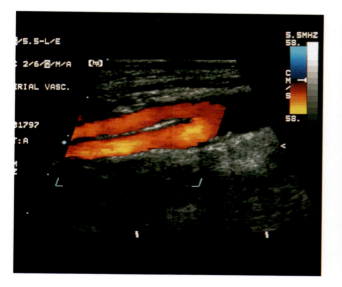

Figure 7.5 *Carotid bifurcation. In this longitudinal view, the internal and external carotid arteries are seen for approximately 3 cm distal to the bifurcation. Such views are not always possible. Note the small amount of plaque on the posterior wall of the carotid bulb, a common site of early disease.*

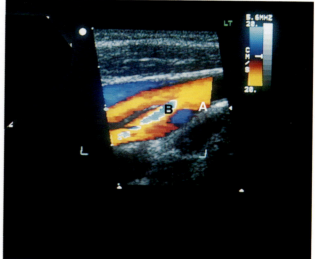

Figure 7.6 *Carotid bifurcation, longitudinal view. The B-mode has been steered to the right to optimize reflections from the vessel walls. The color flow beam has been steered to the left to improve the Doppler beam/flow angle. The color image shows a region of flow separation at the posterior wall of the bulb (A) and high velocities at the dividing wall of the ICA (B), a common feature caused by the geometry of the undiseased bifurcation. The vessel coded blue, anterior to the ECA, is the jugular vein.*

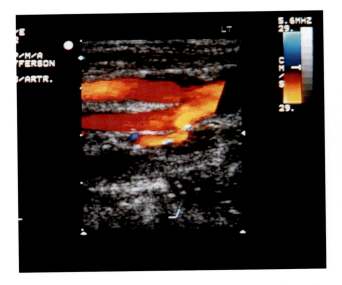

Figure 7.7 *Carotid bifurcation. In this image, a branch artery is seen just distal to the origin of the ECA. The presence of branching arteries is an aid in distinguishing the ECA from the ICA (which has no branches at this level).*

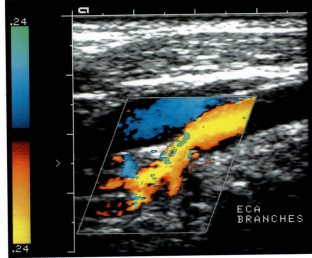

Figure 7.8 *ECA and branches. Several early branches of the ECA may be visible as in this longitudinal view.*

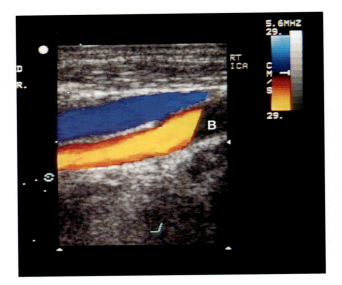

Figure 7.9 *ICA, longitudinal view. The ICA lies posterior to the jugular vein. The carotid bulb is to the right of the image (B). The color shows high velocities in the center of the artery, with slower flow near the walls.*

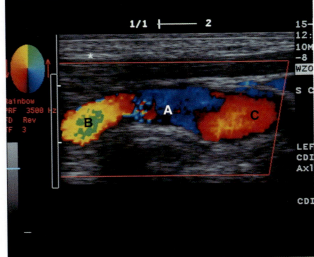

Figure 7.10 *Change in color hue in an ICA. The change in flow direction relative to the CFI beam in this ICA results in flow coded blue (at A) and red (at B and C). At B the flow is more aligned to the ultrasound beam and aliasing occurs.*

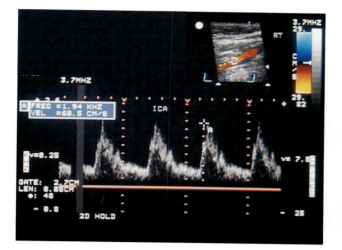

Figure 7.11 *ICA flow waveform. The ICA flow waveform shows gentle transition from systole to diastole. With a small pulsed wave sample volume placed centrally in the lumen, there is little spectral broadening.*

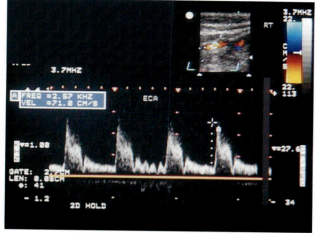

Figure 7.12 *ECA flow waveform. When compared to the ICA waveform, ECA waveforms have steeper acceleration and lower diastolic flow. The fluctuations during the second cardiac cycle are caused by manual oscillations of the superficial temporal artery.*

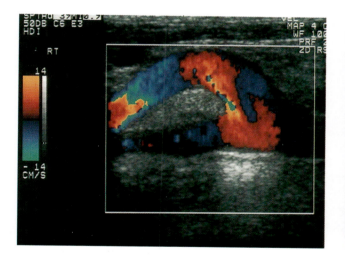

Figure 7.13 *Tortuous arteries. There is great variation in the appearance of the carotid arteries. This large superficial ICA turns through nearly 90°. The color image shows a range of hues reflecting the different ultrasound beam/flow angles that result.*

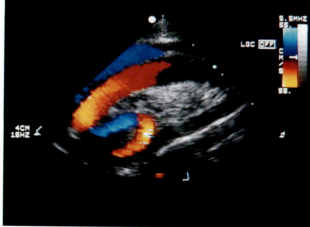

Figure 7.14 *Tortuous arteries. This longitudinal scan of an ICA demonstrates the high degree of tortuosity that can arise in the carotid arteries. The color image displays a range of hues. Local velocity increases due to tight curvature can occur.*

branches (Figs 7.4–7.7) into the more medial and anterior external carotid artery (ECA) which has multiple branches (Figs 7.7 and 7.8), and the larger more postero-lateral ICA (Figs 7.9 and 7.10) which continues cephalad inside the skull eventually entering the dura, giving rise to the ophthalmic artery and the basal arter-

ies of the anterior circle of Willis. Apart from anatomic variations, the ICA can be identified by the increased diastolic flow when compared to the ECA (Figs 7.11 and 7.12).

Kinking, coiling and tortuosity of the ICA is not uncommon in the adult (Figs 7.13 and 7.14). These authors have scanned neonatal carotids and noted the ICA often to be redundant and S-shaped in the neonate, becoming less tortuous as the infant grows.

High-frequency (5.0–10.0 MHz) linear transducers are the transducers of choice for cerebrovascular examinations in most cases. Sector transducers are helpful in angling up under the mandible in patients with high bifurcations, or below the clavicle when proximal stenosis is suspected. While CFI has not been shown to improve the accuracy of this examination, it may reduce examination times as a result of the spatial flow map created over the scan field. CFI is also useful for extending the scope of the examination in deep vessels or vessels which are at angles to the ultrasound beam which result in poor gray scale visualization, but high color frequency shifts (flow directly toward or away from the probe). The pictorial summary of primary and secondary flow events at a stenosis which color creates is no doubt an interpretive advantage in the hands of an experienced operator, and may reduce examination time by reducing the necessity to 'walk' the spectral Doppler cursor throughout the vessel. Finally, velocity increases which are not focal, such as increased carotid flow contralateral to a high-grade stenosis or occlusion, are readily appreciated in color images.

The North American Symptomatic Carotid Endarterectomy Trial (NASCET) has demonstrated that carotid endarterectomy is the treatment of choice for symptomatic patients with carotid artery lesions greater than 70%. In this study a 2-year overall risk reduction of 17% and 10% was noted in the surgical group as compared to the medically treated group for any ipsilateral stroke and major or fatal stroke respectively. Even before the results of this large randomized multicenter trial, carotid duplex sonography enjoyed widespread application and was well correlated with angiography.

While several different diagnostic schemes for determining percentage of stenosis in the ICA have been suggested, probably the most popular is the one developed at the University of Washington, in which B-mode appearance as well as peak systolic and diastolic velocities of the ICA were used to place stenoses in the categories of normal, 1–15%, 16–49%, 50–79%, 80–99% diameter stenosis and total occlusion (Table 7.2). These categories reflect the presumed clinical relevance of flow- and pressure-reducing lesions (those greater than 50%), particularly those which are more severe (greater than 80%) and are more often associated with tertiary flow effects. In this scheme, stenosis is defined in terms of minimum

Table 7.2   Color flow and spectral velocity criteria for diagnosis of internal carotid artery disease.

Category	*Criterion*
Normal	No increase in peak systolic velocity (PSV)
	No spectral broadening
	Normal bulb flow separation
1–15% stenosis	No increase in PSV
	Minimal spectral broadening during diastole
16–49% stenosis	No increase in PSV, marked spectral
	broadening (sample volume in center stream)
50–79% stenosis	PSV greater than 125 cm/s (4 kHz @ 60° and 5 MHz)
	End diastolic velocity (EDV)
	less than 140 cm/s (4.5 kHz @ 60° and 5 MHz)
80–99% stenosis	PSV greater than 250 cm/s
	EDV greater than 140 cm/s
Total occlusion	No flow
70%–99% stenosis (cervical ICA)	ICA PSV/CCA PSV ratio > 4.0[a] (Moneta et al)
	ICA PSV >230 cm/s (Patel et al)

[a]Sensitivity 91%, specificity 87%, positive predictive value (PPV) 76%, negative predictive value (NPV) 96%, overall accuracy 88%.
ICA stenosis defined as narrowest ICA diameter/distal cervical ICA diameter × 100.

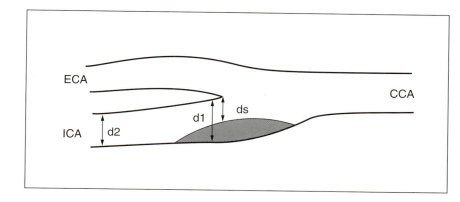

Figure 7.15 *Definitions of percentage stenosis. The dimension (ds) is the residual lumen diameter at the stenosis site. d1 is the diameter of the internal carotid artery (ICA) at the stenosis site, in this case in the carotid bulb. d2 is the ICA diameter distal to the bulb. The percentage diameter stenosis has been described both as follows:*
% stenosis = (d1 − ds)/d1 × 100
% stenosis = (d2 − ds)/d2 × 100.

diameter of ICA lumen/bulb diameter, which is different from the angiographic criterion of minimum lumen ICA/lumen of distal cervical ICA used in the NASCET trial, and will underestimate stenosis if compared to such angiographically defined lesions (Fig. 7.15). The results of the NASCET trial prompted Moneta et al to generate duplex criteria for identifying lesions of 70% or greater (corresponding to the selection criterion for endarterectomy in symptomatic patients), as defined by a ratio of the peak systolic velocity ICA/peak systolic velocity CCA of 4.0 or greater. More recently other studies have endeavoured to determine peak systolic velocity and end diastolic velocity criteria for this category of stenosis.

Although the natural history of asymptomatic high-grade lesions and the efficacy of carotid endarterectomy in this population is less clear, Strandness has reported that in his experience lesions that are

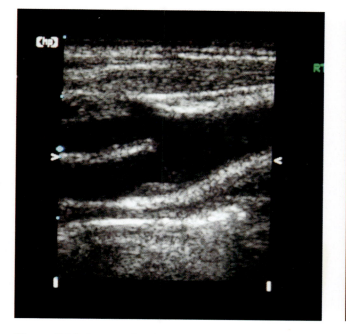

Figure 7.16 *Low grade ICA stenosis. The gray scale shows a plaque at the entrance to the ICA on the posterior wall of the carotid bulb indicating a <15% diameter reduction.*

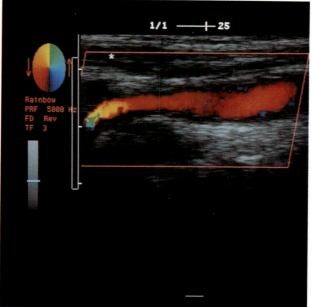

Figure 7.17 *Low grade ICA plaque. Plaque is visible on the posterior wall of the artery. Color changes do not indicate the presence of disease, but are caused by flow/beam angle changes.*

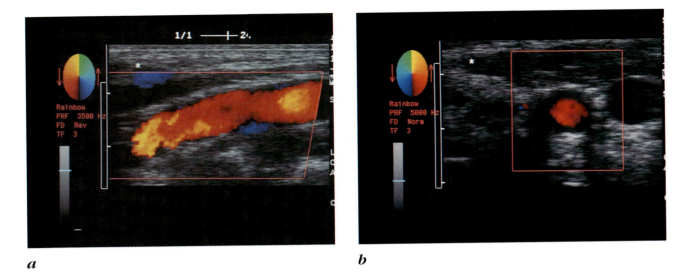

a   *b*

Figure 7.18 *Intimal thickening. (a) In the longitudinal view, flow fluctuations caused by the disease are shown on the color image, distal to the stenosis. Color resolution is not as good as gray scale resolution. The color image can obscure plaque detail. (b) Transverse view. The vessel wall shows uniform thickening. The residual lumen is narrowed but circular in section.*

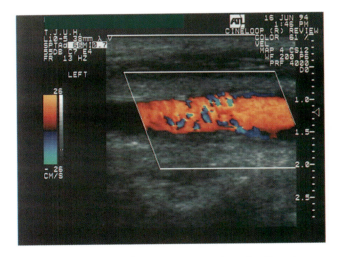

Figure 7.19 *Post-endarterectomy patch, color flow image. Flow fluctuations lead to non-uniform color flow in the image.*

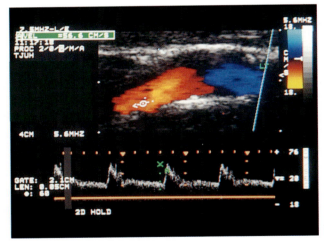

Figure 7.20 *Low grade plaque, Doppler image. There is <15% plaque. Flow is relatively unaffected as seen in the color image. Pulsed wave Doppler ultrasound shows normal velocities and no spectral broadening.*

categorized as greater than 80% using University of Washington criteria prove to be the most dangerous in terms of outcome in such patients. Certainly, aggressive treatment would be more likely for asymptomatic lesions contralateral to high-grade stenosis or occlusion.

A representative sample from a range of stenoses is shown in Figs 7.16–7.48. In low-grade stenoses (<50%), the gray scale image is usually a reliable means of estimating the degree of stenoses; peak velocities are relatively unchanged through the stenosis. In higher grade stenoses, the gray scale image may be less

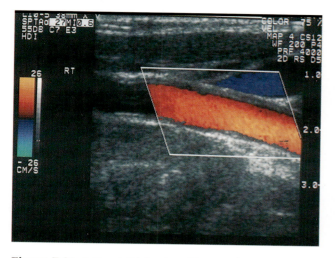

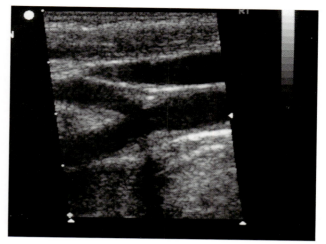

Figure 7.21 *Intimal thickening. The vessel wall shows thickening throughout the scanned length. Flow vectors are uniform, as shown in the color image.*

Figure 7.22 *Carotid bulb stenosis. There is plaque on both the anterior and posterior walls.*

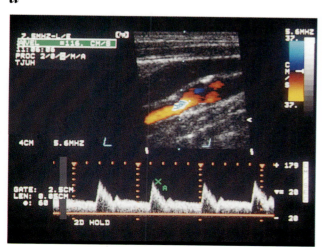

a

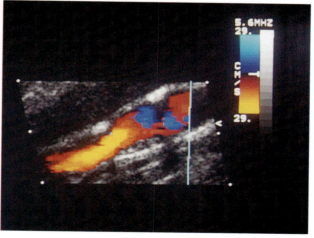

b

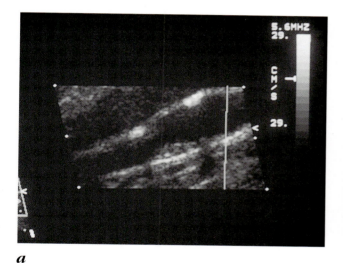

c

Figure 7.23 *ICA stenosis, 15–49%. (a) Gray scale. In this image, the B-mode is steered orthogonally to the vessel wall in order to optimize images. There is evidence of calcification on the anterior wall and smooth plaque along the posterior wall. (b) Color flow. The color shows a range of velocity vectors as flow direction changes. Nevertheless, a stenotic jet appears, coded yellow. (c) Pulsed wave Doppler. The Doppler cursor is placed in the stenotic jet and a peak systolic velocity of 116 cm/s is measured.*

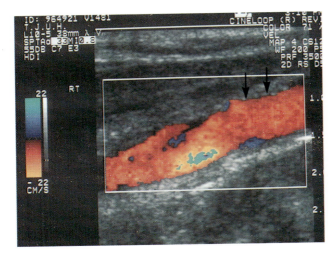

Figure 7.24 *ICA showing sutures from an arteriotomy (arrows).*

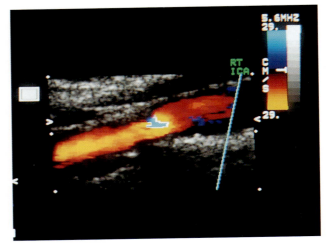

Figure 7.25 *Flow in an artery following endarterectomy. There is concentric narrowing with increased velocity but no flow disturbances.*

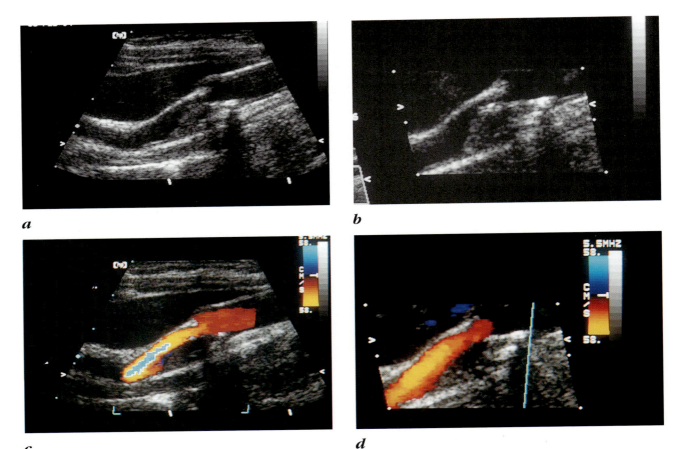

Figure 7.26 *Smooth plaque ICA. (a) With the trapezoidal image, the carotid bulb is seen to the right of the image. There is smooth plaque at the entrance to the ICA. (b) With the image of the stenosis magnified and the gray scale steered, the plaque is seen more clearly. The surface of the plaque reflects more strongly than its interior. (c) The color flow image shows increased velocity through the stenosis lumen. There is aliasing where the stenotic jet is more aligned to the Doppler beam direction. (d) In diastole, the velocities are reduced but the jet remains (there is no longer any aliasing). Because of the smooth shape, distal flow is not disorganized (despite the high grade lesion).*

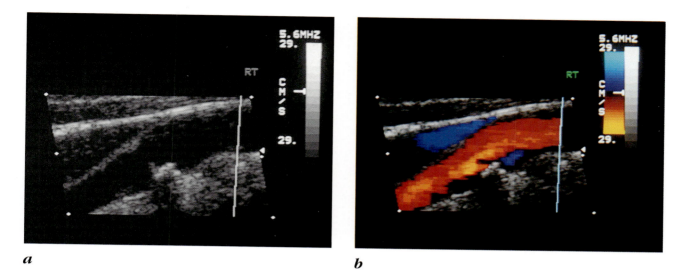

a　　　　　*b*

Figure 7.27 *Irregular plaque, ICA. (a) In the gray scale image, the plaque is irregular in shape and has a region of calcification. (b) The color flow shows the range of velocity vectors in the region of the stenosis. The protrusion of the irregular shape into the flow stream produces regions of sudden flow direction changes upstream, and of separation downstream.*

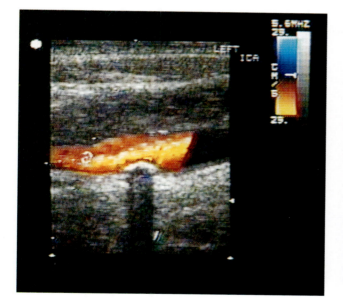

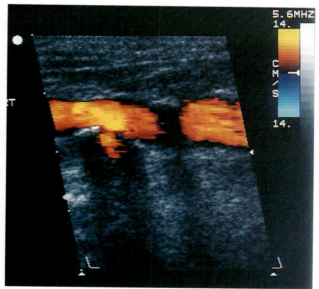

Figure 7.28 *ICA stenosis: calcification. The high reflectivity of a calcified plaque on the posterior wall shows as a bright area on the gray scale image. Poor transmission beyond it produces an 'acoustic shadow'.*

Figure 7.29 *ICA stenosis: calcification. Calcification on the anterior wall produces color and B-mode signal loss.*

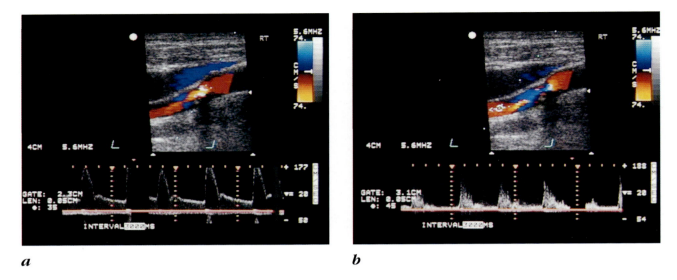

a   *b*

Figure 7.30 *ICA stenosis, 50–79%. (a) CFI shows high velocities within the stenosis and disturbed flow distally. In the stenosis, pulsed wave Doppler detects velocities >180 cm/s. Note the lack of spectral broadening in the stenotic jet. (b) Distally, velocities are lower and flow disturbances are evident.*

reliable and greater emphasis should be placed on the hemodynamic changes resulting from the narrowing.

While determining the percentage of stenosis is clearly accepted as a predictor of patient outcome, attempts have been made to identify plaque types which may give rise to embolic disease. It has been postulated that emboli are generated from active areas of plaque such as those which are ulcerated or hemorrhagic. Attempts have been made to identify ulceration by irregular plaque surfaces and intraplaque hemorrhage by plaque heterogeneity. To date, correlating systematic plaque characterization with pathology specimens obtained at endarterectomy has been disappointing, due to false-positive results caused by pits in fibrotic plaque, atheromatous debris and calcified plaque shadowing. Correlation has also been hampered by errors in handling histologic specimens, and variability in ultrasound and histology reporting methods.

In addition to atherosclerotic disease, CFI can be used in the diagnoses of carotid artery dissection, (Fig. 7.49) and pseudoaneurysms (Fig. 7.50). Again, the combination of high resolution B-mode and specific flow characteristics clearly identifies the anatomy and morphology of these conditions. In a similar way, the rare but readily apparent characteristics of a carotid body tumor (Fig. 7.51) are seen if color flow sensitivity is adequate to detect the low flow velocities in tumors.

VERTEBRAL ARTERIES

Although a benign course is common in patients with vertebral basilar insufficiency, duplex examination of the vertebral arteries should be included in all cerebrovascular ultrasound evaluations. The reasons for this are twofold:

- the vertebrobasilar system may function as an important collateral pathway in cases of severe carotid artery stenosis or occlusion;
- some patients are referred to the vascular laboratory for TIAs and CVAs which appear by symptomatology to be from the posterior circulation.

Vertebrobasilar embolic phenomena are less common than fixed atherosclerosis, presumably due to the small caliber and acute angles of the vertebral arteries. Furthermore, vertebral artery occlusion may be well tolerated and last for a short segment only due to the rich collateral network of the muscular neck branches. Vertebrobasilar symptoms often arise from global ischemia as well as the lipohyalinosis seen in hypertensives which may lead to pontine or internal capsule lacunar infarcts. Congenital anomalies such as vertebral artery hypoplasia or aplasia, dissection due to trauma, and compression by osteophytes with head rotation or hyperextension, are

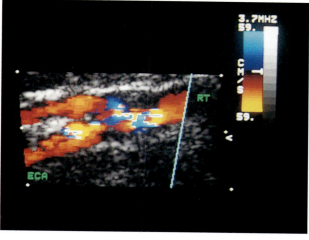

a

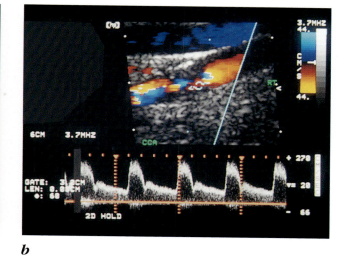

b

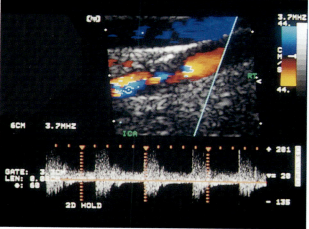

c

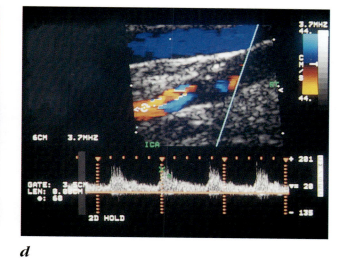

d

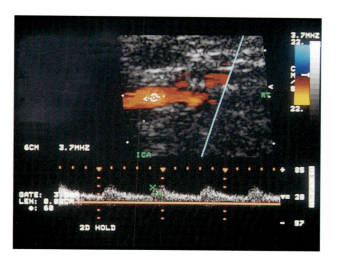

e

Figure 7.31 *Heterogeneous plaque (50–79%) in the carotid bulb. (a) There is plaque visible on the anterior and posterior walls of the carotid bulb. The course of the lumen is tortuous and the lumen walls irregular, causing non-uniform flow as displayed on the color image. (b) In the stenosis, velocities are high (peak systolic velocity >250 cm/s) and the waveform shows no flow disturbances. (c) Distal to the stenosis, there are flow disturbances in the expansion region. (d) Further downstream, flow disturbances are less severe. (e) Distally, there is a damped flow waveform in the ICA as a result of the proximal stenosis.*

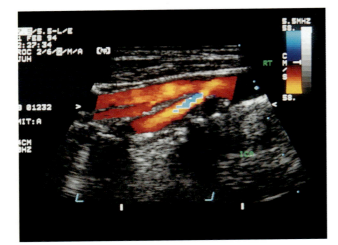

Figure 7.32 *Carotid bifurcation: 50–79% stenosis of the ICA. The image shows a stenosis at the posterior wall of the carotid bulb leading to the ICA. This is a common site of disease. A branch of the more superficial artery identifies it as the ECA.*

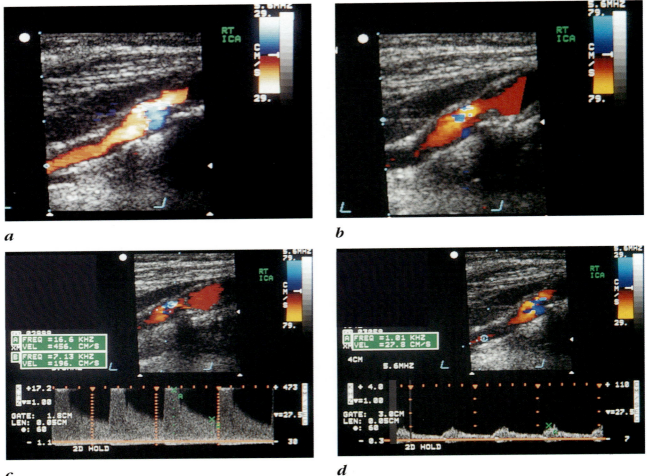

Figure 7.33 *High grade (80–99%) ICA stenosis. (a) Inappropriate use of low-velocity scale results in a confusing color image with aliasing and color 'bleeding' which obscures image detail. (b) A higher velocity scale (increased pulse repetition frequency) shows aliasing in the stenosis jet. Note, however, that the low flow velocities in the distal artery do not register at this setting. (c) Pulsed wave Doppler in the stenosis shows a peak systolic velocity of >456 cm/s, and an end diastolic velocity of 196 cm/s. Spectral broadening can occur due to multiple direction vectors in a stenosis depending on the geometry or from insonating the immediate post-stenotic region. (d) Distally, the ICA flow waveform is dampened.*

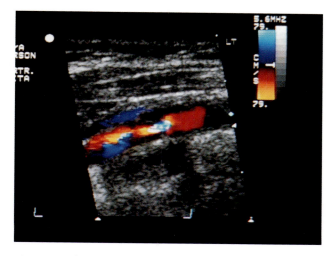

Figure 7.34 *High-grade (80–99%) ICA stenosis. This color image depicts the classical features of flow through a stenosis. To the right of the image, pre-stenotic flow is uniform and low velocity. In the stenosis, high velocities lead to aliasing. Post stenosis, the jet gradually dissipates and there are regions of eddies (coded blue) in the expansion region.*

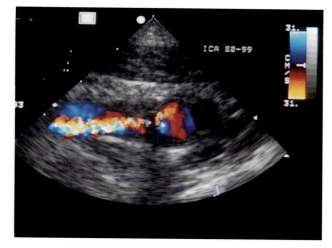

Figure 7.35 *High grade stenosis (80–99%), sector scanner. The phased array transducer produces ultrasound beams radiating from a point or surface (as opposed to linear arrays, where the individual beams are of uniform direction). The complex velocity vectors through the stenosis combine with the geometry of the phased array scan to produce an image which may be difficult to interpret. This image does show, however, the presence of a stenotic jet.*

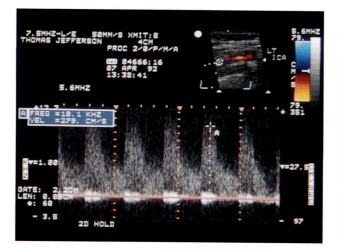

Figure 7.36 *Carotid bruit, spectral display. The spectral display shows high velocities (peak systolic velocity 279 cm/s) associated with an 80–99% ICA stenosis. Within the spectrum, there is a low-frequency, high-amplitude signal resulting from vibrations associated with a carotid bruit.*

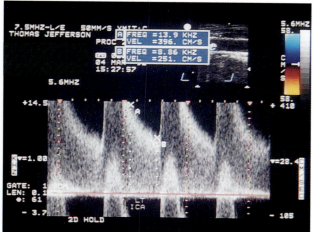

Figure 7.37 *ICA stenosis, spectral aliasing. In very tight stenoses, flow velocities may exceed the depth/range limits for pulsed wave Doppler ultrasound. In this example, peak systolic velocity is over 600 cm/s. Although the spectral display shows aliasing, in this case it is clearly visible and the correct velocity can be assessed by adding the aliased portion of the waveform to the maximum of the velocity scale.*

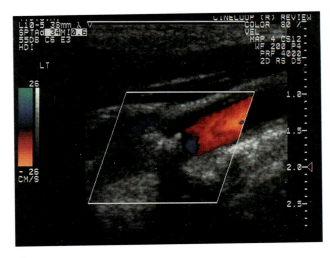

a

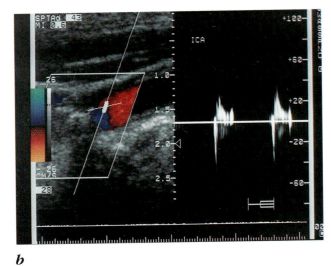

b

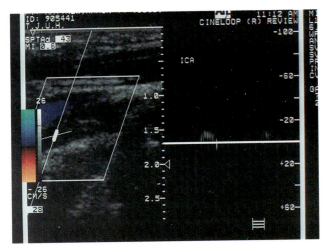

c

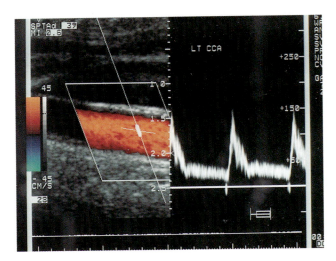

d

e

Figure 7.42 *ICA occlusion. Color and spectral indications. (a) The color image shows a stump of the ICA with distal plaque and no flow signal. (b) Pulsed wave Doppler of the arterial stump shows sudden flow reversal. (c) There are no detectable flow signals from the ICA. (d) The ipsilateral CCA has a high-resistance flow waveform with no diastolic flow. (e) The contralateral CCA has a low-resistance waveform with high diastolic flow.*

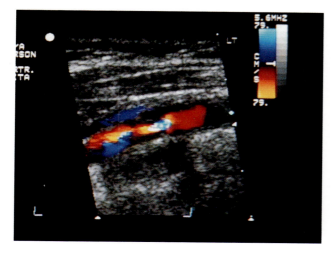

Figure 7.34 *High-grade (80–99%) ICA stenosis. This color image depicts the classical features of flow through a stenosis. To the right of the image, pre-stenotic flow is uniform and low velocity. In the stenosis, high velocities lead to aliasing. Post stenosis, the jet gradually dissipates and there are regions of eddies (coded blue) in the expansion region.*

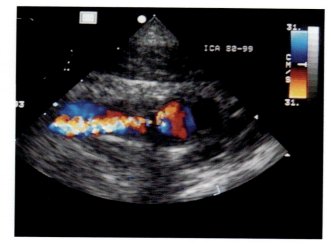

Figure 7.35 *High grade stenosis (80–99%), sector scanner. The phased array transducer produces ultrasound beams radiating from a point or surface (as opposed to linear arrays, where the individual beams are of uniform direction). The complex velocity vectors through the stenosis combine with the geometry of the phased array scan to produce an image which may be difficult to interpret. This image does show, however, the presence of a stenotic jet.*

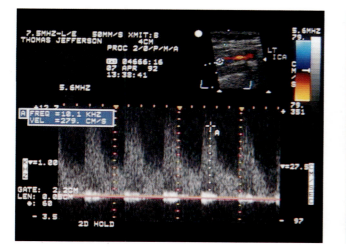

Figure 7.36 *Carotid bruit, spectral display. The spectral display shows high velocities (peak systolic velocity 279 cm/s) associated with an 80–99% ICA stenosis. Within the spectrum, there is a low-frequency, high-amplitude signal resulting from vibrations associated with a carotid bruit.*

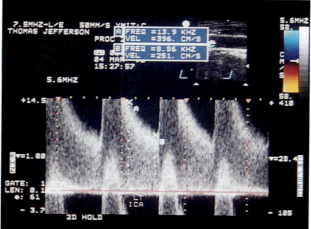

Figure 7.37 *ICA stenosis, spectral aliasing. In very tight stenoses, flow velocities may exceed the depth/range limits for pulsed wave Doppler ultrasound. In this example, peak systolic velocity is over 600 cm/s. Although the spectral display shows aliasing, in this case it is clearly visible and the correct velocity can be assessed by adding the aliased portion of the waveform to the maximum of the velocity scale.*

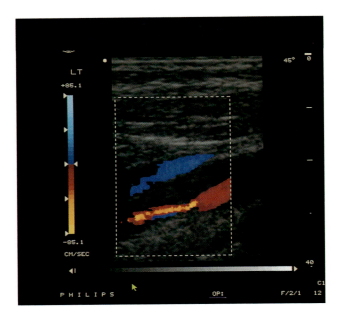

Figure 7.38 *Color Velocity Imaging, 80–99% ICA stenosis. Although the artery is deep and the flow/beam angle is poor, the contrasting yellow indicates high-velocity vectors in the stenosis.*

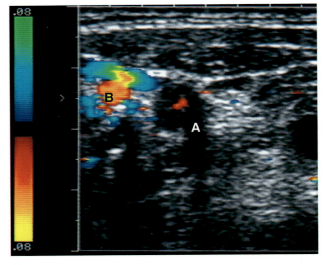

a

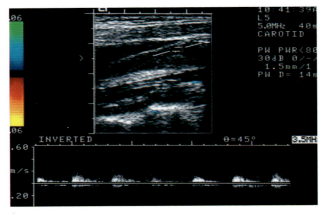

b

Figure 7.39 *ICA >95% stenosis. (a) A tight stenosis is imaged in the ICA (A) in a transverse view. The ECA is seen at B. Velocities through this stenosis are very low and the color flow pulse repetition frequency is reduced for increased sensitivity to low velocities. (b) In a longitudinal view, pulsed spectral Doppler shows a low-velocity flow waveform which is typical of a pre-occlusive stenosis.*

other etiologies of vertebrobasilar ischemia. The latter has been successfully evaluated with 'blind' transcranial Doppler.

Duplex evaluation of the cervical portion of the vertebral arteries for fixed disease is more limited and less sensitive (65%) than in carotid evaluation; however, its relatively high specificity (88%) warrants attempting evaluation. Stenosis or occlusion of the proximal subclavian or brachiocephalic artery may cause reversed flow in the ipsilateral vertebral artery, providing collateral bloodflow to the affected arm. This condition, known as subclavian steal, may be associated with arm claudication (pain with exercise), and is easily documented with CFI or duplex sonography. It may be treated with vertebral implantation

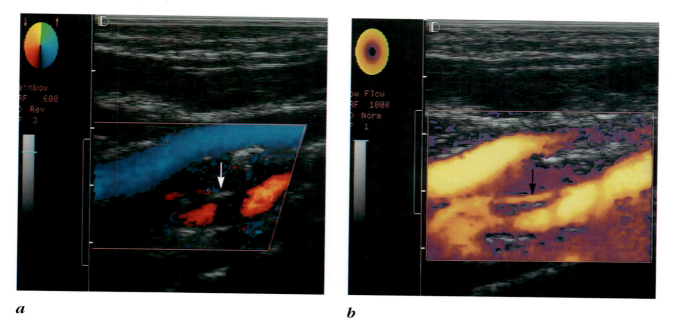

a   *b*

Figure 7.40 *(a) Conventional (mean Doppler frequency shift) image of a pre-occlusive stenosis. There is evidence of flow in the ICA (arrow) but visualization is generally poor. (b) Color amplitude imaging of the same stenosis. A string 'sign' is seen (arrow) indicating patency. Some color flow artifact occurs from the tissue. These findings were confirmed on a subsequent MRA examination.*

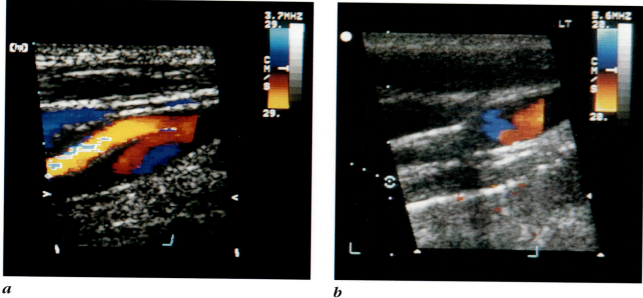

a   *b*

Figure 7.41 *ICA occlusion—CFI characteristics. (a) The image shows the ECA lying superficial to the ICA. Flow in the bulb appears normal but there are no flow signals from within the ICA lumen. (b) The carotid bulb ends in a stump with swirling flow in the bulb but no signals in the ICA. The lumen of the ICA is more echogenic than normal, suggesting plaque/thrombus.*

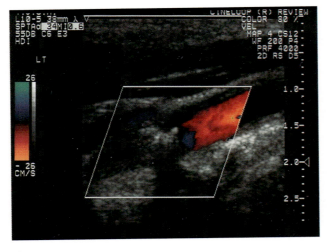

a

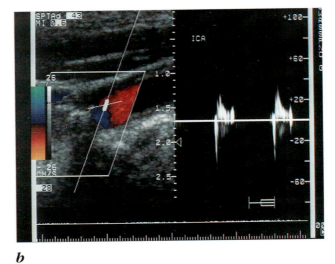

b

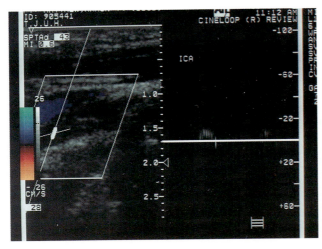

c

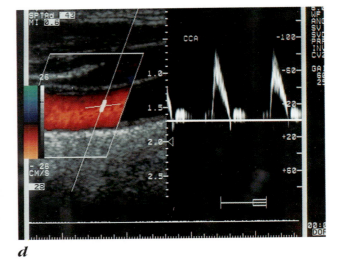

d

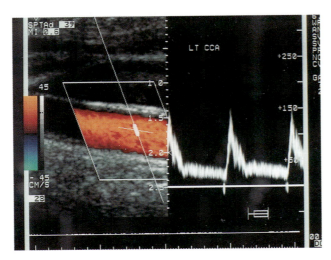

e

Figure 7.42 *ICA occlusion. Color and spectral indications. (a) The color image shows a stump of the ICA with distal plaque and no flow signal. (b) Pulsed wave Doppler of the arterial stump shows sudden flow reversal. (c) There are no detectable flow signals from the ICA. (d) The ipsilateral CCA has a high-resistance flow waveform with no diastolic flow. (e) The contralateral CCA has a low-resistance waveform with high diastolic flow.*

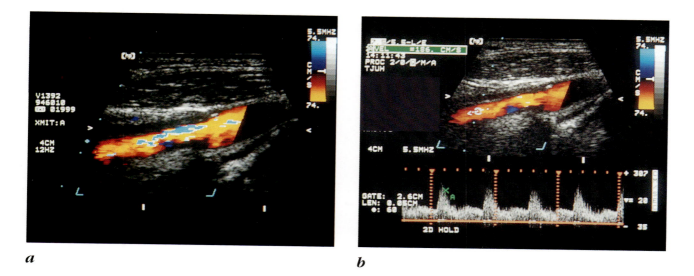

a   *b*

Figure 7.43   *Flow in an ICA contralateral to an ICA occlusion. (a) Flow in the patent ICA is high to compensate for the contralateral occlusion. Note that there is aliasing despite a high pulse repetition setting for the color flow image. (b) Pulsed spectral Doppler shows high velocities throughout this ICA despite only minor disease. Occluded arteries (especially an ICA) can render normal hemodynamic criteria in arteries providing collateral flow unreliable because of compensatory flow changes.*

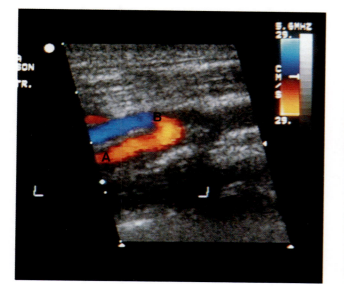

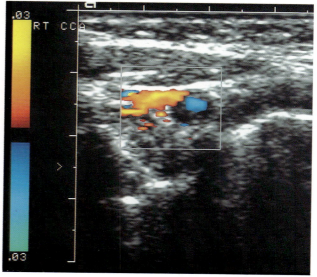

Figure 7.44   *CCA occlusion. Flow to the ICA (A) is from the ECA through the bulb (B) as demonstrated by the color image.*

Figure 7.45   *CCA sub-occlusive stenosis. A rare finding, this small flow channel was found 30 years following surgical ligation of the CCA. The color flow sensitivity is at its maximum setting; flow velocities (coded blue) through the remaining lumen are very low.*

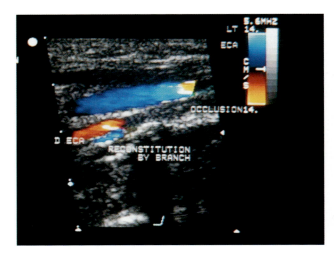

Figure 7.46 *Common and internal artery occlusion. In this case, ECA flow is from retrograde flow in a small arterial branch.*

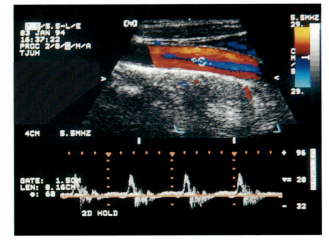

Figure 7.47 *CCC flow reversal in diastole. Reversed flow is seen on the sonogram caused by aortic insufficiency. CFI shows flow reversal in the center of the vessel. This can occur in cases of sharp acceleration or deceleration due to differences in fluid momentum across the bloodstream.*

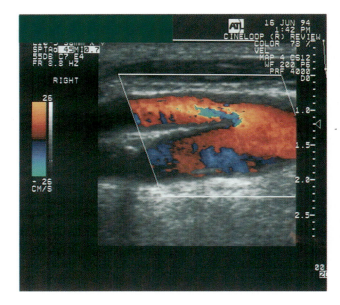

Figure 7.48 *ECA focal stenosis. The color box is steered to optimize the color flow image of the ECA. A stenotic jet is seen at the origin of the artery.*

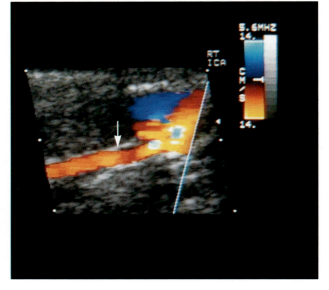

Figure 7.49 *Carotid artery dissection. The anterior wall of the ICA is dissected (arrow). Thrombus lies between the dissected wall and the adventitia.*

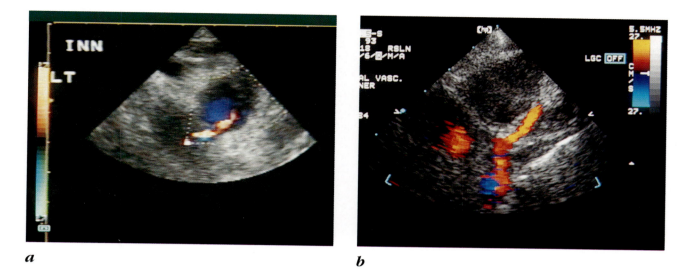

a *b*

Figure 7.50 *CCA pseudoaneurysm. (a) A misplaced venous line has resulted in iatrogenic injury to the CCA and a pseudoaneurysm has resulted. (Note the bi-directional flow in the pseudoaneurysm with the high flow velocities leading to it.) (b) The pseudoaneurysm has now thrombosed. (The artery lying posteriorly in this view is the subclavian artery.)*

or various bypasses. The vertebrals, however, are not frequently approached surgically, even in the case of subclavian steal, as symptomatology tends to be non-specific and may resolve spontaneously (or with carotid endarterectomy in the case of severe bilateral carotid artery disease), while persistence of symptoms postsurgery is common.

The vertebral artery usually originates as the first branch of the subclavian artery. The proximal (pre-osseous) segment of the vertebral artery at the vertebral origin from the subclavian artery may be evaluated sonographically in 81–88% of individuals on the right and in 25–67% of individuals on the left. The increased incidence of failure on the left side is due to the deeper and more variable location of the vertebral artery on this side (the vertebral artery may arise from the arch in 8% of cases). The origin is the most common site of fixed disease, and is best located by scanning proximally down the vertebral artery from its interosseous portion where the shadows of the transverse processes verify its identity. A 5 MHz sector transducer is most appropriate for examination of this segment. The intraosseous segment can be seen intermittently as it passes the transverse processes with a 5.0–7.5 MHz linear transducer in almost all individuals (Fig. 7.52). Color is not always necessary, but is very helpful in locating these small, deep vessels, and may be required in many cases. The intracranial portion as well as portions of the basilar artery may be seen using color flow imaging with low-frequency (2.0 MHz) phased array transducers in approximately 87% of an age-appropriate population (Figs 7.53 and 7.54). The transforamenal approach is used for evaluation of this segment.

While the interosseous or cervical portion of the vertebral artery tends to have a peak systolic flow velocity of approximately 40 cm/s with a standard deviation of 10 cm/s, individual variation is common, particularly the presence of one vertebral artery which appears 'dominant'. Thus diagnosis is more qualitative than quantitative. Hypoplasia/aplasia can be defined as a small or absent vertebral artery, often with a high-resistance spectral waveform. When stenoses are visualized they should reveal a jet with diminished distal flow. A blunted waveform suggests proximal disease, a high-resistance waveform suggests intrinsic vertebral artery disease, and the absence of flow in a visualized artery suggests occlusion if technical factors can be excluded. In the case of subclavian steal a reverse or to and fro (transient steal) waveform in the vertebral artery is observed (Fig. 7.55), with a diminished ipsilateral brachial

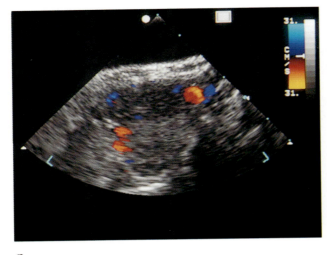

a

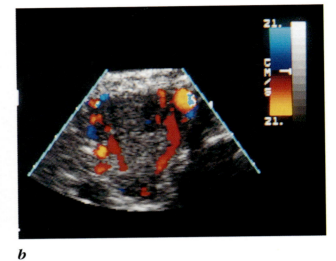

b

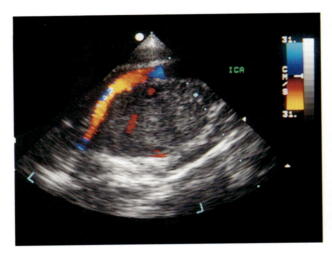

c

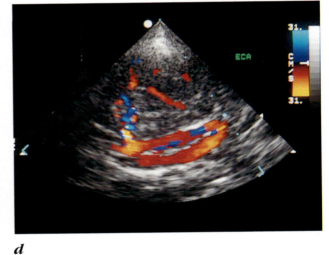

d

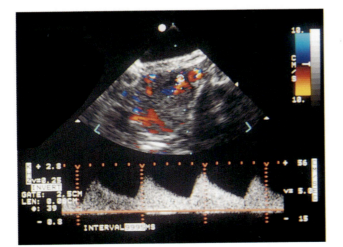

e

Figure 7.51 *Carotid body tumor. (a) In this transverse view with pulse repetition frequency (PRF) set high, the ICA is seen laterally (to the right of the image) and superficially. The ECA and a branch are medial. The tumor lies between them. (b) In the same plane with the PRF reduced, flow is seen within the tumor. (c) In a longitudinal scan, the ICA curves around the tumor. (d) In another longitudinal scan the ECA is seen posterior to the tumor. As a consequence, the ECA lies deeper than normal. Note that the mass is supplied by a branch of the ECA. (e) Flow waveforms in the tumor vessels show a low distal resistance.*

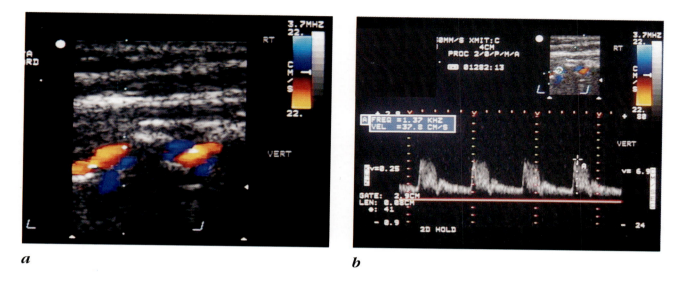

a   *b*

Figure 7.52 *Vertebral artery and vein. (a) As these vessels pass through the transverse processes of the vertebrae, acoustic shadowing leads to loss of image and flow signals. (b) The pulsed wave Doppler sonogram shows a flow waveform similar to those obtained from the ICA.*

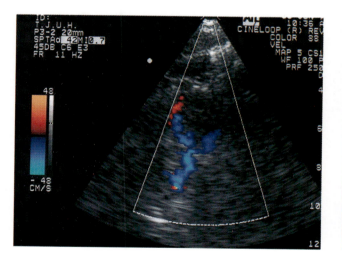

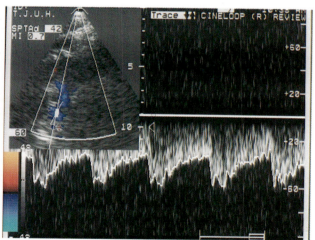

Figure 7.53 *Transforamenal CFI of the basilar and vertebral arteries.*

Figure 7.54 *Basilar artery waveform. Like the ICA and vertebral artery waveforms, this has low resistance with high diastolic flow.*

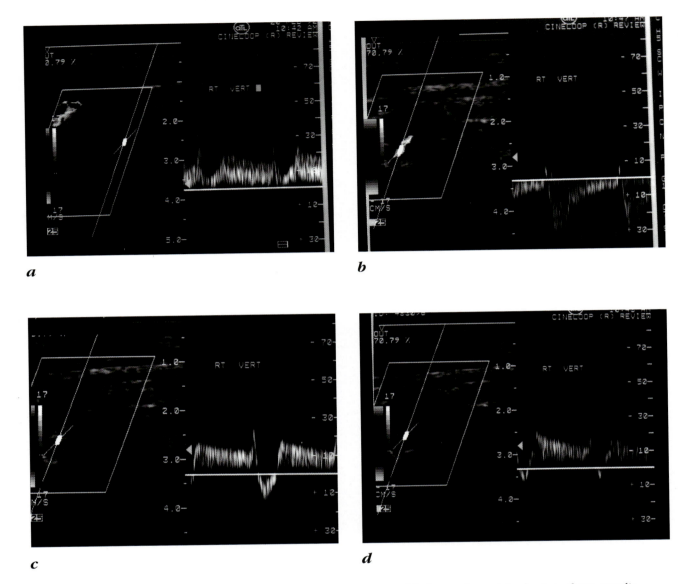

Figure 7.55 *Vertebral/subclavian steal—effect of hyperemic response. (a) At rest the vertebral artery shows systolic hesitation, suggesting a steal. (b) Following exercise of the ipsilateral hand, there is a hyperemic response and flow is reversed in the vertebral artery throughout the cardiac cycle. (c,d) As the hyperemic response diminishes, recovery of the diastolic flow commences (c) and later the reversed flow in systole reduces (d).*

blood pressure. Jet-like or monophasic ipsilateral subclavian waveforms (see peripheral arteries, upper extremity in this section) may be observed.

INTRACRANIAL IMAGING

Transcranial duplex and CFI has enjoyed recent popularity as a result of instrument modification and the development of manufacturer presets which optimize settings for penetration and insonation of the small, deep vessels of the circle of Willis. Introduced by Rune Aaslid in 1982, transcranial Doppler was originally performed in a 'blind' fashion using a pulsed wave 1.0–2.5 MHz Doppler transducer without the benefit of B-mode imaging. Vessels were identified by depth, probe angulation, identification of landmark

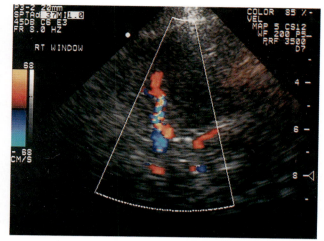

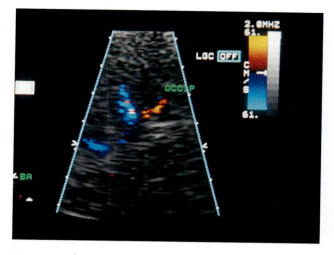

Figure 7.56 *Transforamenal CFI of a steal. Flow in the left vertebral artery is reversed.*

Figure 7.57 *Transcranial image of a middle cerebral stenosis. The color image shows aliasing at the site of narrowing.*

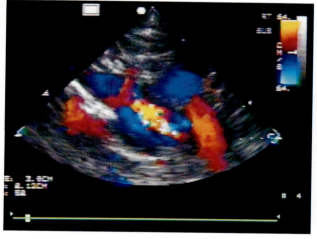

a

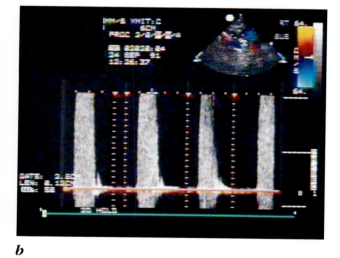

b

Figure 7.58 *Subclavian artery stenosis. (a) The color image shows the presence of a stenotic jet (coded yellow) at the origin of the subclavian artery. (b) The pulsed wave Doppler sonogram shows a high velocity jet. (c) The ipsilateral vertebral artery shows flow reversal in systole. There is a steal into the subclavian artery.*

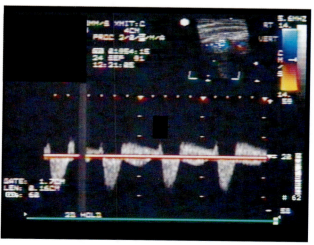

c

bifurcation points and with compression and oscillation maneuvers. The addition of B-mode imaging and CFI to the examination allows the visualization of bony and soft tissue landmarks, as well as color flow display of vessels to aid in vessel identification. While this is a learning and interpretive aid, it should be noted that a full transtemporal examination (middle cerebral artery, anterior cerebral artery and posterior cerebral artery) can be obtained in only approximately 52% of cases in an age-appropriate population; as opposed to a success rate of 72% using the 'blind' probes. These differences reflect an increased attenuation using the imaging probe, and suggest that in individuals in whom an acoustic window cannot be obtained using imaging, a blind examination should be attempted.

The utility of transcranial Doppler has been argued in the literature. Its most well-accepted application is monitoring for vasospasm after subarachnoid hemorrhage, an examination which is done with the more portable and less expensive 'blind' instruments. Transcranial imaging may be used as an extension of the cerebrovascular examination, however, and may provide information on the downstream effects of lesions seen proximally (cervical ICA, vertebral artery) (Fig. 7.56), including collateral flow through the circle of Willis, as well as to detect intracranial stenosis in patients with lateralizing TIAs, but a normal extracranial examination (Fig. 7.57).

The transcranial examination is performed using a 2.0 MHz phased array transducer. It is advisable to use software specifically designed for transcranial imaging. The temporal window is located superior to the zygomatic arch and just anterior to the conch of the ear. The majority of the examination is done in the transaxial plane. However, longitudinal views are also possible. The cerebral peduncles and the sphenoid bone serve as landmarks, the posterior cerebral arteries lying adjacent to and wrapping around the peduncles, while the middle cerebral artery passes through the temporal lobe in the middle fossa just posterior to the sphenoid bone. The examination is extremely operator dependent, whether done blindly or with imaging. Normal values for angle-corrected peak systolic velocities of the basal cerebral arteries in an age appropriate population are included in Table 7.3. The bulk of the transcranial literature is based on blind transcranial Doppler (TCD), which uses time average peak velocities (mean of the peaks), assuming an angle of insonation of 0°. A comparison of angle corrected and non angle corrected peak systolic velocities obtained by transcranial imaging suggests that angle correction was only potentially clinically significant 7% of the time (the most frequently affected vessels being the vertebral arteries, the anterior cerebral artery, followed by the posterior cerebral artery). Thus, established norms obtained with blind instruments can probably be applied to information obtained with imaging with angle correction (or with the cursor set at 0°) (see Table 7.3).

TRANSORBITAL

Blind evaluation of the carotid siphon, ophthalmic artery and periorbital vessels has been well described in the literature. While the carotid siphon is a likely area for atherosclerotic disease, imaging of the siphon has not enjoyed as widespread application as transforamenal and transtemporal imaging, presum-

Table 7.3 Normal velocity values of the basal cerebral arteries (from Fujioka et al 1994).

Vessel	Normal PSV TCI (transcranial imaging) (imaging angle corrected) (cm/s)	Normal averaged PSV TCD (transcranial Doppler) TCD (blind) (cm/s)
Middle cerebral artery	78 ± 26	55 ± 12
Anterior cerebral artery	71 ± 19	50 ± 11
Posterior cerebral artery	57 ± 14	39 ± 10
Basilic artery	55 ± 16	41 ± 10
Vertebral arteries	48 ± 19	38 ± 10

ably due to concerns regarding exposure of the retina to high intensities of acoustic energy, and difficulty with acoustic access. The ophthalmic artery and its branches, however, can be readily imaged with higher frequency probes (5.0–10.0 MHz) using minimal power output settings to minimize patient exposure. Excellent CFI angles of insonation are available in the vessels in question. The ophthalmic artery can be evaluated to determine whether it is functioning as a collateral source for a carotid stenosis or occlusion (reversal of direction). The information which this adds to the examination will probably be purely descriptive.

The ophthalmic artery passes through the optic foramen inferior to the optic nerve, but then moves upward, crossing the nerve superiorly, running medially across the retro-orbital space. In its proximal portion it gives rise to the ciliary arteries, which supply the orbit, the lacrimal artery, which runs along the lateral aspect of the orbit to the lacrimal gland, and the central retinal artery, which is easily identified by its location in the optic nerve. The ophthalmic artery is most confidently identified as it crosses the optic nerve, and in its segment proximal to that, prior to branching.

We have seen many cases in which severely reduced ophthalmic artery flow was seen on CFI contralateral to a high grade carotid stenosis or occlusion. As some of these patients were experiencing loss of vision in the eye in question, the potential of this method for evaluating visual symptoms which may be of vascular origin is raised. It is interesting also to note that in a series of 54 patients correlated with angiography, we noted three cases of ophthalmic artery occlusion.

Other pathologies which have been described using CFI in this anatomic region include carotid cavernous fistulas, orbital masses, varices, arterial-venous malformations and superior ophthalmic vein thrombus (see Chapter 6).

UPPER AND LOWER LIMB ARTERIAL AND VENOUS FLOW

UPPER EXTREMITY—ARTERIAL

Atherosclerosis of the major arteries of the upper extremity occurs far less frequently than in the lower extremity and is rarely associated with symptoms of claudication or ischemia. The proximal subclavian artery, however, has a moderate frequency of

Table 7.4 Diagnostic criterion for LIMA at the third intercostal space (from Strauss et al 1991).

	Diameter	Velocity	Resistive index
Preop.	2.2 ± 0.2	54 cm/s	1.0 or greater
Postop.			0.5 or less

atherosclerotic involvement (an example is given in Fig. 7.58). Arterial disease at this site may cause subclavian steal (Fig. 7.55) or be of concern when it occurs on the left side and a left internal mammary artery (LIMA) graft to the coronary arteries is being contemplated (the LIMA is a branch of the subclavian). In the latter case, duplex ultrasound of the subclavian arteries and the LIMA as it courses down the chest wall can be performed pre- and postoperatively for surveillance (Table 7.4 and Fig. 7.59).

Other cases in which non-invasive upper extremity ultrasound evaluation may be indicated include preoperative evaluation prior to dialysis fistula or graft placement, evaluation of iatrogenic (usually catheter-induced) or traumatic injuries, evaluation for compression at the thoracic outlet (thoracic outlet syndrome or TOS) and evaluation of obstructive and vasospastic disorders of the digital arteries. The latter is usually evaluated with non-imaging modalities such as plethysmography, pressure assessment and high-frequency continuous wave Doppler.

The subclavian artery exits the thoracic outlet (Fig. 7.60) and runs peripherally through the axilla, where it is called the axillary artery, down the upper arm to the humerus, where it is called the brachial artery (it may be duplicated in this segment). The brachial artery is accompanied by two or more brachial veins, and may be approximated by the basilic vein, particularly as this superficial vein nears its confluence with the brachial vein. At the antecubital fossa the brachial artery divides into the radial and ulnar arteries, each running adjacent to their analogously named forearm bone to the level of the wrist, continuing into the hand and forming the deep and superficial palmar arches that give rise to the digital arteries. The radial and ulnar arteries are accompanied by paired veins. Occasionally the radial and ulnar arteries may arise from separate paired brachial arteries.

Spectral waveforms of the normal upper extremity arteries are usually triphasic with a rapid systolic

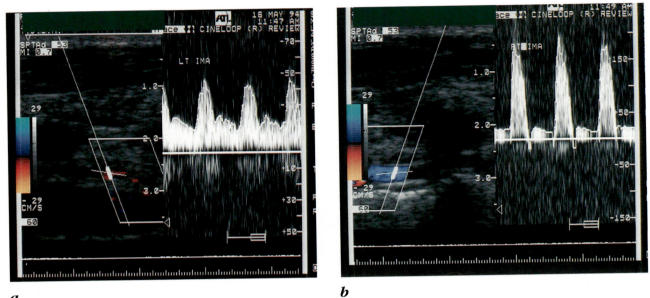

a *b*

Figure 7.59 *Subclavian stenosis—effect on the internal mammary artery. (a) The internal mammary artery is imaged in a parasternal long axis view. A proximal subclavian stenosis causes reduced peak systolic velocity and dampened flow with a reduced resistive index. (b) The contralateral internal mammary artery has a normal triphasic flow waveform.*

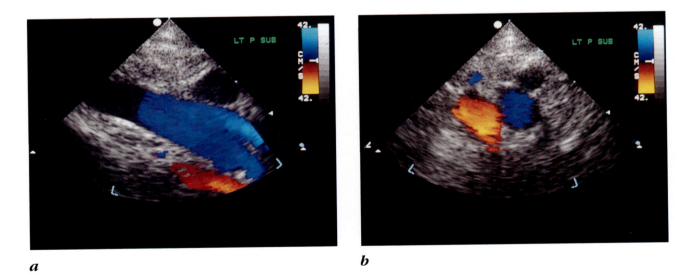

a *b*

Figure 7.60 *Subclavian artery and vein. (a) In this longitudinal view the vein lies anteriorly. The echoluscent region anterior and to the right of the image is a lymph node. (b) Transverse view.*

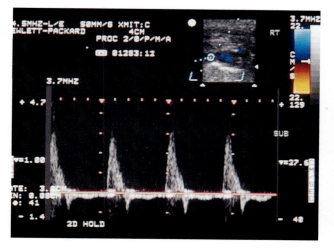

Figure 7.61 *Normal subclavian artery waveform. In contrast to the arteries supplying the cerebral circulation, the subclavian artery shows a high-resistance waveform typical of arteries supplying at-rest striated muscle.*

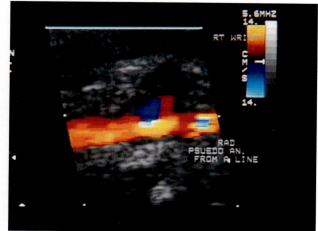

Figure 7.62 *A small pseudoaneurysm of a radial artery which occurred following insertion of an arterial line. Color in the pseudoaneurysm is bi-directional, resulting from swirling flow.*

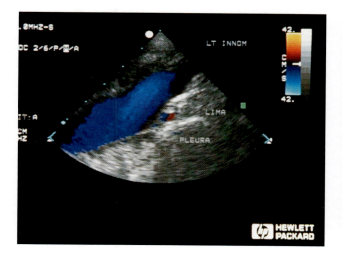

Figure 7.63 *Left innominate vein, coronal plane. The clavicle restricts ultrasound access to this and adjacent arteries and veins. Phased array transducers are helpful for these scans because of their wide field of view from a limited contact area. Note the echogenic pleura posterior to the vein and the internal mammary artery between the pleura and vein.*

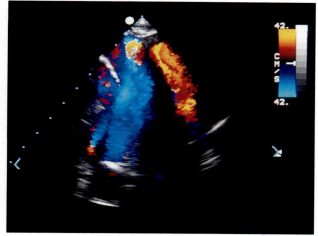

Figure 7.64 *Right innominate vein and brachiocephalic artery, coronal plane.*

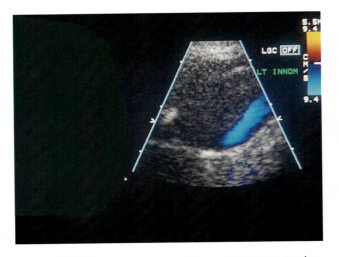

Figure 7.65 *Thrombus surrounding a pacer wire in the left innominate vein. There is a residual flow channel around the thrombus.*

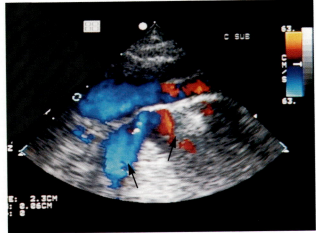

Figure 7.66 *Mirror image of the subclavian vein. The color 'ghost image' (arrows) arises from the strong ultrasound reflections from the pleura. Ghost images of the vein and artery can be very convincing.*

upstroke (Fig. 7.61). Distal to an obstruction, waveforms may be monophasic or demonstrate continuous positive bloodflow. Patients with vasospasm may exhibit an oscillating type of waveform with five or more phases. Stenosis of the upper extremity arteries is categorized as <50% or ≥50% by documenting an increase of 100% or more in peak systolic velocity at the stenotic site as compared to the prestenotic segment (see discussion on lower extremity arteries for further explanation).

Examining the potential inflow vessels of a dialysis access placement is often done in conjunction with venous mapping of the upper extremity. This is particularly true in the diabetic population, in which a higher incidence of stenosis/occlusion and or vessel calcification in the forearm has been noted. Poor inflow vessels may lead to a low-flow fistula which provides inadequate dialysis and is likely to thrombose.

Vascular injuries in the upper extremity are varied. Areas of penetrating (gunshot or stab wound) or blunt trauma or previous catheterization may be evaluated to rule out pseudoaneurysm (Fig. 7.62), fistula or intimal tear. Repetitive or vibration trauma of the hand has been reported to cause thrombosis of the ulnar artery.

A dynamic color/duplex Doppler evaluation can be performed to assess for subclavian artery compression (TOS), a condition which most often

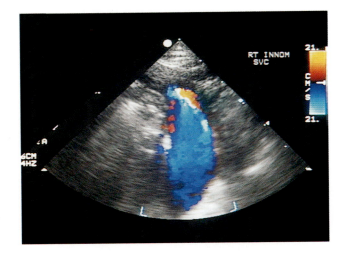

Figure 7.67 *Right innominate vein draining into the superior vena cava, coronal plane.*

occurs in conjunction with a cervical rib and is most common in young women. The artery can become compressed in the interscalene, costoclavicular or subcoracoid triangles. Flow jets in the medial subclavian artery demonstrating a 100% increase from

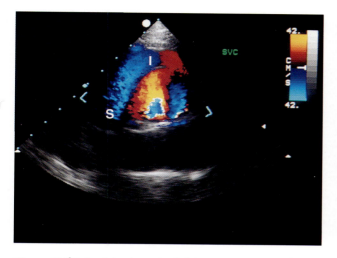

Figure 7.68 *In this view, the left innominate vein (I) crosses over the aorta seen in cross-section, and drains into the superior vena cava (S). In the far field, the pulmonary artery can be seen.*

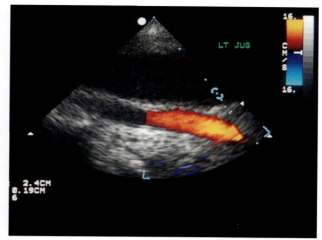

Figure 7.69 *Jugular vein thrombus. The jugular vein lies anterior to the CCA. The enlarged lumen contains echogenic material and no flow signals are detected from it.*

baseline, or diminished, monophasic or absent flow with the arm fully adducted may be indications of compression. It is important to note that compression may occur in asymptomatic individuals, and that the symptoms of TOS are rarely vascular in origin.

UPPER EXTREMITY—VENOUS

The most common mechanism for thrombus formation in the upper extremity veins is some form of intimal disruption, such as injury due to the mechanical irritation from a catheter rubbing against the venous wall, peripheral injection or trauma. The increased usage of central venous appliances such as catheters and pacemakers has caused an increase in the incidence of upper extremity venous disease in recent years. Prior to this increase the most common etiologies of upper extremity venous disease were compression at the thoracic outlet area (subclavian vein), effort-induced thrombosis (axillary vein), and thromboses as a result of poor venous return, such as with congestive heart failure or hypercoaguable states.

In patients with indwelling appliances, duplex Doppler and color flow imaging can be performed to rule out thrombosis in an attempt to keep access sites patent and catheters functional as well as to prevent pulmonary embolism. Upper extremity venous imaging may also be used to evaluate symptoms of venous thrombosis, such as swelling, redness and warmth, in the general patient population. This can occur in patients after mastectomy or following radiation therapy for breast malignancy (radiation-induced venous fibrosis) and post-traumatically, particularly in the setting of first stage reflex sympathetic dystrophy (RSD). Imaging of the infraclavicular subclavian vein with stress maneuvers (see discussion upper extremity arteries) can be done to rule out venous compression which is estimated to occur in 1.5% of individuals with TOS.

The forearm has three sets of two or more veins which run adjacent to their corresponding arteries. These are the radial, ulnar and interosseous veins, their locations being indicated by their names. At the antecubital fossa these vessels join to form the brachial vein, which is often paired, and runs parallel to the humerus, becoming the axillary vein in the axilla, and the subclavian vein in the deltoid fossa, where it enters the thoracic outlet. The subclavian vein forms a confluence with the jugular vein which runs down the neck lateral to the carotid artery to form the innominate or brachiocephalic vein (Figs 7.63–7.66). The right and left innominate veins join to form the superior vena cava on the right side of the heart (Fig. 7.67) which empties into the right atrium. The left innominate must

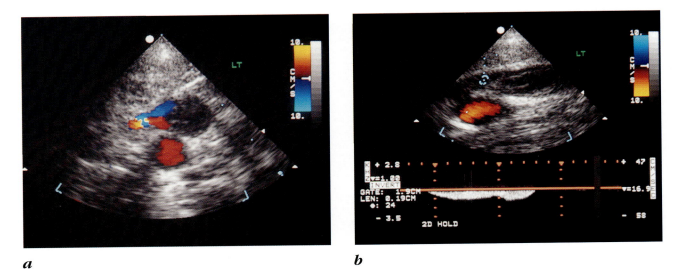

a *b*

Figure 7.70 *Partial thrombus—jugular vein. (a) Transverse view. The jugular vein lies superficial to the CCA. Most of the lumen is filled with thrombus but a small channel has flow. (b) In a longitudinal view, the lumen contains material of mixed echogenicity. The spectral display shows a phasic venous waveform with only minimal pulsatility.*

pass across the mediastinum superior to the aorta to reach the superior vena cava (Fig. 7.68). The superficial veins of the upper extremity, although variable, most commonly include the cephalic vein, which is located in the lateral aspect of the arm in the radial distribution running centrally, joining the subclavian vein just prior to its entry into the thoracic outlet. The basilic vein runs up the medial aspect of the arm, joining the brachial vein or axillary vein in the upper arm. Both of these superficial veins may have multiple tributaries, and often communicate with the deep veins at the antecubital fossa.

Venous thrombi of the central veins of the upper extremity tend to start centrally and propagate peripherally. Thrombus formation usually begins at sites of trauma. This simplifies the ultrasound examination by focusing it at these sites. Catheter-induced thrombi tend to begin at insertion sites (jugular or central subclavian veins) (Figs 7.69 and 7.70), venous confluences where catheters bend and rub against vein walls (right central subclavian and left central innominate vein) (Fig. 7.71) and in the superior vena cava, where infusate may irritate the intima (Fig. 7.72). Thrombus and fibrin may also 'sleeve' catheters (Figs 7.73 and 7.74). To detect thrombi in this patient population, before they have progressed to the point where there is extensive mural involvement and the

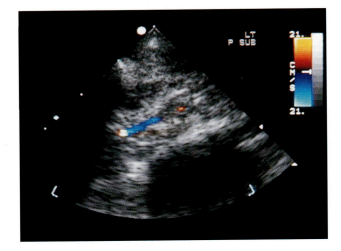

Figure 7.71 *Chronic thrombus in the left innominate vein.*

access site is lost to chronic venous thrombosis, it is necessary to perform a central venous evaluation using a mid-frequency (3.0–5.0 MHz) small footprint sector transducer to image around bony impediments such as the clavicle, sternum and ribs.

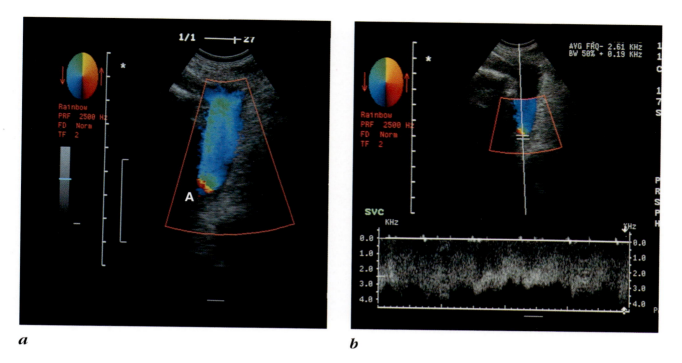

a   *b*

Figure 7.72 *Partial thrombus—superior vena cava. (a) A thrombotic obstruction which partially occludes the lumen causes aliasing in the superior vena cava (A). (b) Pulsed Doppler spectral display shows a venous jet at the site of obstruction.*

Compressive ultrasound is not possible central to the clavicle. However, thrombi can be detected through direct visualization or by observing a flow void with CFI. Duplex Doppler is also performed, examining for pulsatile flow (Fig. 7.75) with a super-imposed phasic variation, and comparing signals qualitatively from side to side. As with the lower extremity, asymmetry in the venous signal or a loss of pulsatility (phasicity in the lower extremity) unilaterally or bilaterally is suggestive of a compression or obstruction more centrally (Fig. 7.76). However, to determine if the pathology is thrombotic further testing must be done, including more central examination for a stenotic jet (Figs 7.77 and 7.78). Due to the inability to use compressive ultrasound, and areas of non visualization due to the clavicle, sternum and ribs, the sensitivity and accuracy of central upper extremity venous imaging is lower than that of the lower extremity (sensitivity 81%, accuracy 85%). However, specificity remains somewhat high (90%).

Isolated thrombus in the peripheral upper extremity is not frequently seen. These authors have encountered it on multiple occasions as the result of peripheral venous injection, presenting as a red,

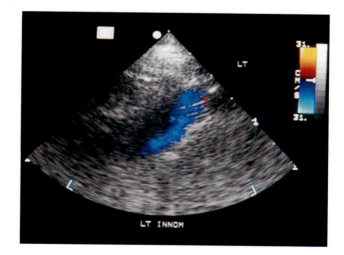

Figure 7.73 *Acute thrombus surrounding a venous catheter in the left innominate vein.*

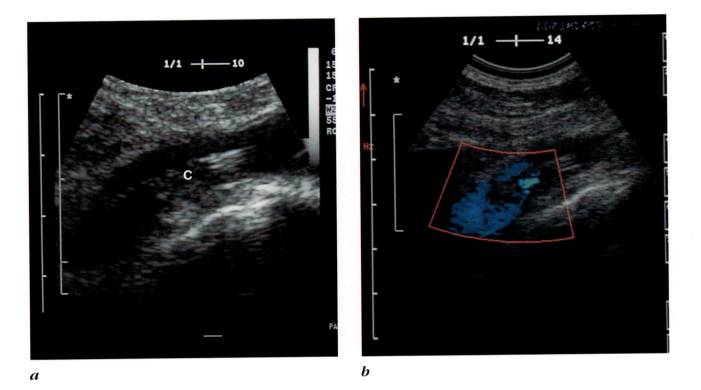

a   *b*

Figure 7.74 *Pericatheter thrombus—left subclavian vein. (a) The gray scale image shows material of mixed echogenicity in the vicinity of the catheter (C). (b) Color flow image of the vein shows flow around the thrombus which partially obstructs the lumen.*

warm streak on the skin. In such cases attention may be focused on the symptomatic area. Compressive ultrasound can be performed quite successfully in the arm. The superficial veins of the peripheral arm are also of interest as surgical bypass conduits for the lower extremity and the coronary arteries, and for use as a dialysis access in an arteriovenous fistula. The cephalic and basilic veins can be mapped; however, the investigator needs to keep in mind that the superficial veins of the upper extremity are variable in their presence and formation. They may be absent or ultrasonically undetectable, particularly in smaller women.

DIALYSIS GRAFTS AND FISTULAS

Dialysis access circulations would seem to provide almost ideal conditions for CFI: high flows and velocities combined with superficial arteries, grafts and veins. These circulations are artificially created, however, and the very high velocities that can result have made it difficult to establish diagnostic criteria,

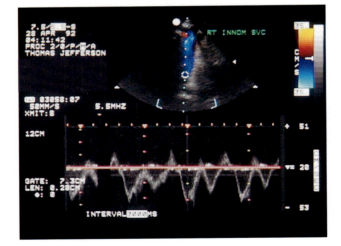

Figure 7.75 *Spectral display from the superior vena cava showing normal fluctuations arising from the pressure changes from the right atrium.*

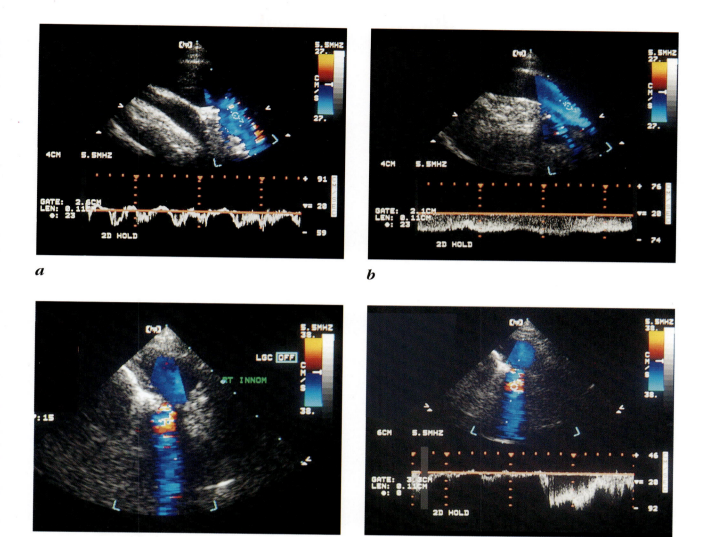

Figure 7.76 *Innominate vein stenosis. Primary and secondary effects. (a) Left jugular vein. The spectral waveform shows fluctuations from breathing and right heart pressure changes. (b) Right jugular vein. The spectral waveform shows only slight velocity variation over time. (c) A tight stenosis is seen in the color image of the right innominate vein (note the color aliasing). The central venous pressure fluctuations are not transmitted so well to the right jugular vein as they are to the left, leading to the difference in the jugular vein waveforms. (d) The spectral jet through the stenosis shows fluctuations with time due to the varying pressure difference across it.*

for example in the identification of a significant arterial or venous stenosis (Figs 7.79 and 7.80).

There are a wide range of surgical constructions for dialysis access, usually a fistula or graft in the arm, although the femoral arteries and veins are also used when necessary. Ultrasound investigation is sometimes requested as a preassessment of the arterial supply and venous drainage. In combination with pressure measurements, the arterial supply can be examined for disease and the superficial veins identified. It is difficult, however, to determine whether a venous stenosis (for example at subclavian level) will cause future difficulties when the investigation is conducted at normal physiologic flow levels (typically under 40 ml/min) but flow in excess of 500 ml/min following surgery is predicted.

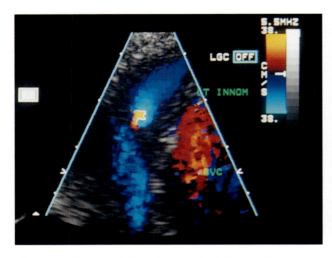

Figure 7.77 *Partial thrombus in the left central innominate vein with a stenotic jet.*

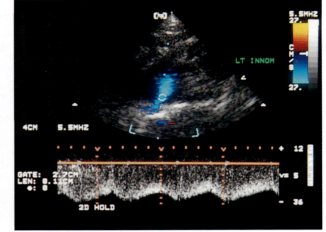

Figure 7.78 *Spectral Doppler, left innominate vein stenosis. The flow waveform shows a velocity jet with a concentration of high velocities in the spectral display.*

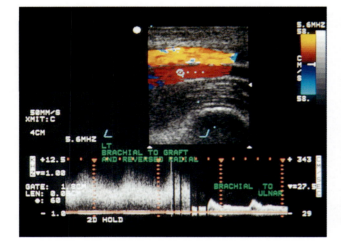

Figure 7.79 *A double brachial artery. In this example, the anterior artery is supplying a radial artery arteriovenous fistula for dialysis. Flow velocities are high as seen by color aliasing and the left side of the spectral display. The posterior artery supplies the ulnar artery and, from there, the palmar arch and, by retrograde flow, the radial fistula. Flow velocities are in general lower (right side of the spectral display) although they still show moderately low resistance.*

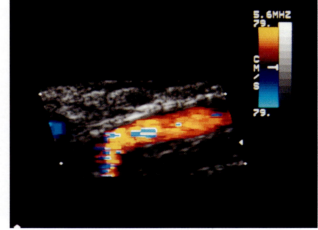

Figure 7.80 *Normal arterial anastomosis of an arteriovenous dialysis graft. The low resistance of the circuit produces high velocities which lead to aliasing despite high pulse repetition frequencies.*

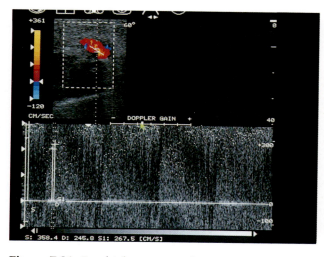

Figure 7.81 *Brachial artery—graft anastomosis. High volume flow combines with local flow conditions to produce exceptionally high velocities—in this case exceeding 700 cm/s.*

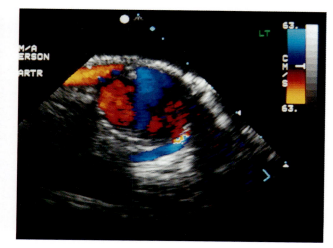

Figure 7.82 *Aneurysm of an arterial anastomosis of a radial artery/prosthetic dialysis graft. A stand-off pad is being used to provide a large field of view with a phased array transducer.*

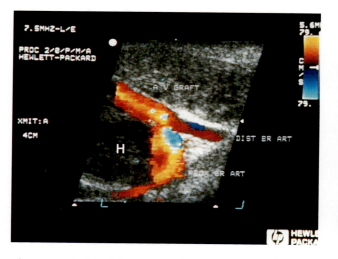

Figure 7.83 *Arterial anastomosis from a brachial artery to a prosthetic arteriovenous dialysis graft. There is a hematoma (H) adjacent to the artery.*

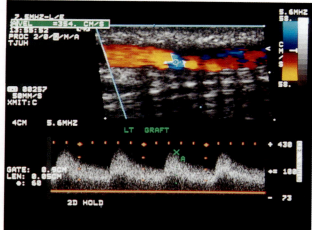

Figure 7.84 *A stenosis in the mid-portion of a prosthetic arteriovenous graft. The site of the stenosis is shown by aliasing. Note the shadowing of both the gray scale and color image arising from the banding around the graft.*

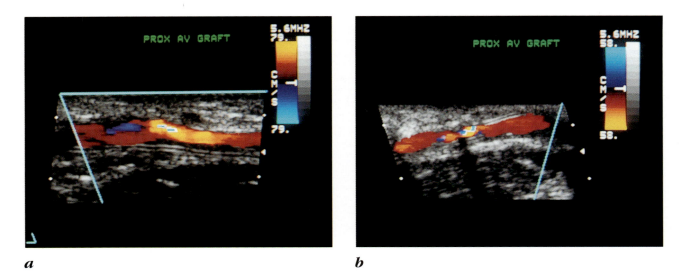

a   *b*

Figure 7.85 *Multiple stenoses—prosthetic arteriovenous dialysis access graft. (a) Residual thrombus in the arteriovenous graft post lysis. Flow is from right to left. The posterior wall of the graft shows evidence of thrombus. The narrowed lumen increases velocities at this point. (b) In the same graft, there is narrowing without thrombus at the distal anastomosis.*

More frequently, patients are referred for investigation for follow up of the graft/fistula circulation or following difficulties during dialysis. The circuit is investigated for indications of hyperplastic stenosis using gray scale, CFI and measurement of velocity increases (Figs 7.81–7.88). High velocities often occur at anastomoses due to normal graft tapering. It is therefore important to visualize the narrowing on color or gray scale to measure the diameter of any suspected stenoses. Stenoses occur most often at the venous anastomosis or in native veins central to the graft (Fig. 7.89), but may also be found in the graft body (especially at cannulation sites), in the donor artery and, rarely, at the arterial anastomosis. The presence of pseudoaneurysms (Figs 7.90 and 7.91) and/or thrombus (Fig. 7.92) is recorded. The flow characteristics associated with pseudoaneurysms have been shown to be associated with clotting of dialysis needles. Since arterial and venous stenoses both cause a reduction in volume flow, accurate calculation of this parameter may be a guide to impending graft/fistula failure (Figs 7.93 and 7.94). Volume flow is best measured in the supplying artery, where flow velocities are most likely to be axial.

Since individual circuits may exhibit markedly different or unusual flow characteristics (e.g. Fig.

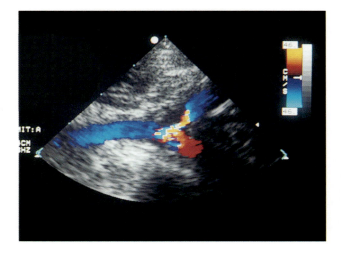

Figure 7.86 *Venous anastomoses—prosthetic dialysis grafts. A common site of narrowing, in this example the stenosis is clearly visible as a focal reduction in lumen size with severely aliased flow.*

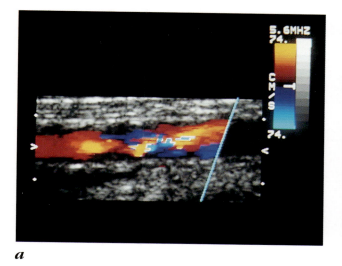

a

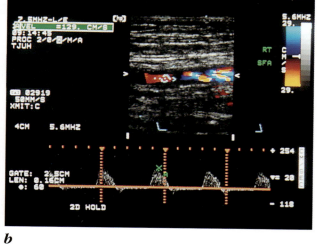

b

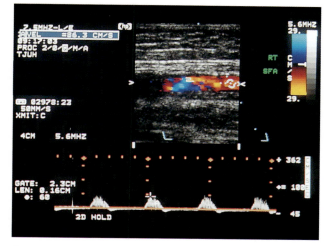

c

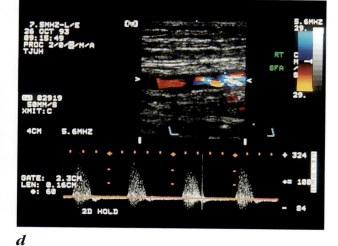

d

e

Figure 7.101 *Superficial femoral artery stenosis. (a) CFI shows a wide range of velocity vectors within the artery with a color aliasing in the jet and areas of flow separation poststenosis. (b) Pulsed wave Doppler—prestenotic flow. The peak systolic velocity is measured as 129 cm/s. (c) Pulsed wave Doppler—in-stenosis flow. The sample volume is placed in the stenosis. The peak systolic velocity is approximately 360 cm/s, nearly a threefold increase caused by the reduced lumen size. (d) Pulsed wave Doppler—poststenotic flow. The spectral display shows features typical of flow in the expansion region with a dissipating flow jet, disturbed flow and evidence of flow separation. (e) Pulsed wave Doppler—distal flow. Flow is reorganized and peak systolic velocities are low.*

7.95), it is advantageous to scan the access circulation while it is functioning well to obtain baseline velocities prior to any developments which may cause dialysis problems later.

LOWER EXTREMITY—ARTERIAL

CFI, used with spectral Doppler, has several direct applications in the investigation of arterial circulation in legs. In the evaluation of peripheral arterial disease causing rest pain or intermittent claudication, it is complementary to other non-invasive tests, particularly the measurement of ankle/brachial pressure indices. Once the presence of disease is identified by a reduction in pressure at the ankle, CFI may be employed to locate sites of narrowing.

Follow-up of arterial bypass grafts by CFI, either routinely or in response to evidence of impending failure, is routinely employed in management of the postsurgery patient. The technique is also useful in identifying suitable host and recipient arteries prior to surgery. Lastly, CFI has proved invaluable in the evaluation of masses of suspected vascular origin. In all these examinations the addition of CFI has contributed greatly to speed and accuracy by allowing a color survey to direct the spectral Doppler examination of the large territories which require investigation.

The common iliac arteries are formed by the branching of the aorta at the umbilicus. This artery divides into the internal and external iliac arteries, the former supplying pelvic organs, and the latter continuing caudally, passing under the inguinal ligament to become the common femoral artery. The common femoral artery bifurcates into the deep or profunda femoris, which perfuses the thigh, and the superficial femoral artery (Fig. 7.96) which runs caudally, passing through the adductor hiatus into the popliteal fossa. Here this conduit is called the popliteal artery (Fig. 7.97); it branches to form the anterior tibial artery, which runs between the tibia and fibula to perfuse the anterior compartment, and the tibial peroneal trunk, which bifurcates into the posterior tibial artery and the peroneal artery, which perfuse much of the calf musculature. The posterior tibial artery runs parallel to the tibia past the medial malleolus into the foot, while the peroneal artery runs closer to the fibula. All three calf vessels communicate in the foot via the pedal arch, which gives rise to the digital vessels. The deep femoral artery and the geniculate arteries (around the knee) are important collaterals in the case of superficial femoral disease.

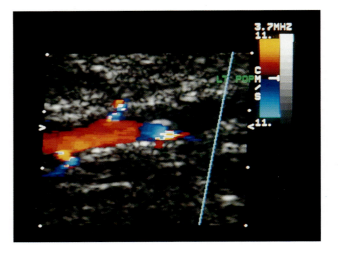

Figure 7.102 *Popliteal artery occlusion. The popliteal artery is occluded at the right of the image. Two small collaterals are seen branching from the patent portion of the artery.*

COLOR FLOW IMAGING OF NATIVE VESSELS

CFI is being used increasingly in the diagnosis of peripheral arterial disease. Following clinical assessment and continuous wave Doppler evaluation of ankle pressures and flow waveforms, CFI can be used to locate sites of narrowing. The stenosis is identified by evidence of narrowing on the gray scale image and increases of velocity in the color and pulsed wave Doppler image. Scanning is, however, a time-consuming process. If the arteries are scanned from the aorta to the ankle, the time required may be well over 30 min. If scanning is undertaken only to popliteal level, the time is considerably reduced, but with a corresponding reduction in information obtained. In large patients, image quality may be poor in the pelvic arteries, at the adductor canal level, and in the tibioperoneal trunk. In severe disease, poor flows and calcification may reduce the clarity of the images, especially in the calf vessels.

Because of the range of depths of the scans from the common iliac vessels to the arteries at the ankle, several transducers may be used during the scan. In the pelvic vessels, a curvilinear or phased array, in the 3–5 MHz range, usually provides adequate penetration. From common femoral to popliteal level,

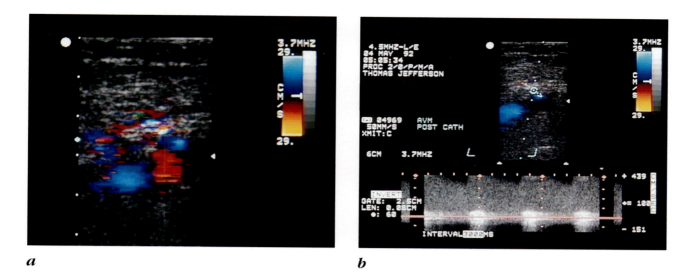

a   *b*

Figure 7.103 *Arteriovenous malformation (fistula). (a) The femoral artery and vein are imaged in a transverse view. CFI shows a flow channel not normally seen at this site. (b) Pulsed wave Doppler shows a very high velocity dampened pulsatility waveform in the abnormal flow channel. The waveform is typical of flow in a small conduit with very low distal resistance—in this case forming part of an arteriovenous shunt.*

linear arrays in the 5–7 MHz range are preferred. Below knee level, higher frequency linear arrays may provide better sensitivity to low flows as well as improved gray scale resolution of the calf arteries. Manufacturers increasingly offer multifrequency (or multi-Hertz) transducers. While this does provide some improvement in transducer versatility, it should be remembered that each transducer is tailored for specific applications (for instance in setting the minimum slice thickness at a specific depth). A good range of transducers offers an operator the best chance of obtaining optimum images.

In the absence of disease, peripheral arteries exhibit high resistance triphasic waveforms while the patient is resting (Figs 7.98–7.100). Because the flow waveform has high acceleration, the flow profile is blunt at peak systole and, consequently, a reduction in lumen area is accompanied by a corresponding increase in peak systolic velocity. Some authors have equated a doubling of peak systolic velocity with a 50% reduction in vessel diameter. This, however, depends on the morphology of the stenosis. An eccentric stenosis of 50% may result in an area decrease of 50%. A concentric stenosis results in an area decrease of 75%. Since it is the reduction in area which corresponds to the increase in mean velocity, these two different types of stenoses will produce different veloc-

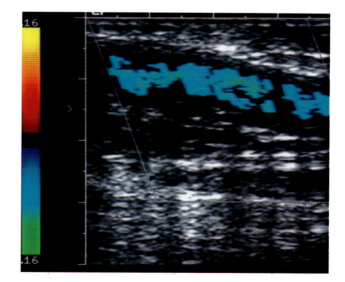

Figure 7.104 *Artificial graft—ultrasound attenuation. The weave of the graft causes variation in attenuation in both the gray scale and color flow image.*

ity increases. It is fair to say that peripheral artery stenoses are not as well defined in terms of velocity increases as are carotid artery stenoses. The situation

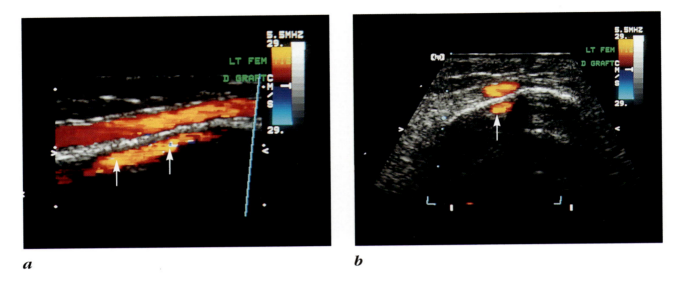

a   *b*

Figure 7.105 *Mirror image artifact in a lower extremity graft. (a) Longitudinal view. Strong reflections from the surface of the tibia cause a mirror image (arrows) of flow in the graft to be shown apparently within the tibia. (b) Transverse view.*

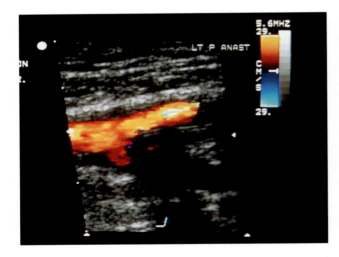

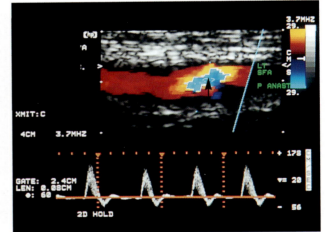

Figure 7.106 *Color flow image of the proximal anastomosis of an artificial graft arising from a common femoral artery.*

Figure 7.107 *Graft anastomosis—color and pulsed wave Doppler ultrasound. The color image shows a graft anastomosed to a superficial femoral artery. The change in color is at least partly caused by the better alignment of flow to the beam direction at that point (arrow). Anastomoses are often the site of velocity increases which can be quantified by the pulsed wave Doppler spectrum.*

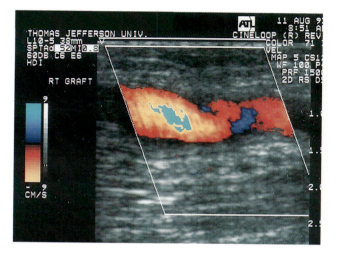

Figure 7.108 *Graft-vein anastomosis of a lower extremity composite graft. Changes in flow direction at anastomoses can result in a range of colors as velocity vectors change.*

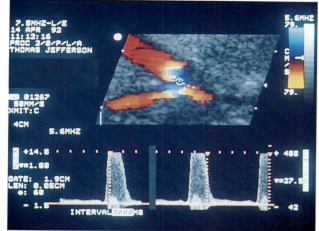

Figure 7.109 *Stenosis of the distal anastomosis in a lower extremity bypass graft. Peak systolic velocities exceed 500 cm/s.*

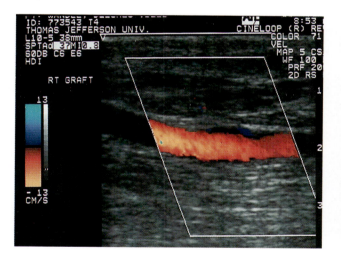

Figure 7.110 *Venous segment of a composite graft.*

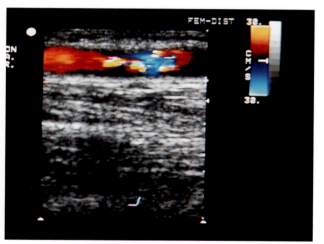

Figure 7.111 *Stenosis of a lower extremity bypass graft. Despite being superficial, the stenosis does not show clearly on the gray scale image. CFI clearly shows the lack of filling at the stenosis site. The color hues clearly show increased velocities and post-stenotic flow disturbances.*

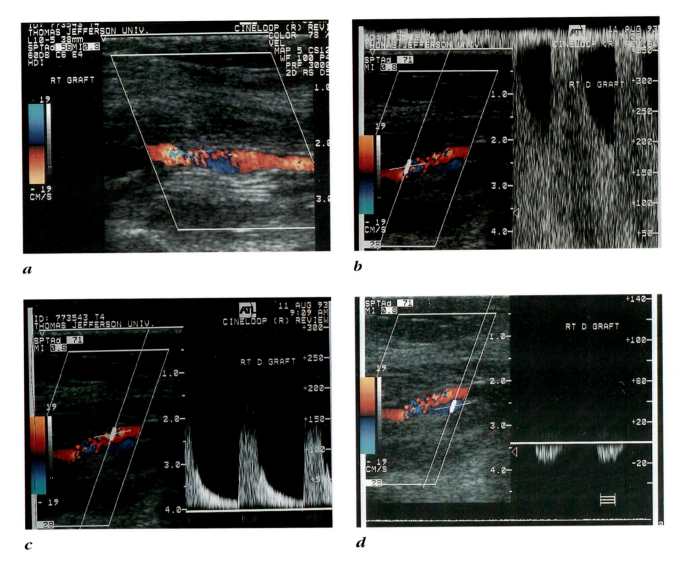

Figure 7.112 *Stenosis in a venous segment of a lower extremity bypass graft. (a) CFI shows high velocities in the stenosis and poststenotic flow disturbances. (b) Spectral Doppler is used to quantify the severity of stenoses. Peak systolic velocity exceeds 400 cm/s. (c) In the velocity jet dissipation region, flow velocities decrease. There is still evidence of spectral broadening caused by the range of velocity vectors in the expansion region. (d) In the lee of the stenosis, there is evidence of flow reversal at the wall in the area of flow separation.*

is further complicated in the presence of proximal disease, which may affect both velocity waveform and profiles. However, large increases in velocity (Fig. 7.101) do indicate narrowing. Features of increased velocity in the stenosis and disturbed flow distally are apparent in the color image. Pulsed wave spectral Doppler is used to quantify the velocity increases.

Occlusion is apparent from flow voids in the artery. Bloodflow may be visualized in collateral vessels (Fig. 7.102).

CFI readily identifies the presence of arteriovenous malformations. The malformation itself is displayed as a flow channel between a larger artery and vein. High velocity, reduced pulsatility waveforms indicate abnormally low resistance typical in these arterial-venous shunts which are usually post-traumatic (Fig. 7.103).

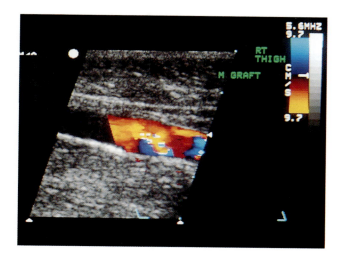

Figure 7.113 *Retained valve cusp causing a stenosis in an in situ bypass graft. The gray scale image is steered to obtain the best reflections/scattering from the vessel walls, while the color flow is steered to optimize the beam/flow angle. The flow through the valve cusp shows characteristics similar to those through a stenosis.*

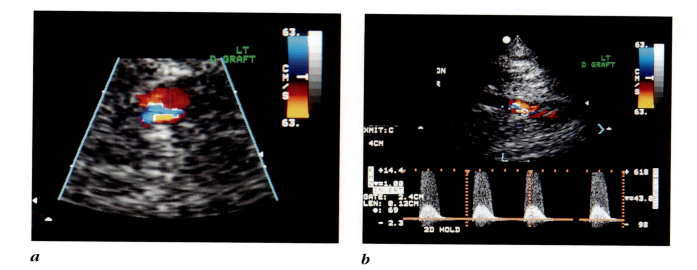

a   *b*

Figure 7.114 *Dissection in a graft. (a) Transverse view of a dissection in the distal portion of a lower extremity bypass graft. The graft shows two distinct regions of flow, one of low velocity (coded red – uppermost) and the other with aliasing showing high flow velocities. (b) Longitudinal view with spectral Doppler. The sample volume encompasses both the true and false lumens in the dissection with high- and low-flow velocity waveforms.*

ARTERIAL GRAFTS

The mechanisms of graft failure can be summarized as thrombosis, hemodynamic failure and structural failure. Short-term failure (less than 30 days) is usually due to poor inflow or (more commonly) poor outflow, infection or technical error (e.g. raised intimal flap). In the medium term (up to 2 years),

failure usually results from lesions developing in the graft, at retained valve cusps, or at anastomoses. In the longer term, failure usually results from progression of atherosclerosis.

CFI is employed extensively in the follow-up of grafts. The large diameter and superficial location of grafts make them an ideal subject for ultrasound investigation, although in artificial grafts attenuation

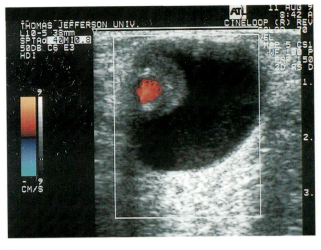

a

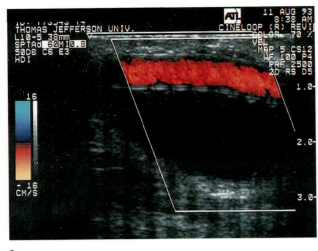

b

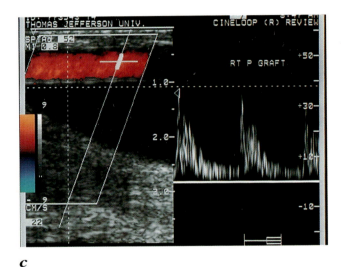

c

Figure 7.115 *Arterial graft surrounded by a fluid collection. (a) Transverse scan. (b) Longitudinal scan. (c) Pulsed wave Doppler sonogram of flow within the graft. In all three images, the color flow image quickly indicates which regions of the image contain flow and which do not.*

of the graft material may prevent imaging of the graft lumen in the first few days postoperatively (Fig. 7.104). Thereafter, investigation of the graft can be made from the proximal artery to the run-off vessels. Strong ultrasound reflections may lead to artifacts where the graft lies adjacent to bone (Fig. 7.105).

Velocities at the arterial, venous and in-graft anastomoses may rise due to mismatch in the cross-sectional area of the artery and graft (Figs 7.106–7.110). If there are sudden changes in flow direction (e.g. Fig. 7.107), local flow changes can give rise to regions of flow separation and high flow velocities at the dividing wall. Baseline measurements can be made with pulsed wave spectral Doppler for comparison at a later date.

Stenosis of a graft produces ultrasound characteristics similar to those in native arteries. The void in flow at the stenosis combined with high flows around it are accompanied by distal flow disturbances (Fig. 7.111) and these can be quantified by spectral Doppler (Fig. 7.112). Similar findings can be seen in retained valve cusps (Fig. 7.113). Severe stenoses can limit flow and give rise to flow conditions in which thrombosis may occur.

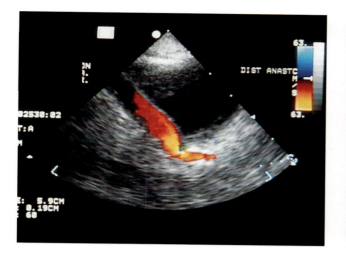

Figure 7.116 *Seroma at the distal anastomosis of a lower extremity bypass graft. The color flow image shows the absence of flow in the collection.*

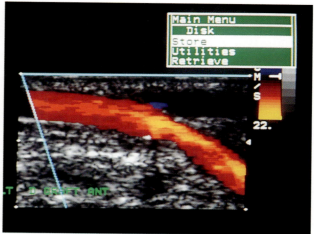

Figure 7.117 *A lower extremity bypass graft with an occluded distal limb (anechoic region, upper right in the image) and a patent jump graft.*

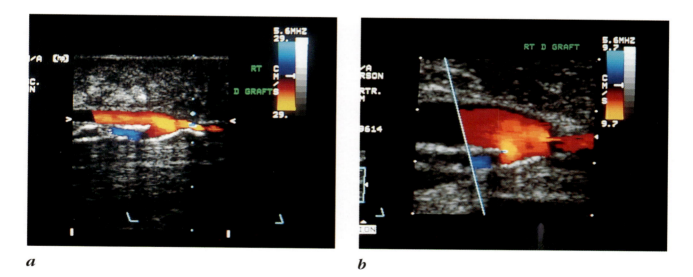

a

b

Figure 7.118 *Distal anastomosis of lower extremity bypass grafts. (a,b) These images (of different patients) show flow from grafts to recipient arteries with retrograde flow in the proximal portion of the recipient artery. This is a result of high pressure in the graft and a lower pressure in the recipient artery as a result of proximal disease. Note the large difference in graft diameters between these two patients. The wide range of graft diameters makes velocity criteria for critical stenoses difficult to establish.*

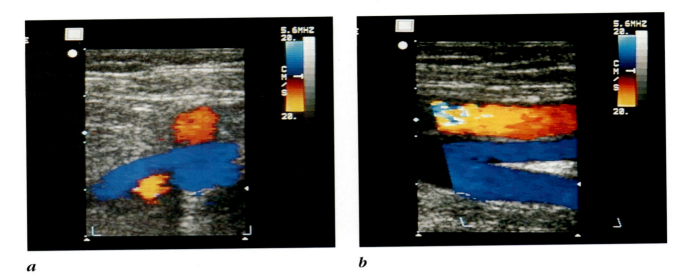

a   *b*

Figure 7.119 *Confluence of the deep and superficial femoral veins. (a) Transverse view. The confluence is normally distal to the femoral artery bifurcation, and in this view the two arteries are visible. (b) Longitudinal view. Note the low velocities compared with those in the superficial femoral artery.*

Dissection in grafts is a rare complication. The dissection is usually visible on the gray scale image and the flow characteristics in the true and false lumens are evident on CFI (Fig. 7.114). CFI also aids in the rapid assessment of areas which do not contain flow, whether they are collections around the graft (Figs 7.115 and 7.116) or in occluded grafts or artery segments (Fig. 7.117). Lastly, CFI provides a rapid assessment of altered bloodflow patterns in arterial reconstructions, resolving ambiguities such as retrograde flow in the recipient artery proximal to the anastomosis (Fig. 7.118).

LOWER EXTREMITY—VENOUS

As with the peripheral arteries, the quality of gray scale and color flow ultrasound in the peripheral veins has meant that scanning even small veins with low flow is a practical proposition. Extensive use of CFI has been made for the investigation of thrombus, where color flow complements gray scale imaging of venous compression, and venous insufficiency.

The deep veins of the leg accompany the arteries described above. The common and superficial femoral (Fig. 7.119) and popliteal veins may be duplicated and the posterior tibial, anterior tibial and peroneal veins are paired, running either side of the corresponding artery. The greater (also called the long or internal) saphenous vein runs from the

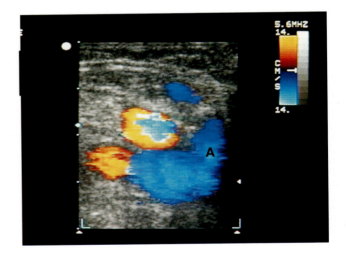

Figure 7.120 *Saphenofemoral junction, transverse view. The femoral arteries (superficial and deep) are color coded red. The greater saphenous vein (A, also called the internal or long saphenous vein) enters the common femoral vein.*

medial malleolus up the medial aspect of the thigh and joins the common femoral vein (Fig. 7.120). The lesser (or short or external) saphenous vein runs directly along the posterior aspect of the calf. In

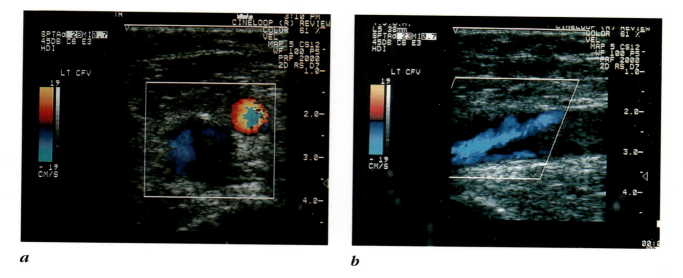

Figure 7.121 *Thrombus partly occluding a femoral vein. (a) Transverse view. (b) Longitudinal view.*

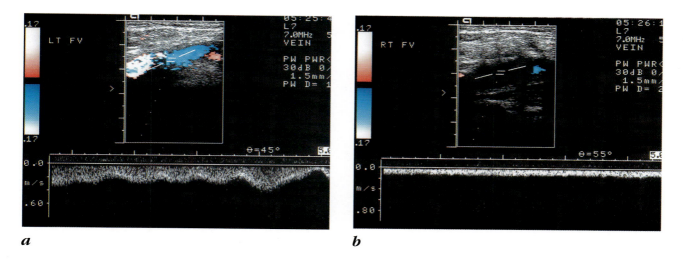

Figure 7.122 *Partial thrombus in a femoral vein. (a) In the limb without thrombus, the femoral vein waveform shows normal periodic velocity fluctuations. (b) In the contralateral limb, partial thrombus reduces the venous lumen. The venous stenosis prevents transmission of the subtle pressure fluctuations through the stenosis. Venous velocities appear constant.*

approximately 60% of cases, it enters the popliteal vein just above knee crease level. The most common variant is for the vein to continue up the thigh and enter the deep system and/or the greater saphenous vein in the upper thigh.

Imaging of the veins from common femoral vein level to ankle is usually conducted using a linear array transducer, most usually at 5 or 7 MHz imaging frequency. For the pelvic veins, it is useful to have a sector format transducer (3–5 MHz). The success of

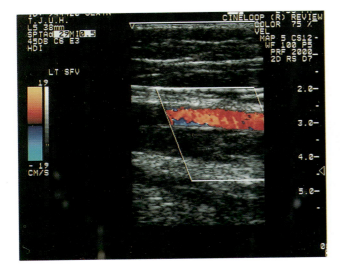

Figure 7.123 *Occluded superficial femoral vein. The artery is patent but there is no flow visible in the vein and the lumen contains echogenic thrombus.*

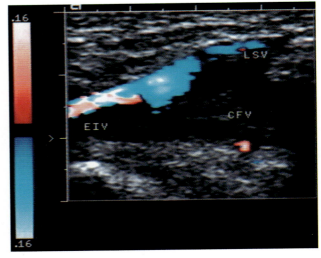

Figure 7.124 *Occluded common femoral vein, longitudinal view. Flow returns to the external iliac vein from the long saphenous vein.*

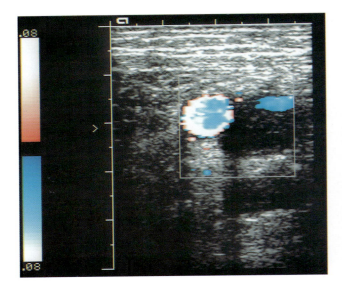

Figure 7.125 *Occluded common femoral vein, transverse view. The common femoral artery shows aliasing. To the right in the image, the common femoral vein contains echogenic material and is occluded. The small area of flow is from the long saphenous vein, which is patent and drains into the proximal patent common femoral vein.*

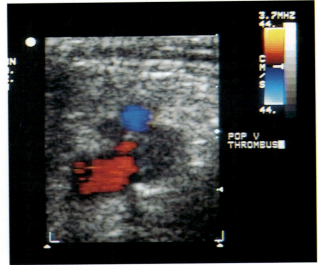

Figure 7.126 *Popliteal vein thrombus. The popliteal artery shows flow but the adjacent vein is occluded with echogenic thrombus. A small vein superficial to the popliteal vein is patent.*

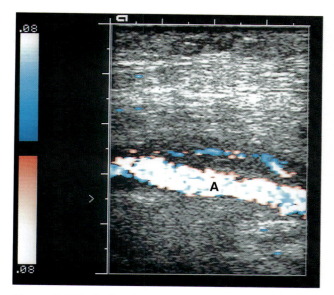

Figure 7.127 *Popliteal vein—partial thrombus. The vein contains echogenic material but a small flow channel remains. The color pulse repetition frequency is set low to image the low venous velocities. High velocities cause aliasing in the popliteal artery (A).*

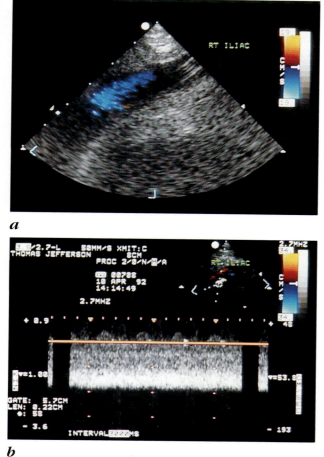

a

b

Figure 7.128 *Iliac vein—pericatheter thrombus. (a) In this longitudinal view, there is evidence of thrombus around the catheter with partial occlusion of the iliac vein. (b) Pulsed wave Doppler ultrasound. Because the thrombus reduces the effective lumen, flow through the remaining lumen shows high velocities and a jet-like distribution of velocities. There is no variation during the cardiac or respiration cycles.*

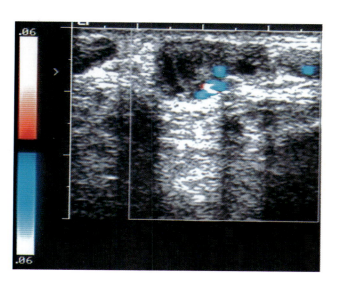

Figure 7.129 *Recannalized superficial vein thrombus. Thrombus in a superficial vein secondary to chronic venous insufficiency. A small channel remains through which there is flow.*

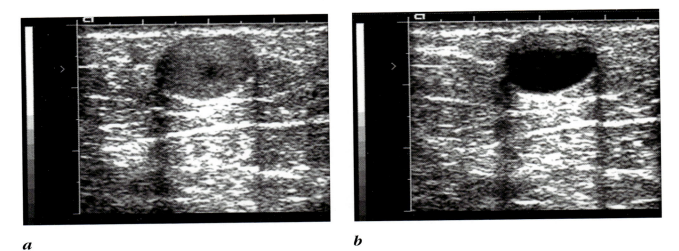

a   *b*

Figure 7.130 *Superficial vein—changes in blood echogenicity. Slow moving blood sometimes appears to have greater echogenicity than normal. In this case, hemostasis in a varicose vein leads to increased scattering (a), giving the impression of thrombus. The velocities may be too low to register on CFI. Following a calf squeeze (b), blood circulates and the lumen has normal echogenicity.*

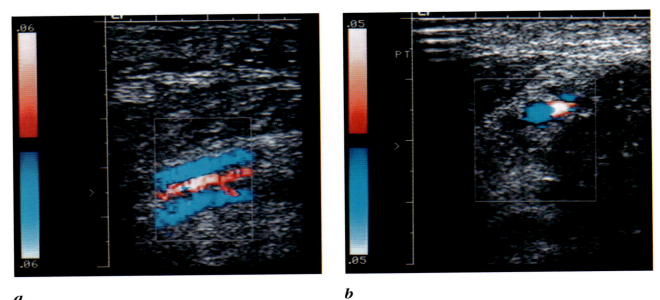

a   *b*

Figure 7.131 *Calf vein visualization. (a) Posterior tibial veins. Despite the superficial cellulitis, the posterior tibial veins are imaged with CFI during squeezing of the foot. The lack of flow voids suggests that there is no major thrombus in this segment. (b) Transverse view of posterior tibial veins. The high systolic velocities in the corresponding artery are helpful in identifying the course of the deep veins. With augmentation, flow in the veins is detected.*

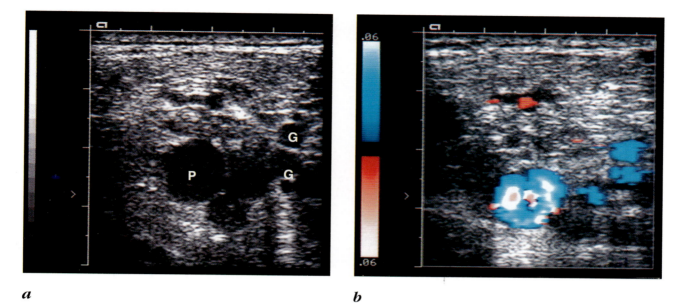

a   *b*

Figure 7.132 *Gastrocnemius veins. (a) The image shows the presence of gastrocnemius veins (G) adjacent to the popliteal vein (P). These can be a site of early deep vein thrombosis. (b) By squeezing the calf, flow is detected with CFI, indicating vein patency.*

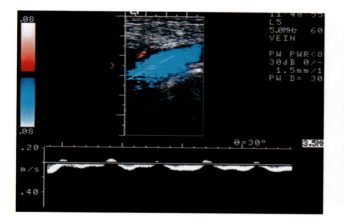

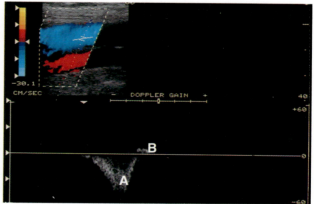

Figure 7.133 *Femoral vein, normal flow waveform. Flow fluctuations occur spontaneously due to pressure changes from the right heart and breathing.*

Figure 7.134 *Flow changes in the femoral vein caused by distal augmentation on the calf. During calf squeezing blood flows towards the heart at high velocity (A). Upon release, there is a very slight return of blood (B) before the venous valves close.*

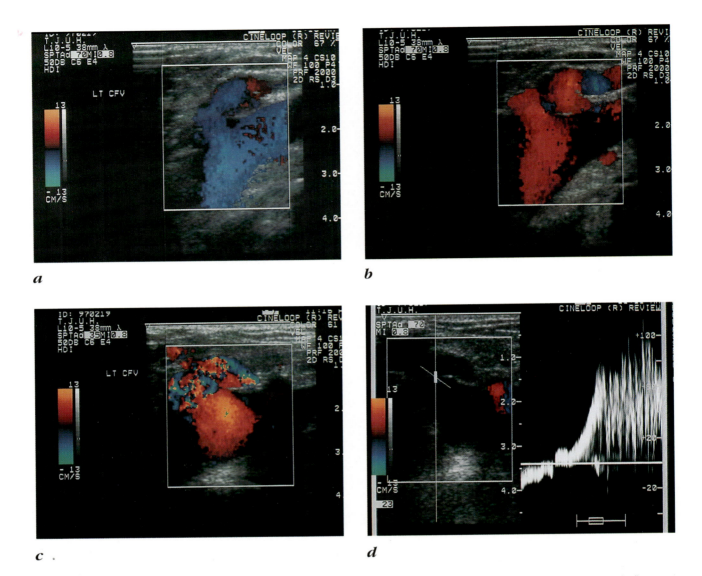

Figure 7.135 *Reflux at a saphenofemoral junction. (a) Longitudinal view of the saphenofemoral junction with flow from the greater saphenous vein into the common femoral vein resulting from squeezing of the thigh. (b) Upon release of the thigh, reflux is checked in the femoral vein by the venous valves. The valves in the greater saphenous vein are incompetent and reflux occurs in this vein as demonstrated in the image by the flow from common femoral vein to saphenous vein. (c) Transverse view of the saphenofemoral junction with reflux. (d) Pulsed wave Doppler ultrasound of reflux. At the beginning of the sonogram, flow is from the saphenous vein to the femoral vein but after releasing the thigh, gross reflux occurs.*

imaging of the veins is, in part, dependent on the size of the patient. In obese patients, it may not be possible to image the pelvic vessels successfully, although information may be inferred from the flow waveforms more distally. For imaging of reflux in the superficial veins, a high-frequency linear array with a high color flow frequency is advantageous in identifying the sometimes low-velocity flows.

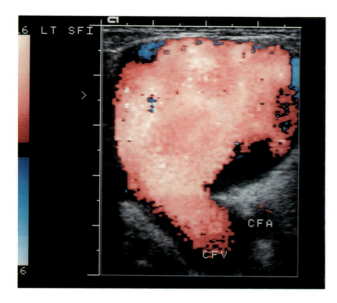

Figure 7.136 *Gross reflux at a saphenofemoral junction. The lumen size of the superficial vein greatly exceeds that of the common femoral vein.*

THROMBOSIS

Ultrasound transducer compression of the femoral and popliteal veins is now employed by many centers as the imaging modality of choice in the investigation of suspected lower limb deep vein thrombosis. Rapid investigation of the major deep veins from common femoral vein level to popliteal level is almost always possible and accuracy is reported to be 95% or greater. Imaging of the major calf veins takes longer; detection of thrombus is specific although sensitivity is very operator-dependent.

The initial investigation is conducted in transverse section using the transducer to compress the vein. In the absence of thrombus, collapse of the lumen is usually seen on the display. In deeper veins the addition of color can help identify the course of the vein and the extent of venous patency in difficult-to-scan areas such as the adductor canal. Thrombus is manifest by the inability of the vein to collapse fully and by incomplete color flow filling of the apparent lumen. The clarity of the image of thrombus is dependent on the age of thrombus and normal ultrasound considerations, especially intervening attenuation.

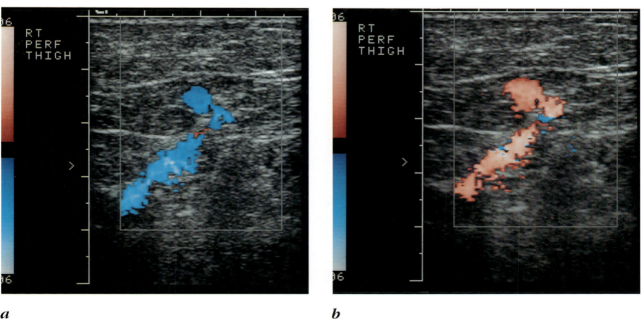

a

b

Figure 7.137 *Reflux in a thigh-perforating vein. (a) During a thigh squeeze, blood flows from the superficial vein towards the superficial femoral vein (which is not seen in the image). (b) On calf release, flow returns through the incompetent perforating vein to the long (inner) saphenous vein.*

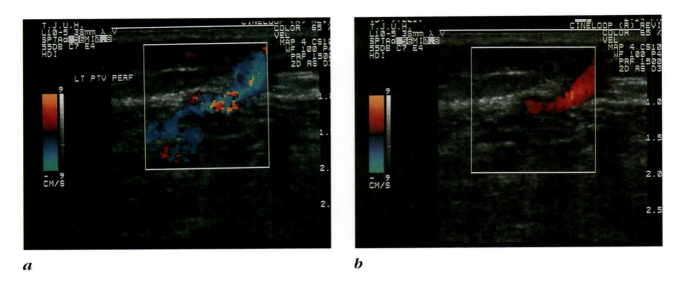

a *b*

Figure 7.138 *Reflux in a calf-perforating vein. (a) During a calf squeeze, there is flow from a superficial vein to the posterior tibial vein. (b) Upon release of the calf, blood returns to the superficial vein due to an incompetent valve in the perforating vein.*

Acute thrombi may appear as a free floating 'tail' or totally obstructive and distending the vein. Chronic thrombi often appear contracted or as synechiae. Examples of thrombus in deep veins are given in Figs 7.121–7.128 and in a superficial vein in Fig. 7.129. Slow-moving blood may lead to increased echogenicity, giving the impression of thrombus. Augmentation of flow reduces blood echogenicity (Fig. 7.130).

In the calf veins, the smaller vein size may cause problems in gray scale visualization. Flow augmentation by squeezing the calf can induce flow velocities detectable by CFI as an aid to identification and to check patency (Figs 7.131 and 7.132).

Additional information is obtained from the flow waveform in and distal to thrombus. If thrombus is extensive but not occlusive, the residual channel may exhibit abnormally high velocities (Figs 7.127 and 7.128). The reduced lumen can prevent transmission of the subtle pressure fluctuations caused by the right heart and respiration (Fig. 7.133). A continuous non-fluctuating venous flow gives cause for suspicion of partial or complete thrombus between the site of measurement and the right heart.

REFLUX—VENOUS INCOMPETENCE

CFI is invaluable in specifying the exact site of reflux from the deep veins into incompetent veins. The most common sites for reflux are the saphenofemoral and saphenopopliteal junctions. In both cases, the junction is identified with the patient standing and the investigated leg relaxed. Flow is generated in the superficial veins by a distal squeeze (Fig. 7.134). Upon release, incompetence is immediately apparent as reflux in either color or spectral Doppler (Figs 7.135 and 7.136).

Incompetent perforating veins are identified by transverse scanning. Any veins visibly connecting the superficial and deep systems are investigated for reflux (Figs 7.137 and 7.138). Normal perforating veins are small, typically <2 mm, and are usually not apparent on the gray scale image.

CFI is particularly useful in identifying the source of recurrent varicose veins. These can occur from recurrent incompetence at the saphenofemoral junction, from incompetent perforating thigh veins or from superficial abdominal vein or pudendal vein tributaries, as well as from unsuccessful surgery.

VASCULAR INJURIES

CFI has proved to be an accurate method for the diagnosis of vascular injuries following arterial or venous puncture. These occur most commonly as

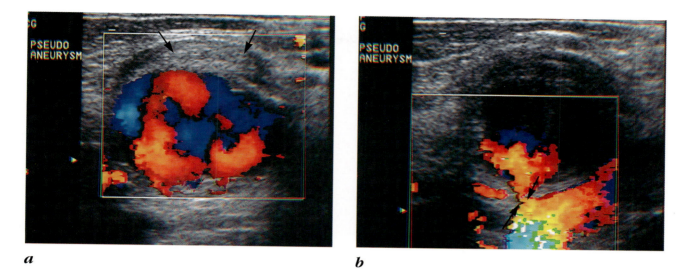

Figure 7.139 *Subclavian artery pseudoaneurysm. (a) The color identifies swirling flow within the pseudoaneurysm. Mural thrombus is evident (arrows). (b) In another plane, the site of leak (i.e. tract) from the subclavian artery is seen clearly (arrows). Images courtesy of DA Merton.*

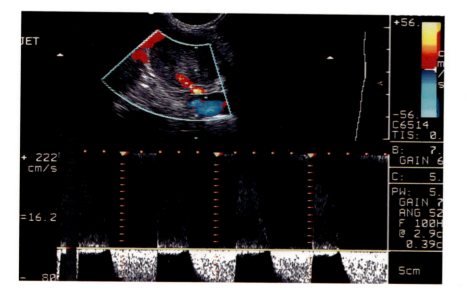

Figure 7.140 *In the communicating tract of this subclavian pseudoaneurysm there is high velocity bidirectional flow shown on the spectral display. Note that movement during the cardiac cycle results in a periodic change in spectral amplitude.*

iatrogenic injuries following invasive diagnostic or therapeutic procedures, and more rarely as a result of gunshot, blunt trauma or stab wounds. The most common complication is a pseudoaneurysm; others include arteriovenous fistula, hematoma, thrombosis or an intimal flap.

Pseudoaneurysms appear as an abnormal echoluscent region adjacent to the artery. Flow within a pseudoaneurysm appears as a swirling motion containing multidirectional velocities which are often low (Fig. 7.139a). Sequential imaging can determine whether the pseudoaneursym is expanding or contracting. Flow velocities in the communicating tract from the injured artery are usually high (Fig. 7.139b) with a characteristic to-and-fro motion apparent on pulsed wave spectral Doppler (Fig. 7.140).

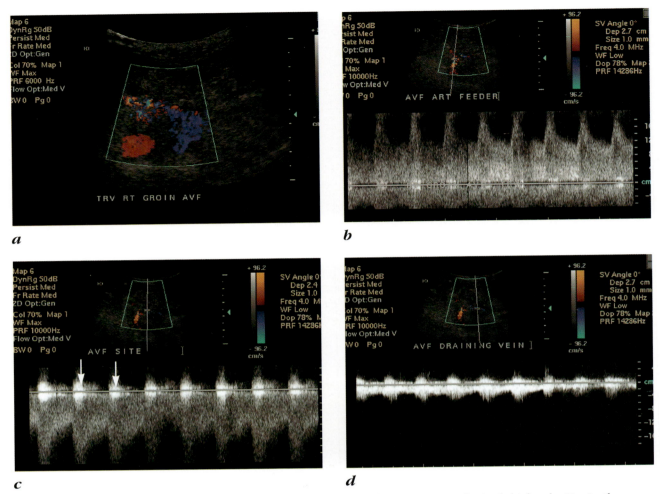

Figure 7.141 *Iatrogenic arteriovenous fistula. (a) The color image shows a region of mixed, high velocities in the vicinity of the common femoral artery and vein. (b) Pulsed spectral Doppler shows a small common femoral artery branch with high velocity, low pulsatility flow consistent with reduced downstream resistance. (c) At the site of the fistula, there is a high amplitude low frequency signal (arrows) consistent with a bruit. (d) In the draining vein, flow shows arterial pulsations. Images courtesy of DA Merton.*

The color image can be used to direct compression for repair of the puncture site, permitting immediate determination of its success.

Arteriovenous fistula results from a puncture of artery and vein with a corresponding large pressure gradient and consequent high flows. The supplying artery shows a low resistance waveform with high velocities. The draining vein (Fig. 7.141) may show arterial-like pulsations. Again, CFI may be used to aid compression repair.

CONCLUSION

Color flow imaging plays a pivotal role in the diagnosis of peripheral vascular disease. In the past few years, CFI has significantly reduced the need for more invasive procedures for evaluation of extracranial disease, deep vein thrombosis and peripheral arterial disease. It is highly effective in pre-surgical assessment of venous incompetence.

Its mobility and non-invasiveness makes it a versatile method for evaluating circulation in many situations which preclude the use of other imaging modalities.

In the future new developments, particularly high frequency ultrasound, will extend the range of tests offered to include examination of small vessels in the hand and feet and, eventually, tissue perfusion. New scanning and signal processing techniques will enhance sensitivity to low flows and flow in deep vessels, improving confidence in current vascular applications and enabling new ones. Three-dimensional ultrasound will extend the role that CFI already has in the planning of interventional radiology and surgery and will permit measurement of true flow vectors in three-dimensional space. CFI will continue to be an essential diagnostic tool for an increasingly wide range of vascular applications.

FURTHER READING

GENERAL

Bernstein EF (ed.), *Vascular Diagnosis* 4th edn (Mosby-Year Book: St Louis, 1993).

Jager K, Frauchiger B, Eichlisberger R: Vascular ultrasound. In: Tooke JE, Lowe GDO (eds), *A Textbook of Vascular Medicine* (Arnold: London, 1996) 81–99.

Strandness DE, *Duplex Scanning in Vascular Disorders* (Raven Press: New York, 1990).

Zweibel WJ, *Introduction to Vascular Ultrasonography*. 3rd edn (WB Saunders, Philadelphia, 1992).

CAROTID ARTERIES

Barry R, Pienaar C, Nel CJ, Accuracy of B-mode ultrasonography in detecting carotid plaque hemorrhage and ulceration. *Ann Vasc Surg* (1990) **4**:466–70.

Bluth EI, Wetzner SM, Stavros AT et al, Carotid duplex sonography: a multicenter recommendation for standardized imaging and Doppler criteria, *RadioGraphics* (1988) **8**:487–506.

Bock, RW, Gray-Weale AC, Mock PA et al, The natural history of asymptomatic carotid artery disease, *J Vasc Surg* (1993) **17**:160–9.

Burnham CB, Ligush JL, Burnham SJ, Velocity criteria redefined for the 60% carotid stenosis, *J Vasc Tech* (1996) **20**: 5–11.

Carpenter JP, Lexa FJ, Davis JT, Determination of duplex Doppler ultrasound criteria appropriate to the North American Symptomatic Carotid Endarterectomy trial, *Stroke* (1996) **27**:695–9.

European surgery Trialists' Collaborative Group. MRC European carotid surgery trial: interim results for symptomatic patients with severe (70–99%) and mild (0–29%) carotid stenosis. *Lancet* (1991) **337**:1235–43.

Hobson RW, Weiss DG, Fields WS et al, Efficacy of carotid endarterectomy for asymptomatic carotid stenosis. The veterans affairs co-operative study group. *N Engl J Med* (1993) **328**:221–27.

Moneta GL, Edwards JM, Chitwood RW et al, Correlation of North American Symptomatic Carotid Endarterectomy Trial (NASCET) angiographic definition of 70 to 99% internal carotid artery stenosis with duplex scanning. *J Vasc Surg* (1993) **17**: 152–7; discussion 157–9.

North American Symptomatic Carotid Endarterectomy Trial Collaborators. Beneficial effect of carotid endarterectomy in symptomatic patients with high grade carotid stenosis, *N Engl J Med* (1991) **325**:445–53.

Patel MR, Kuntz KM, Klufas RA et al, Preoperative assessment of the carotid bifurcation. Can magnetic resonance angiography and duplex ultrasonography replace contrast arteriography? *Stroke* (1995) **26**:1753–8.

Primozich J, Color flow in the carotid evaluation, *J Vasc Tech* (1991) **15**:112–22.

Tanganelli P, Bianciardi G, Centi L et al, B-Mode imaging and histomorphometric evaluation of atherosclerosis, *Angiology* (1990) **41**:908–14.

VERTEBRAL ARTERIES

Bartels E, Fuchs HH, Flugel KA, Duplex ultrasonography of vertebral arteries: examination technique, normal values, and clinical applications, *Angiology* (1992) **43**:169–80.

Fujioka KA, Ernsberger AM, Nicholls SC, Spencer MP, Transcranial Doppler Assessment of mechanical compression of the vertebral arteries, *J Vasc Tech* (1991) **15**:254–9.

Jak, JG, Hoeneveld H, van der Widt JM, van Doorn JJ, Ackerstaff RG, A six year evaluation of duplex scanning of the vertebral artery. A non-invasive technique compared with contrast angiography, *J Vasc Tech* (1989) **13**:26–30.

Schoning M, Walter J, Evaluation of the vertebrobasilar-posterior system by transcranial color duplex sonography in adults, *Stroke* (1992) **23**:1280–6.

Trattinio S, Hubsch P, Schuster H, Polzleitner D, Color coded Doppler imaging of normal vertebral arteries, *Stroke* (1990) **21**:1222–5.

Tschammler A, Landwehr P, Hohman M, Moll R, Wittenberg G, Lacknaer K, Color coded duplex sonography of the extracranial arteries supplying the brain: diagnostic significance and sources of error in comparision with intraarterial DSA, *Rofo Fortschr Geb Rontgenstr Neuen Bilgeb Verfahr* (1991) **155**:452–9.

TRANSCRANIAL AND OCCIPITAL

Erickson SJ, Hendrix LE, Massaro BM et al, Color Doppler flow imaging of the normal and abnormal orbit, *Radiology* (1989) **173**:511–16.

Foley D, *Color Doppler flow imaging.* (Andover Medical Publishers: Boston, 1991).

Fujioka KA, Gates DT, Spencer MP, A comparison of transcranial color Doppler imaging and standard static pulsed wave Doppler in the assessment of intracranial hemodynamics, *J Vasc Tech* (1994) **18**:29–36.

Lieb WE, Cohen SM, Merton DA, Shields JA, Mitchell DG, Imaging of intraocular and orbital vessels using angiodynography, *Fortschr der Ophthalmol* (1990) **87**:537–9.

UPPER EXTREMITY—ARTERIAL

Greenwold D, Sessions EG, Haynes JL, Rush DS, Bynoe RP, Miles WS, Duplex ultrasonography in vascular trauma, *J Vasc Tech* (1991) **15**:79–82.

Strauss AL, Soeparwate R, Is preoperative evaluation of the internal mammary artery for suitability in coronary artery bypass surgery possible? *Vasa* (1991) **33** (suppl):212–13.

van de Wal HJCM, van Asten WNJC, Wijn PFF, Skotnicki SH, Value of Doppler spectral analysis in the diagnosis of ischemic disease in the upper extremities. *J Vasc Tech* (1992) **16**:252–5.

UPPER EXTREMITY—VENOUS

Grassi CJ, Polak JF, Axillary and subclavian venous thrombosis: follow-up evaluation with color Doppler flow US and venography, *Radiology* (1990) **175**:651–4.

Horattas MC, Wright DJ, Fenton AH et al, Changing concepts of deep venous thrombosis of the upper extremity: Report of a series and review of the literature, *Surgery* (1988) **104**:561–7.

Knudson GJ, Wiedmeyer DA, Erickson SJ et al, Color Doppler sonographic imaging in the assessment of upper-extremity deep venous thrombosis. *AJR* (1990) **154**:399–403.

Nack TL, Needleman L, Comparison of duplex ultrasound and contrast venography for evaluation of upper extremity venous disease. *J Vasc Tech* (1992) **16**:69–73.

DIALYSIS GRAFTS AND FISTULAS

Middleton WD, Picus DD, Marx MV, Melson GL, Color Doppler sonography of hemodialysis vascular access: comparison with angiography, *AJR* (1989) **152**:633–9.

Tordoir JH, Hoeneveld H, Eikelboom RC, Kitslaar PJ, The correlation between clinical and duplex ultrasound parameters and the development of complications in arteriovenous fistulas for hemodialysis, *Eur J Vasc Surg* (1990) **4**:179–84.

Walters GK, Jones CE, Color duplex evaluation of arteriovenous access for hemodialysis, *J Vasc Tech* (1994) **18**:295–8.

LOWER EXTREMITY—ARTERIAL

Burnham CB, Color Doppler duplex scanning for arterial occlusive disease, *J Vasc Tech* (1991) **15**:129–38.

Cato R, Kupinski AM, Graft assessment by duplex ultrasound scanning. *J Vasc Tech* (1994) **18**:307–10.

Hatsukami TS, Primozich J, Zierler RE, Strandness E: Color Doppler characteristics in normal lower extremity arteries. *Ultrasound Med Biol* (1992) **18**:167–71.

Jager KA, Phillips DJ, Martin RL, Hanson C, Roederer GO, Langlois YE, Noninvasive mapping of lower limb arterial lesions, *Ultrasound Med Biol* (1985) **11**:515–21.

Papanicolaou G, Zierler RE, Beach KW, Isaacson JA, Strandness DE, Hemodynamic parameters of failing infrainguinal bypass grafts, *Am J Surg* (1995) **169**:238–44.

Taylor T, Stonebridge PA, Allan PL et al, Duplex ultrasound surveillance of infrainguinal bypass grafts: auditing the process, *J R Coll Surg Edinb* (1994) **39**:297–300.

Vandenberghe NJ, Duplex scan assessment of arterial occlusive disease, *J Vasc Tech* (1994) **18**:287–93.

LOWER EXTREMITY—VENOUS

Blackburn DR, Venous anatomy, *J Vasc Tech* (1988) **12**:78–81.

Bradbury AW, Stonebridge PA, Callam MJ et al, Recurrent varicose veins: assessment of the saphenofemoral junction, *Br J Surg* (1994) **81**:373–5.

Foley WD, Middleton WD, Lawson TL, Color Doppler ultrasound imaging of lower extremity venous disease, *AJR* (1989) **152**:371–6.

Lensing AWA, Levi MM, Buller HR et al, An objective Doppler method for the diagnosis of deep-vein thrombosis, *Ann Intern Med* (1990) **113**:9–14.

Mattos MA, Londrey GL, Leutz DW et al, Color-flow duplex scanning for the surveillance and diagnosis of acute deep venous thrombosis, *J Vasc Surg* (1992) **15**: 366–75.

Nix ML, Troillett RD, The use of color in venous duplex examination, *J Vasc Tech* (1991) **15**:123–8.

Polak JF, Culter SS, O'Leary DH, Deep veins of the calf: assessment with color Doppler flow imaging, *Radiology* (1989) **171**:481–5.

Rose SC, Zweibel WJ, Nelson BD et al, Symptomatic lower extremity deep venous thrombosis: accuracy, limitations, and role of color duplex imaging in diagnosis, *Radiology* (1990) **175**:639–44.

van Bemmelen PS, Bedford G, Strandness DE, Visualization of calf veins by color flow imaging, *Ultrasound Med Biol* (1990) **16**:15–17.

White RH, McGahan JP, Daschbach MM, Hartling RP, Diagnosis of deep-vein thrombosis during duplex ultrasound, *Ann Intern Med* (1989) **111**:297–304.

VASCULAR INJURIES

Bynoe RP, Miles WS, Bell RM et al, Noninvasive diagnosis of vascular trauma by duplex ultrasonography, *J Vasc Surg* (1991) **14**:346-52.

Fellmeth BD, Roberts AC, Bookstein J et al, Postangiographic femoral artery injuries: nonsurgical repair with ultrasound guided compression, *Radiology* (1991) **178**:671–5.

Igidbashian VN, Mitchell DG, Middleton WD, Schwartz RA, Goldberg BB, Iatrogenic femoral arteriovenous fistula: diagnosis with color Doppler imaging, *Radiology* (1989) **170**:749–52.

Knudson MM, Lewis FR, Atkinson K, Neuhas A, The role of duplex ultrasound arterial imaging in patients with penetrating extremity trauma, *Arch Surg* (1993) **128**:1033–7.

Merton DA, Ultrasound examination of invasive procedure puncture site complications. A review of scan techniques and benefits of color Doppler imaging, *J Diag Med Sonography* (1993) **9**:297–305.

Mitchell DG, Needleman L, Bezzi M et al, Femoral artery pseudoaneurysm: diagnosis with conventional duplex and color Doppler ultrasound, *Radiology* (1987) **165**:687–90.

Chapter 8 Contrast-enhanced color flow imaging

Ji-Bin Liu, Flemming Forsberg and Barry B Goldberg

INTRODUCTION

Investigations of ultrasound contrast agents continue to develop more than 27 years after Gramiak and Shah first described the echocardiographic contrast effect in 1968. Since then, there has been considerable development of ultrasound contrast agents that can increase the reflectivity of tissue as well as bloodflow. Many attempts have been made to establish effective ultrasound contrast agents for both cardiac and non-cardiac applications.

With the introduction of gray scale ultrasound imaging, it has become possible to visualize differences between and within tissue structures. However, echotexture differentiation of normal from abnormal tissue is sometimes difficult. Even when tissues are pathologically different, their ultrasonic properties may be quite similar. It is reasonable to suspect that uptake of certain materials in the abnormal tissue (such as a tumor) would be different from that of normal tissue. Two approaches have been followed in the development of ultrasound contrast agents. In one type, the agent increases the echogenicity of the blood and enhances the Doppler signals. In the other type, the agent is organ or tumor specific, collecting within or around abnormalities in such structures as the liver and spleen and increasing the difference in reflectivity (echogenicity) between the normal and adjacent abnormal tissue.

CONTRAST AGENTS

We have undertaken investigation of several types of contrast agent, including non-gas-containing agents. The principle of these agents is the difference in their density compared to the tissue and fluid in which they are located, which leads to increased reflection of ultrasound imaging. The most extensive investigations into non-microbubble-containing contrast agents have been those using perfluorochemicals. These particles are much smaller than red blood cells and, thus, they easily pass through the capillary circulation. They have been shown to increase the reflectivity of both the gray scale and Doppler signals due to their relative high density (1.9 g/ml) and low acoustic velocity (600 m/s) resulting in an acoustic impedance difference of 30% between them and the adjacent tissues. In animal experiments, we have used a perfluorochemical injected into a peripheral vein and demonstrated an instantaneous increase in the reflectivity of the blood utilizing both gray scale and Doppler ultrasound techniques. These perfluorochemicals are removed from the circulation by the reticuloendothelial system, resulting in a progressive increase in liver echogenicity over time. This increase in the reflectivity of the normal liver tissue improved the visualization of tumors which had destroyed the normal liver cells. Thus, this agent can help identify tumors due to the development of a hyperechogenic ring around the tumors.

We have also utilized several microbubble-containing agents, evaluating their effectiveness in increasing Doppler signal intensity in both normal and abnormal vessels within the abdomen and other areas of the body. The first agent was an albumin-coated microbubble agent (Albunex®, Molecular Biosystems Inc., San Diego, CA). Human albumin is sonicated, resulting in microbubbles of air being trapped within the albumin. This coating allows for their circulation beyond the right side of the heart and lungs. Their size, from 1 to 8 μm with a mean of 3.8 ± 2.5 μm, allows for their easy passage through capillaries. The half-life of this contrast agent, when injected into blood, has been shown to be less than 1 minute. After 3 minutes, more than 80% of the contrast agent was found to be deposited in the liver. These microspheres are phagocytized by the reticuloendothelial system, with byproducts returned to the blood and, within 24 hours, excreted in the urine.

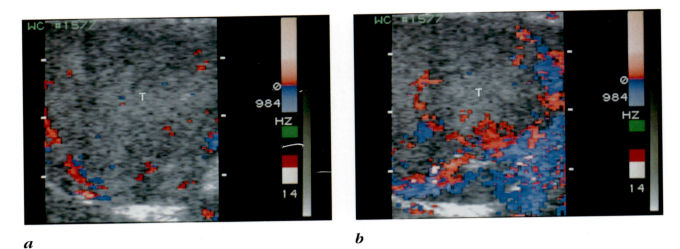

a   *b*

Figure 8.1 *The differences in the color flow imaging just before (a) and after (b) peripheral intravenous injection of air-filled albumin (Albunex). The color flow signal enhancement is seen around the periphery of the woodchuck hepatocellular tumor (T).*

Investigations using naturally occurring hepatocellular tumors in woodchucks have shown that intravenous injections of Albunex produced immediate Doppler signal enhancement within the inferior vena cava, followed by enhancement within the abdominal aorta and hepatic artery and its branches. While the two-dimensional ultrasound images showed no perceivable change in tissue reflectivity of the normal parenchyma, tumor or vessels, Doppler (both spectral and color) ultrasound demonstrated a clear signal enhancement. This effect was found in both normal and tumor vessels. In the larger tumors the greatest increase in Doppler intensity was apparent at the tumor periphery, since the central portion tended to be less vascular and, in some cases, was even necrotic (Fig. 8.1). Preliminary human studies using Albunex were carried out to evaluate patients with upper extremity venous diseases. The value of this agent appears to be in its ability to increase the echogenicity of thrombi, rather than opacifying the venous system. It has been approved for clinical use as an echocardiographic contract agent in Japan and the USA.

Recently, a second generation of the albumin-based agent has been developed (FS069, Molecular Biosystems Inc., San Diego, CA). Preliminary animal studies have shown that this agent has excellent contrast effect on Doppler signals, with very low dose administration, and the capability of recirculation over minutes (Fig. 8.2).

Another type of agent evaluated in our facilities is a galactose-based product consisting of microparticles in which microbubbles of gas have been trapped. The first such agent, Echovist® (Schering AG, Berlin, Germany), has been successfully used in both animals and humans to evaluate the right side of the heart. These particles, however, are too large to pass through the pulmonary capillary system. The agent has been used for direct injection into arteries to visualize the distal organs. A limitation of this agent is that it cannot be injected into a peripheral vein and still produce a significant effect in vessels and organs beyond the heart. It has been clinically evaluated and approved for use as a right heart contrast agent in Europe.

Based on the first generation of the saccharide agent Echovist, a new type of contrast agent (Levovist®, Schering AG, Berlin, Germany) has been developed. This agent is made from galactose but is produced with a slight change in its chemical composition to produce smaller, more stable and uniform bubbles, with diameters ranging from 2 to 8 µm, and with 97% of the bubbles measuring less than 6 µm. As a result, this agent can be injected into a peripheral vein and circulate throughout the body. Experiments in animals and humans have demonstrated that this

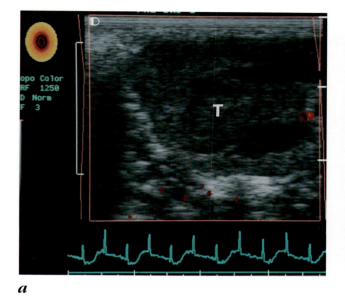

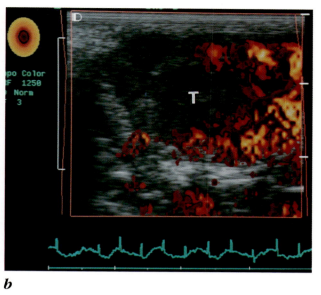

a

b

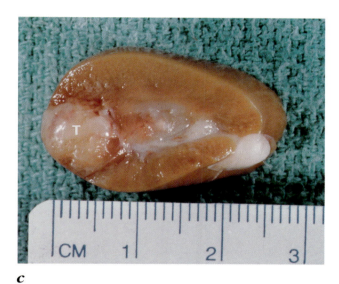

c

Figure 8.2 *Color flow signal enhancement is seen within a rabbit kidney with upper-pole VX2 tumor (T) before (a) and after (b) an intravenous injection of 0.01 ml/kg of perfluoropropane albumin (FS069). Close correlation between the cross-sectional anatomic specimen (c) and contrast-enhanced color flow imaging in (b) can be seen.*

agent can circulate for more than 3–5 minutes. Of particular interest is its ability to enhance Doppler signals in the portal circulation, which means that this agent has passed through two capillary beds and still maintains a significant contrast effect. However, it does not enhance the parenchymal echogenicity of organs. In large animal models this agent produced enhancement of the Doppler signals in the vessels of the retina of the eye as well as in the gallbladder, urinary bladder and bowel walls (Fig. 8.3). Within the

kidney there is enhancement of both the large and the small parenchymal vessels. Our experiments with VX2 tumors in rabbits and hepatomas in woodchucks have shown that this agent, when injected into a peripheral vein, will enhance both pulsed and color flow signals, demonstrating small tumor vessels as well as displacement of normal vessels. As expected, there was an increasing effect with increasing dose.

We have also carried out human trials to evaluate the effect of this agent in enhancing both normal

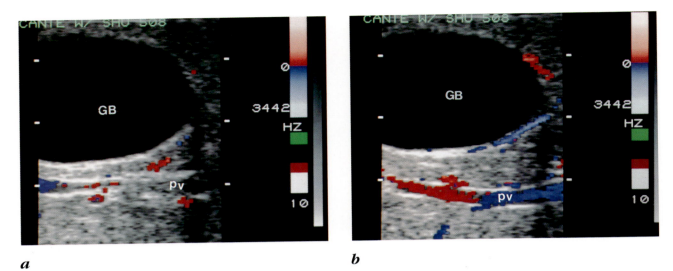

Figure 8.3 *Color flow imaging of the canine gallbladder (GB) and portal vein (PV) is enhanced after injection of 1 ml (0.04 ml/kg) air-filled microspheres Levovist: (a) preinjection; (b) postinjection. (Reprinted with permission from Goldberg et al 1993.)*

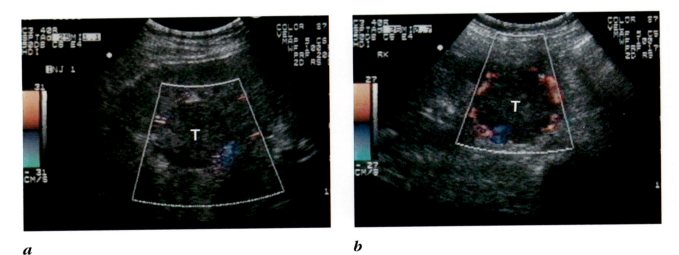

Figure 8.4 *In a patient with a renal mass, color flow imaging demonstrated tumor flow enhancement after an intravenous injection of 16 ml of Levovist: (a) preinjection; (b) postinjection. T, tumor.*

and abnormal vessels throughout the body. Ten to sixteen milliliters of Levovist injected into an antic-ubital vein have resulted in significant improvement in the signal-to-noise ratio within vessels, with effects lasting in excess of 3–5 minutes, similar to results reported in animals. A variety of tumors were evaluated, including malignant tumors in the liver,

kidney, ovary, pancreas and breast. In these studies, enhancement of both color and spectral Doppler signals within tumor and normal vessels was clearly demonstrated (Figs 8.4 and 8.5). In a retroperitoneal tumor, it was initially difficult to identify any tumor vessels. However, after intravenous injection of this agent, tumor vessels were clearly demonstrated

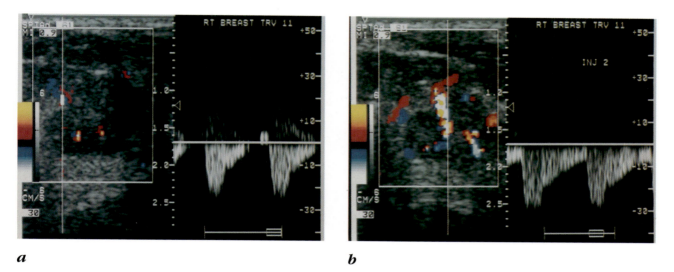

a   *b*

Figure 8.5 *Baseline color flow image (a) of a breast mass shows scattered areas of color signals within the tumor and poor-quality spectral waveforms. After Levovist injection, additional vessels are visible at the center and periphery of the tumor (b). The spectral waveform of tumor vessels is clearly demonstrated.*

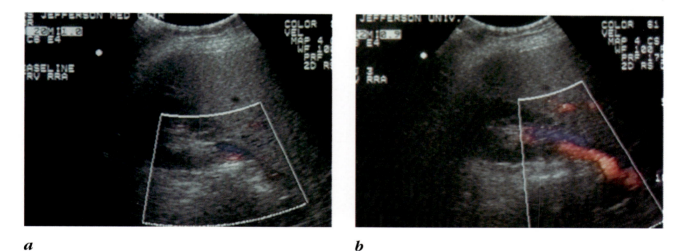

a   *b*

Figure 8.6 *In a patient with suspected right renal artery stenosis, color flow enhancement of the normal renal artery after injection of 16 ml of Levovist intravenously is clearly visible. With this information renal artery stenosis was ruled out: (a) preinjection; (b) postinjection. (Reprinted with permission from Goldberg et al 1994.)*

using color flow imaging. In addition, pulsed Doppler could identify a typical malignant flow pattern of high diastolic flow due to low peripheral resistance probably arising from tumor arteriovenous shunts. Color flow enhancement proved useful for localizing sample volume placement for spectral analysis. In the vascular studies, the agent was able to improve the reliability of vascular diagnosis by better demonstrating the presence or absence of high-velocity jets, by improving delineation of collateral or run-off vessels, by showing longer segments of vessels or by detecting flow through regions with absent or weak Doppler signals (Fig. 8.6).

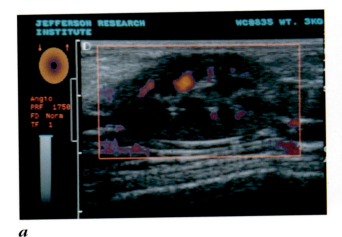

a

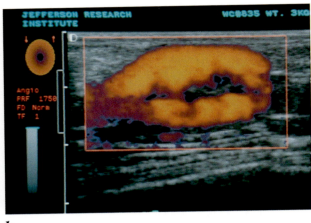

b

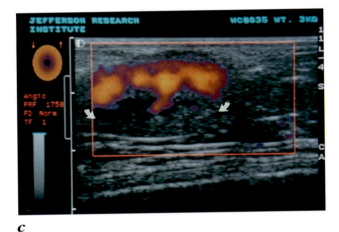

c

Figure 8.7 *Color amplitude signal enhancement can be seen in a woodchuck kidney following intravenous injection of 0.3 ml/kg of EchoGen: (a) baseline color amplitude imaging; (b) enhanced color amplitude imaging after injection; and (c) after injection with ligation of a segmental renal artery. Note the lack of flow in the ischemic region (arrows).*

The effectiveness of ultrasound contrast agents in enhancing vessels has been quantitatively evaluated by the placement of Doppler flow cuffs around both normal and abnormal vessels in animal models. It has been shown that the enhancement of the Doppler signals in a celiac vessel was as much as 24 dB and in a tumor vessel within a woodchuck hepatoma as much as 14 dB. The possibility of measuring the uptake and the outflow of this contrast agent within masses, helping to differentiate benign from malignant tumors, has also been demonstrated in work reported by Kedar and Duda for the evaluation of breast masses using Levovist. A similar study has been reported with gadolinium used with magnetic resonance imaging to differentiate benign from malig-

nant breast masses. The uptake and washout of these contrast agents appears to vary between malignant and benign breast tumors, with a much faster washout seen in malignant tumors. More research is being conducted to confirm these initial reports and to evaluate their potential in other areas of the body.

A newly developed contrast agent EchoGen™ (Sonus Pharmaceuticals, Bothell, WA) has the ability to undergo a PhaseShift™ change from an emulsion containing a water-immiscible liquid to echogenic gas bubbles upon injection into the bloodstream. The microbubbles are 1–5 µm in diameter. In animal evaluations, this temperature-dependent contrast medium has shown the capability of enhancing not only Doppler signals (both pulsed and color) but also

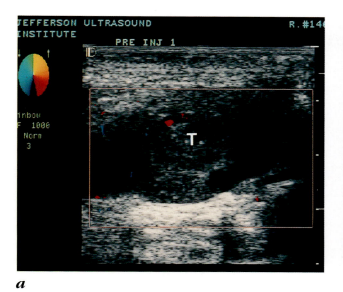

a

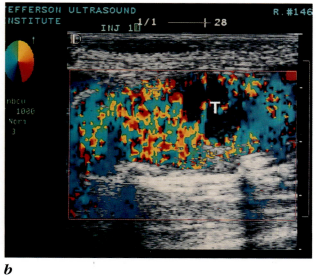

b

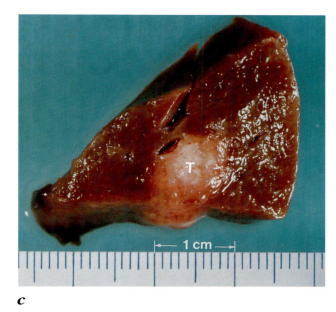

c

Figure 8.8 *(a) Baseline color flow image of a VX2 liver tumor (T) in a rabbit. (b) Fifteen minutes after injection of 0.2 ml/kg Sonovist, color flow signals are displayed in the normal parenchyma of the liver. The tumor (T) is clearly demonstrated because no agent is taken up by the tumor. Close correlation between the anatomic specimen (c) and contrast-enhanced color flow imaging (b) can be seen.*

the parenchyma on gray scale imaging in such organs as the kidney and liver. Increased echogenicty of bloodflow could also be identified. Delineation of areas of ischemia produced within the kidney by tying off a segmental renal artery has been demonstrated using both gray scale and Doppler ultrasound imaging (Fig. 8.7). In addition, there was enhancement of the color and pulsed Doppler signals within both normal and tumor vessels. This agent can recirculate, the effect lasting in excess of 5 min. Clinical trials in normal volunteers have shown enhancement of vessels within the abdomen utilizing pulsed Doppler and color flow imaging.

More recently, a new type of ultrasound contrast agent (Sonovist®, Schering AG, Berlin, Germany) has been produced. This agent, after being injected intravenously, is taken up by the reticuloendothelial system of the liver, spleen and lymph nodes. Contrast enhancement using color flow imaging is produced in all normal areas of the parenchyma, resulting in

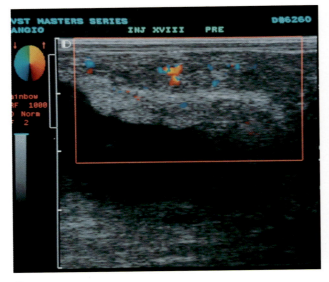

a

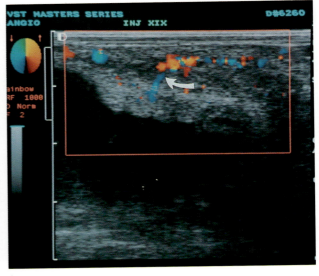

b

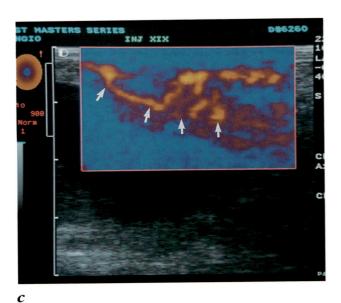

c

Figure 8.9 *(a) Baseline color flow imaging of a canine bladder wall. (b) Color flow signal enhancement is seen after a peripheral intravenous injection of 1 ml of Levovist. A feeding vessel (arrow) into the bladder wall is demonstrated. (c) With the use of color amplitude imaging, additional vessels (arrows) are clearly documented.*

improved visualization of tumors which do not take up this agent. Initial work using VX2 tumors grown in the liver of rabbits has clearly demonstrated the capability of this agent to detect small tumors which were not clearly seen prior to the injection of the agent (Fig. 8.8). Further experiments are underway to confirm these initial results in improving the detection of tumors in such structures as the liver, spleen and lymph nodes.

INSTRUMENT MODIFICATIONS

The modification of ultrasound equipment to utilize the specific ultrasound qualities of contrast agents is under investigation. One of the concepts being evaluated is harmonic imaging. When ultrasound is transmitted into the body at one frequency, vibrating microbubbles of gas result in harmonics and subhar-

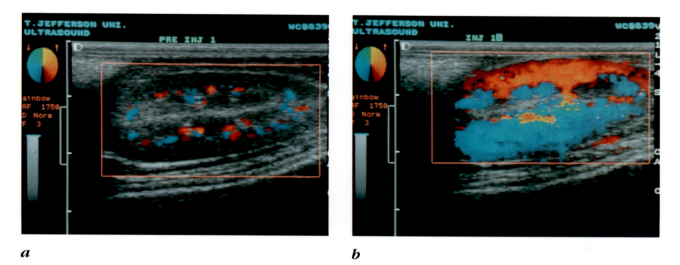

a   *b*

Figure 8.10 *Color blooming artifact is seen obscuring most tissue information after a bolus injection of contrast material: (a) baseline imaging; (b) contrast-enhanced imaging.*

monics being produced. Thus, ultrasound transmitted at 3.5 MHz results in harmonic signals at 7 MHz being returned in those areas where microbubbles of gas are present. Ultrasound instruments have been modified to collect this information and record the harmonic signals produced. While this research is in its early stages, the potential exists for significantly improving the signals, both gray scale and Doppler, from those areas in which microbubbles are present.

Another modification of ultrasound equipment has been to display only the power or amplitude component of the Doppler signal, so-called color amplitude imaging. Since ultrasound contrast agents increase the intensity of Doppler signals, there should be an improvement in the sensitivity of the flow signals to the contrast agent by using this technique. Using this method, an improvement in the signal sensitivity of more than 10 dB can be seen even without the use of an ultrasound contrast agent. Thus, signals from deeper and smaller vessels can be better delineated. It is a non-directional form of color flow display. As a result, vessels are shown in a more anatomically true manner in the plane of the image, similar to the distribution of vascularity demonstrated by X-ray angiography. Initial work in a variety of organs in the abdomen has shown the capabilities of more easily following the course of blood vessels as well as delineating smaller vessels in such areas as the renal cortex. The usefulness of this approach with ultra-

sound contrast agents has been demonstrated in animal models (Fig. 8.9). In a study with a woodchuck hepatoma, color amplitude imaging clearly demonstrated small tumor vessels after an intravenous injection of a contrast agent which were not seen using standard color flow imaging. The capability of following branching vessels and displaying small vessels has been documented. Thus, this technique improves the capabilities of recording the effectiveness of ultrasound contrast agents.

ARTIFACTS

There are a number of artifacts associated with contrast-enhanced Doppler ultrasound, including color blooming, increased maximum Doppler shift and spectral bubble noise. The color blooming artifact occurs immediately after the bolus injection of contrast agent arrives at the imaging site. It appears as contrast-enhanced color display filling up entire gray scale pixels in regions where flow is not possible (Fig. 8.10). Color blooming is an artifact caused by contrast-induced increase in Doppler signal strength and the color reject threshold. This artifact can be eliminated by a reduction in color Doppler gain setting or by a continuous infusion of a contrast

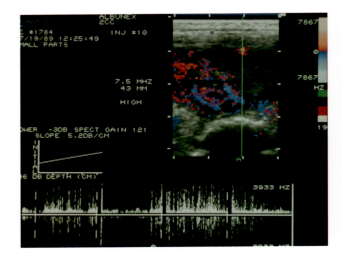

Figure 8.11 *Spectral bubble noise is seen on duplex Doppler imaging following an intravenous injection of an ultrasound contrast agent.*

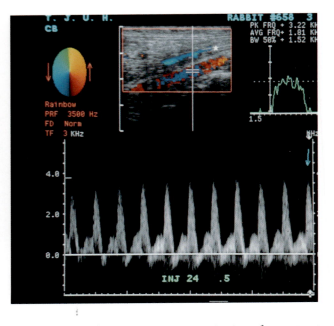

Figure 8.12 *Before an intravenous injection of a contrast agent, an arriving bolus of the agent produces progressive increase in the peak systolic shift.*

material instead of the bolus injection. Spectral bubble noise artifact manifests itself as very large excursions in the spectral display (Fig. 8.11). This artifact is caused by the breakdown of microbubbles, since large bubbles imploding cause momentary very rapid particle movement. The spectral bubble noise is associated with a 'crackling' noise in the audio output. The bubble noise artifact is easy to identify and is of less importance for clinical practice. Finally, ultrasound contrast agents can increase the maximum Doppler shift found in duplex Doppler studies. Generally, the increase in maximum Doppler shift can range from 20% to 45% (Fig. 8.12). Experiments confirmed that this artifact is due to the limited dynamic range of the spectral display available in an ultrasound scanner. Only signals above a certain threshold are detectable. As the Doppler signal power is enhanced by contrast agent, the highest frequency visible also increases. While the color blooming and spectral bubble noise are easy to identify, the increase in peak systolic Doppler shift gives more cause for concern, as it may prevent meaningful quantitative parameters being obtained from the Doppler spectrum under some circumstances.

CLINICAL INDICATIONS

In current clinical practice, Doppler techniques have been extensively used to detect abnormal bloodflow associated with abdominal and pelvic tumors. With small or deep malignant tumors, low signals from moving blood cells are obscured by those of the adjacent stationary solid tissue, and this is a limiting factor in the detection of these small tumors. Ultrasound contrast agents should increase the ability to detect smaller vessels by enhancing backscatter in both tumor and normal vessels. The ability to detect the motion of blood in small vessels is usually limited in deep tissue. By increasing the reflectivity of the blood, a contrast agent will enable better detection of bloodflow in small, deep vessels than is now possible with conventional Doppler techniques. Animal and human experiments suggest that an ultrasound contrast agent could help differentiate between tumor and normal vascularity. The demonstration of normal parenchymal arterial flow within areas that were considered abnormal may help to distinguish tumors from pseudotumors, such as renal columns of Bertin.

Ultrasound contrast agents should also improve the detection of ischemia or occlusion. The introduction of more reflectors should aid in the delineation of a site of vascular narrowing. Ultrasound contrast agents may also aid in the visualization of collaterals caused by occlusion or severe stenosis.

In conclusion, the most effective ultrasound contrast agent would be:

- non-toxic;

- injectable intravenously;
- capable of passing through the pulmonary, cardiac and capillary circulations;
- stable for recirculation.

A variety of potential ultrasound contrast agents have been or are now under development. Modifications to instrumentation will allow for improved display of the effects of ultrasound contrast agents.

FURTHER READING

Duda VF, Rode G, Schlief R, Echocontrast agent enhanced color flow imaging of the breast, *Ultrasound Obstet Gynecol* (1993) **3**:191–4.

Forsberg F, Liu JB, Burns PN et al, Artifacts in intravenous ultrasound contrast agent studies, *J Ultrasound Med* (1994) **13**:357–65.

Goldberg BB, Hilpert PL, Burns PN et al, Hepatic tumors: signal enhancement of Doppler US after intravenous injection of a contrast agent, *Radiology* (1990) **177**:713–17.

Goldberg BB, Liu JB, Burns PN et al, Galactose-based intravenous sonographic contrast agent: experimental studies, *J Ultrasound Med* (1993) **12**:463–70.

Goldberg BB, Liu JB, Forsberg F, Ultrasound contrast agents: a review, *Ultrasound Med Biol* (1994) **20**:317–33.

Gramiak R, Shah PM, Echocardiography of the aortic root, *Invest Radiol* (1968) **3**:356–66.

Kedar RP, Cosgrove D, McCready VR et al, Microbubble contrast agent for color Doppler US: effect on breast masses. Work in progress, *Radiology* (1996) **198**:679–86.

Mattrey RF, Strich G, Shelton RE et al, Perfluorochemicals in US contrast agents for tumor imaging and hepatosplenography: preliminary clinical results, *Radiology* (1987) **163**:339–43.

Ophir J, Parker KJ, Contrast agents in diagnostic ultrasound, *Ultrasound Med Biol* (1989) **15**:319–33.

Schrope BA, Newhouse VL, Second harmonic ultrasonic blood perfusion measurement, *Ultrasound Med Biol* (1993) **19**:567–79.

Index